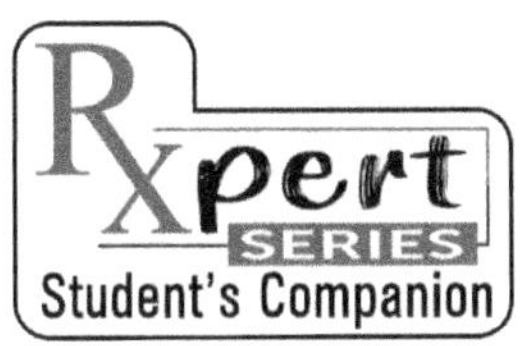

Herbal Drug Technology

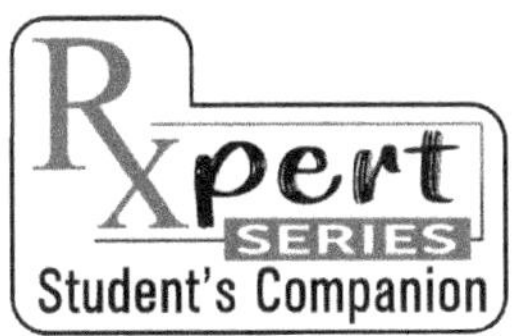

Herbal Drug Technology

Sharada L. Deore

M.Pharm (Pharmacognosy & Phytochemistry),
Ph.D (Pharmaceutical Sciences), PG Diploma in Patent's law
Associate Professor,
Govt. College of Pharmacy,
Amravati-444604
Maharashtra

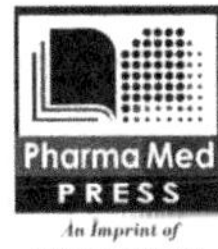

PharmaMed Press

An imprint of BSP Books pvt. Ltd

4-4-309/316, Giriraj Lane,
Sultan Bazar, Hyderabad - 500 095.

Herbal Drug Technology
by **Sharada L. Deore**

Published by:

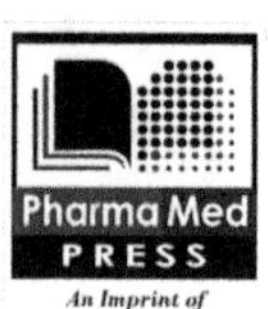

PharmaMed Press

An imprint of BSP Books Pvt. Ltd.

4-4-309/316, Giriraj Lane, Sultan Bazar, Hyderabad - 500 095.
Phone: 040-23445688; Fax: 91+40-23445611
e-mail: info@pharmamedpress.com
www.pharmamedpress.com/pharmamedpress.net

ISBN: 978-93-91910-99-0 (Hardback)

Preface

Increasing demand and fast-growing market of herbal medicines helps to emerge an Herbal drug technology as a new versatile field. Pharmacy council (PCI) of India has appropriately introduced this subject "Herbal Drug Technology" in Undergraduate B.Pharm sixth semester syllabus to inculcate herbal formulations and regulations skills in students.

Herbal cosmetics, nutraceuticals, traditional as well as modern preparations require quality raw materials to claim safety and efficacy by manufacturers. Intellectual property rights of herb derived products and process are increasing day by day. Herbal drug regulations are needed to be updated to make them globally accepted once introduced in specific market.

Experimental skills of qualitative as well as quantitative phytochemical screening, standardised extract preparations and herbal formulations as per Pharmacopeial standards will help student to serve better in herbal industry, academics and research institutes.

Present book is strictly designed as per PCI syllabus to cover theory as well as practical syllabus topics to able students to upgrade the desired theoretical plus practical skills.

Subjective as well as specific and related objective (MCQs) questions are added to analyse the topic understanding of students.

I would first and foremost like to acknowledge the authors and publishers of various books, research articles, journals, websites and other sources that have been referred to for putting together to make this book an fine source of reference.

Author is thankful to all her teachers, students, friends and family for motivation of keeping writing as per the need of time and changing scenario.

Author would like to acknowledge the excellent efforts of Publisher Anil Shah and Editor Naresh Daver for corrections and suggestions to bring out the theory as well as practical syllabus content in the form of semester book.

Sharada Deore-Baviskar

Contents

Part - I

HERBAL DRUG TECHNOLOGY (THEORY)

UNIT 1

UNIT 2

UNIT 3

Part - II

PRACTICAL MANUAL

Part – I

(Theory)

Herbal Drug Technology

Unit 1

1.1 Herbs as Raw Materials

1.1.1 Definition

1.1.2 Selection, Identification and Authentication of Herbal Materials

1.1.3 Processing of Herbal Raw Materials

1.2 Biodynamic Agriculture

1.2.1 Good Agricultural Practices in Cultivation (GACP) of Medicinal Plants

1.2.2 Organic Farming

1.2.3 Pest and Pest Management in Medicinal Plants

1.2.4 Biopesticides/Bioinsecticides

1.3 Indian Systems of Medicine

1.3.1 Basic principles involved in Ayurveda, Siddha, Unani and Homeopathy

1.3.1.1 Ayurveda System

1.3.1.2 Siddha System

1.3.1.3 Unani System

1.3.1.4 Homeopathy System

1.3.2 Preparation and Standardization of Ayurvedic Formulations

1.3.2.1 Bhasma

1.3.2.2 Asava and Arishta

1.3.2.3 Leha (Avaleha/Paka)

1.3.2.4 Churna

1.3.2.5 Gutika/Vati

1.1 Herbs as Raw Materials

1.1.1 Definition

- ***Herbs***: are crude plant materials which may be entire, fragmented or powdered. Herbs include, Example- the entire aerial part, leaves, flowers, fruits, seeds, roots, bark (stems) of trees, tubers, rhizomes or other plant parts.
- ***Herbal medicines***: Herbal medicines include herbs and/or herbal materials and/or herbal preparations and/or finished herbal products in a form suitable for administration to patients
- ***Medicinal herbal products***: finished, labelled pharmaceutical products in dosage forms that contain one or more of the following: powdered plant materials, extracts, purified extracts, or partially purified active substances isolated from plant materials. Medicines containing plant material combined with chemically defined active substances, including chemically defined, isolated constituents of plants, are not considered to be herbal medicines.
- ***Herbal preparations***: are produced from herbal materials by physical or biological processes.

  These processes may be extraction (with water, alcohol, supercritical carbon dioxide (CO2)), fractionation, purification, concentration, fermentation and other processes. They also include processing herbal materials with a natural vehicle or steeping or heating them in alcoholic beverages and/or honey, or in other materials.

  The resulting herbal preparations include, among others, simply comminuted (fragmented) or powdered herbal materials as well as extracts, tinctures, fatty (fixed) or essential oils, expressed plant juices, decoctions, cold and hot infusions.

1.1.2 Selection, Identification and Authentication of Herbal Materials

Authenticated raw material is the basic starting point in developing a botanical product. Conscious efforts must therefore be made to ensure that the botanical identity of test materials is rigorously confirmed and documented through preservation of vouchers, and that their geographic origin and handling are appropriate. Use of material with an associated herbarium voucher that can be botanically identified is always ideal. Indirect methods of authenticating bulk material in commerce, for example use of organoleptic, anatomical, chemical, or molecular characteristics, are not always acceptable for the chemist's purposes. Familiarity with botanical and pharmacognostic literature is necessary to determine what potential adulterants exist and how they may be distinguished.

1.1.3 Processing of Herbal Raw Materials

Introduction

Before using a crude drug for production of herbal formulations, it should be properly processed so that, the active constituents and the appearance of the drug do not deteriorate. The information on the raw material(s) and the solvents/reagents or vehicles used for the Herbal Stock(s) and final dilution preparation should be evaluated. For raw materials of botanical origin, the scientific name -genus, species, variety, chemo type, parts employed and other names should be provided. For raw materials of biological origin, the scientific name (Example-, animal), -genus, species- tissue(s), fluid(s), parts of organ(s) or organ(s) used and other names should be evaluated. For minerals or chemicals, the international non-proprietary name (I.N.N), chemical and other names should be evaluated. For raw materials of botanical origin, the state (Example- fresh, dried) of the material used and, where applicable, information on pharmacological active, toxic constituents or marker compound(s), if applicable, should be analyzed. Additionally a macroscopic and microscopic descri-ption of the raw material should be evaluated. For raw materials of biological origin, information on the physical and/or anatomical and histological state (where applicable) should be evaluated. For minerals or chemicals, physical form, structural formula, molecular formula and relative molecular mass, where applicable, should be evaluated. The preparation of a crude drug for the market depends on the following major processes.

Collection

Collection of drugs from cultivated plants always ensures a true natural source and reliable products. This may or may not be this case when drugs are cultivated from wild plants.

Following are factors to be considered at the time of collection	
Labour	Drugs may be collected from wild or cultivated plants and the task may be undertaken by casual, unskilled native labour. Example- Ipecacuanha
	Drug may be collected by skill worker in a highly scientific manner. Example- Digitalis, Cinchona, Belladona
Season	The season at which each drug is collected is also important, since the amount and sometimes the nature of the active constituents is not constructed through the year. Example- Podophyllum, Ephedra, Rhubarb, Aconite
	Rhubarb contains no anthraquinone derivatives in winter but contain anthranols which on the arrival of warmer weather are converted by oxidation into anthraquinone.
Age	The age of plant is also considerable important and governs not only the total quntity of active constitute produced but also the components of the active mixure. Clove (volatile oil): Cloves contain about 11-21% oil while mother blown cloves contain very little oil. Datura (alkaloids): The hyoscinc/hyoscyamine ratio falls from about 80% in young seedlings to about 30% in mature frutings plants.
Geographical location	Geographical location also affects the cultivation in a certain extent. Location helps in development of the desired type and amount of constitutes. Example- *Ammi vianaga* growing wild in the mediteranean area contains variety of a coumarins and chromones in its seeds, however same plant cultivated in Arizona, found to produce plenty seeds practilly devoid of the desired constituents

Harvesting

Harvesting is the process of collection of the highest quality crude drug from its original source in the appropriate season and time of the day.

- Leaves are collected from plants during the flowering season when the plant is very active.
- Bark is collected in spring or early summer.

- Flowers are collected about the time of pollination in dry weather in the forenoon when the dew has disappeared and dried in shade.
- Roots and tubers are collected in autumn when the plant is inactive and the vegetative process has ceased and contain the maximum active constituents.

Drying

Drying is essential for maintaining the quality of crude drugs after collection to avoid decomposition, microbial growth, enzyme activation and other possible chemical changes. Herbal raw drugs are dried prior to extraction to avoid detoriation on storage and transport as well as to facilitate grinding. In the preparation of crude drugs, drying is usually designed to yield a stable, homogenous product which is easy to manupulate in subsequent operation of storage and packaging.

Drying is defined as the removal of a liquid or moisture contents from a material (herbal drugs) by the application of heat and is accomplished by the transfer of a liquid or moisture content from a surface into an unsaturated vapour phase.

Proper and successful drying depends on control of temperature and regulation of air flow. Drying process is to be done depending upon source of herbal crude drug and its chemical nature.

- If enzymatic action is to be encouraged, slow drying is necessary at moderate temperature. Example- Orris rhizome, Vanilla pods, Cocoa seed, Gentian root.
- If enzymatic action is not desired, drying should take place as soon as possible after collection. Drugs containing volatile oil are liable to lose their aroma if not dried or if the oil is not distilled from them immediately.

Two types of drying are classified as follows:

1. **Natural drying (sun drying)**

   (a) ***Direct sun drying (outdoor drying)***: The crude drugs can be dried directly in sunshine if the contents of crude drugs are quite stable to the temperature and sunlight. Example: Gum acacia, seeds, fruit are dried by direct sun drying method.

   (b) ***Shed drying:*** Shed drying is prepared when the natural colors of the drug (digitalis leaves, clove, senna leaves) and volatile principles of the drug (Example- Peppermint) are to be retained. Drying in the shed at the air temperature is frequently adopted especially for leaves containing oil.

2. **Artificial drying**

   (a) ***Tray dryer: (truck dryer):*** This is most commonly used method in the pharmaceutical plant operatation. Tray dryers are used for drying heat stable plant material. Example- roots, barks. In this process, hot air of desired temperature is circulated through the dryers and this facilitates the removal of water content of the drugs. This is simplest and inexpensive method. Disadvantage of tray dryers is deterioration of material due to high residence time at high temperature.

(b) ***Vaccum dryer:*** In this method, vaccum facilitates drying of plant material at low temperature. It can handle stiky, free flowing, hygroscopic, heat sensitive plant materials. Examples- Tannic acid, Digitalis leaves.

(c) ***Spray dryer:*** This is used for non-hygroscopic products. This is continous, thermally efficient dryer where filtered atmospheric hot air comes in contact with atomized fine mist of the feed and instantly evaporates the water in the feed droplets. The fluidized mixture of air and powder get separted in cyclone separator. This method of drying retains all the original properties of plant material such as color, aroma, efficacy, density etc.

Pulverisation

Pulverisation or comminution is a process of fragmenting a substance into small particles by mechanical forces. It is one of the important process operation and inevitable in very first step of herbal extraction. Comminution of different parts of the herbal drugs can be explained as followed.

Crude Drug	Details and type of mills useful
Leaf drugs	Leaf drugs are predominant in herbal industry. • Shredding mills - medicinal leaves and herbs with high content of stem and stalk • Hammer mills- for resinous and friable leaf drugs • Pin mills – leaf drugs with high fat content or ethereal oil.
Roots and barks	Roots and barks are moderately hard or woody but sometimes brittle and friable also. Example- Cinnamon, Quercus, Ipecacuanha • Shredder mills- cutting and shredding • Hammer mills- grinding
Seeds and fruits	The comminution of seeds and fruits offer proves to be particularly difficult because of their content of fats and ethereal oils. Example- coffee and cocoa beans. • Shredder mills – comminution
Other drug plant materials	These include flowers, part of flowers and products such as alginates, agar, and gelatins • Shredder mills – comminution

Garbling

The next step in preparation of crude drug for market after drying is garbling which is the final step of the preparation of crude drug. The process is desired when sand, dirt and foreign parts of the same plant, not constituents are required to be removed. If extraneous matter to be removed permitted in crude drugs, the quality of crude drugs suffers and at times it doesn't pass pharmacopoeial limits. Example- 1.excessive stem in case of lobelia and stramonium need to be removed. 2. Stalks, in case of cloves are to be detected. 3. Drugs constituting rhizomes need to be separated carefully from roots and rootlets and also stem bases. 4. Pieces of iron must be removed with the magnet in case of caster seeds beforc crushing 5. Shifting in case of vinca and senna leaves. 6. Pieces of bark should be removed by peelings as in gum acacia.

Packing

The morphological and chemical nature of the drug, its ultimate use and effect of climatic conditions during transportation and storage should be taken into consideration while packing of drugs.

- Colophony and balsam packed in kerosene tins.
- Asafoetida is stored in well-closed container to prevent loss of volatile oil.
- Cod liver oil is sensitive to sunlight so it should be stored in such containers, which will not affect the sunlight.
- Leaf drug like senna, vinca are pressed and baled.
- Drug which very sensitive to moisture and costly at the same time need special attention. Example- digitalis, ergot, squills
- Colophony needs to be packed in big masses to control auto oxidation.
- Crude drugs like roots, seeds and other part packed in gummy bags.
- Weight of certain drug in lots also kept constant Example- Indian opium.

Packing material and specific storage of Raw Herbs

1. Woody in nature like stem, heartwood, bark etc. : Gunny bags and woven sacks
2. Soft in nature like creepers, leaves etc. : High gauge HMHD bags, woven sacks with LD liner, High gauge polyethylene bags
3. Fleshy in nature like fruits, rhizomes etc.: High gauge HMHD bags, woven sacks with LD liner, wooden boxes.
4. Flowers, anthers, stigma, petals, seeds etc. : Corrugated box with polypropylene woven sacks, HDPE containers, Fiber board's drums
5. Volatile contents: Air tight HDPE containers, Air tight HDPE carboys, Card board box with polyethylene liners
6. Herbal extracts and compounds: Air tight HDPE containers, corrugated box with polyethylene woven sacks and fiber board's drums with polyethylene bags. HDHM (High molecular weight high density polyethylene), LD liner (Low density liner bags), HDPE (High density polyethylene)

Storage of Herbal Raw Drug

- Proper storage and preservative are important factors in maintaining a high degree of quality of the drug.
- Warehouse should preferably be of fire proof, steel, concrete or brick construction, and unheated and rodent proof.
- Hard packed bales usually reabsorb little moisture. This is also true of barks and resinous drug but leaf, herbs, and roots drugs that are not well packed tend to absorb moisture up to 10%, 15%, or 30% of weight of drug.

- Excessive moisture not only increases the weight of the drug. Thus reducing the % of active constituents but also favours enzymatic activity and facilitates fungal growth. Example-. Digitalis glycoside is deteriorate when moisture in the drug reaches 8% or higher.
- Liquid adversely affects drugs, which are higher colored, rendering them unattractive and possibly causing undesirable changes in constituents. It has been shown that polarized light changes more rapidly the ordinary light.
- The oxygen of the air increase oxidation of the constituent so of the drugs, especially when oxidases (oxidizing enzymes) are present.
- Insects also attack on crude herbal drugs so to prevention of their attacks a number of methods have been employed. The simple method of all being to expose the drug to a temperature of 65°C. They also prevent form determination.
- The fumigation of large lots of crude drugs such as stored in warehoused and manufacturing plants, the use of methyl bromide.
- Small lots of drugs may readily be stored in air-light, moisture proof and lightproof containers.
- If drugs in small quantities are stored in air-tight containers, insect attack can be controlled by the addition of a few drops of chloroform or CCl_4.
- Certain drugs such as biologics must be stored at a temperature between 2° and 10°C

1.2 Biodynamic Agriculture

The term biodynamic, derived from two Greek words "bios" (life) and 'dynamis" (energy), refers to 'working with the energies' which create and maintain life. The concept of biodynamic agriculture, very similar to organic farming, regards the soil as a self-sustained and biologically dynamic and biochemically active environment. Biodynamic agriculture is an alternative farm management mode, free from synthetic inputs. Biodynamic agriculture differs from organic agriculture in as much as it involves specific practices aimed at improving plant vitality by strengthening plant, ground and environmental interactions.

1.2.1 Good Agricultural Practices in Cultivation (GACP) of Medicinal Plants

Section 1: General Introduction and Glossary

Section 2: Good Agricultural Practices (GAP) for Medicinal Plants

- Identification/Authentication of Cultivated Medicinal Plants
- Seeds and Other Propagation Materials
- Site selection
- Personnel
- Ecological Environment and Social Impact
- Soil
- Climate

- Irrigation and Drainage
- Cultivation
- Plant Maintenance and Protection
- Harvest

Section 3: Good Collection Practices (GCP) for Medicinal Plants

- Permission to Collect
- Technical Planning
- Selection of Medicinal Plants for Collection
- Collection
- Personnel

Section 4: Common Technical Aspects of GACP

- Post-harvest Processing
- Inspection and Sorting
- Primary Processing
- Drying
- Specific Processing
- Bulk Packaging and Labelling
- Storage and Transportation
- Equipment
- Quality Assurance
- Documentation
- Personnel (growers, collectors, producers, handlers, processors)

Section 5: Other Relevant Issues

- Ethical and Legal Considerations
- Intellectual Property Rights and Benefits-Sharing
- Threatened and Endangered Species
- Research needs

Annexure

Annex 1. Good Agricultural Practice for Traditional Chinese Medicinal Materials, People's Republic of China

Annex 2. Points to Consider on Good Agricultural and Collection Practice for Starting Materials of Herbal Origin

Annex 3. Good Agricultural and Collection Practices for Medicinal Plants (GACP), Japan

Annex 4. A model structure for monographs on good agricultural practices for specific medicinal plants

Annex 5. Sample record for cultivated medicinal plants

Annex 6. Participants in the WHO Consultation on Good Agricultural and Field Collection Practices for Medicinal Plants

Section 1: General Introduction and Glossary

This section involves following important descriptions.

Need of GACP Guidelines

1. Interest in herbal medicines risen the issues related to safety and quality of herbal medicines
2. Inadvertent use of the wrong plant species
3. Adulteration with undeclared other medicines and/or potent substances
4. Contamination with undeclared toxic and/or hazardous substances
5. Over dosage, inappropriate use by health-care providers or consumers
6. Interaction with other medicines
7. Use of inferior quality raw medicinal plant materials results in poor quality finished products
8. Collection from wild populations leads to global, regional and/or local over-harvesting
9. Protection of endangered species
10. Impact on environment and ecological processes
11. Impact on the welfare of local communities should be considered
12. Respect of intellectual property rights

Objectives

1. Supply of good quality raw material applicablc to national and/or regional quality standards thus improve the quality, safety and efficacy of finished herbal products;
2. guide the formulation of national and/or regional GACP guidelines and GACP monographs for medicinal plants and related standard operating procedures; and
3. encourage and support the conservation of medicinal plants and the environment

Structure

The guidelines are divided into five sections:

- Section 1: provides a general introduction and a glossary for relevant terms
- Section 2: good agricultural practices for medicinal plants
- Section 3: discuss good collection practices for medicinal plants.
- Section 4: outlines common technical aspects of good agricultural practices for medicinal plants and good collection practices for medicinal plants
- Section 5: considers other relevant issues

Following annexures are provided in this guideline:

- Annexure 1: national and regional documents on good agricultural practices for medicinal plants from the China

- Annexure 2: national and regional documents on good agricultural practices for medicinal plants from the European Agency
- Annexure 3: national and regional documents on good agricultural practices for medicinal plants from the Japan
- Annexure 4: model structure for monographs on good agricultural practices for specific medicinal plants
- Annexure 5: sample record for cultivated medicinal plants
- Annexure 6. Participants in the WHO Consultation on Good Agricultural and Field Collection Practices for Medicinal Plants

Section 2: Good Agricultural Practices (GAP) for Medicinal Plants

1. ***Identification/authentication of cultivated medicinal plants:*** The botanical identity – scientific name (genus, species, subspecies/variety, author, and family) – of each medicinal plant under cultivation should be verified and recorded. If available, the local and English common names should also be recorded. Documentation of the botanical identity should be included in the registration file as a specimen.
2. ***Seeds and other propagation materials:*** propagation materials should be from any disease or contamination and provide all necessary information relating to the identity, quality and performance of their products, as well as their breeding history, where possible. Materials used for organic production should be certified as being organically derived.
3. ***Site selection:*** Medicinal plant materials derived from the same species can show significant differences in quality when cultivated at different sites, owing to the influence of soil, climate and other factors. Risks of contamination as a result of pollution of the soil, air or water by hazardous chemicals should be avoided.
4. ***Personnel:*** Growers and producers should have formal or informal practical education and training of the medicinal plant concerned. This should include botanical identification, cultivation characteristics and environ-mental requirements (soil type, soil pH, fertility, plant spacing and light requirements), as well as the means of harvest, storage and personal hygiene, issues relevant to the protection of the environment, conservation of medicinal plant species, and proper agricultural stewardship. Smoking and eating should not be permitted in medicinal plant processing areas.
5. ***Ecological environment and social impact:*** The introduction of non-indigenous medicinal plant species into cultivation may have a detrimental impact on the biological and ecological balance of the region. In terms of local income – earning opportunities, small-scale cultivation is often preferable so that local communities benefit directly from, for example, fair wages, equal employment opportunities and capital reinvestment.
6. ***Soil:*** Optimal soil conditions, including soil type, drainage, moisture retention, fertility and pH, will be dictated by the selected medicinal plant species and/or target medicinal plant part. Green manure should be preferred.
7. ***Climate:*** The duration of sunlight, average rainfall, average temperature, including daytime and night-time temperature differences, also influence the physiological and biochemical activities of plants, and prior knowledge should be considered.

8. ***Irrigation and drainage:*** should be controlled and carried out in accordance with the needs of individual plant.
9. ***Cultivation:*** The conditions and duration of cultivation required vary depending on the medicinal plant materials required. Scientific and if no scientific data available then traditional methods should be used to cultivate medicinal plant.
10. ***Plant maintenance and protection:*** Timely application of measures such as topping, bud nipping, pruning and shading, Integrated pest management should be followed where appropriate
11. ***Harvest:*** The time of harvest depends on the plant part to be used. The best time for harvest (quality peak season/time of day) should be determined according to the quality and quantity of biologically active constituents rather than the total vegetative yield of the targeted medicinal plant parts. No foreign matter, weeds or toxic plants are mixed with the harvested medicinal plant materials. Avoid dew, rain or exceptionally high humidity. If harvesting occurs in wet conditions, the material should be transported immediately to an indoor drying. Use clean devices to harvest as well as to store. Material should be stored in dry and free from insects, rodents, birds and other pests, and inaccessible to livestock and domestic animals. If the underground parts (such as the roots) are used, any adhering soil should be removed from the medicinal plant materials as soon as they are harvested. Medicinal plants should not be collected in or near areas where high levels of pesticides or other possible contaminants are used or found, such as roadsides, drainage ditches, mine tailings, garbage dumps and industrial facilities which may produce toxic emissions.

Section 3: Good collection Practices (GCP) for Medicinal Plants

1. ***Permission to collect:*** In some countries, collection permits and other documents from government authorities and landowners must be obtained prior to collecting any plants from the wild. Sufficient time for the processing and issuance of these permits must be allocated at the planning stage. For medicinal plant materials intended for export from the country of collection, export permits, phytosanitary certificates, Convention on International Trade in Endangered Species of Wild Fauna and Flora (CITES) permit(s) (for export and import), CITES certificates (for re-export), and other permits must be obtained, when required.
2. ***Technical planning:*** Essential information on the target species (the geographical distribution and population Density, taxonomy, distribution, phenology, genetic diversity, reproductive biology and ethnobotany) should be obtained. Data about environmental conditions, including topography, geology, soil, climate and vegetation at the prospective collecting site(s), should be collated and presented in a collection management plan. Transport, personnel, equipments and storage facilities should be ready.
3. ***Selection of medicinal plants for collection:*** select and authenticate plant species for collection.
4. ***Collection:*** same as above given in GAP
5. ***Personnel:*** same as above given in GAP

Section 4: Common Technical Aspects of GACP

1. **Post-harvest processing:**
   (a) **Inspection and sorting:** Raw medicinal plant materials should be inspected and sorted for foreign matter, cross contamination and organoleptic characters prior to primary processing.
   (b) **Primary processing:** Harvested or collected raw medicinal plant materials, prior to processing, should be protected from rain, moisture and any other conditions that might cause deterioration.
   (c) **Drying:** Medicinal plants can be dried in a number of ways: in the open air (shaded from direct sunlight); placed in thin layers on drying frames, wire-screened rooms or buildings; by direct sunlight, if appropriate; in drying ovens/rooms and solar dryers; by indirect fire; baking; lyophilization; microwave; or infrared devices. When possible, temperature and humidity should be controlled to avoid damage to the active chemical constituents. The method and temperature used for drying may have a considerable impact on the quality of the resulting medicinal plant materials.
   (d) **Specific processing:** Common specific processing practices include pre-selection, peeling the skins of roots and rhizomes, boiling in water, steaming, soaking, pickling, distillation, fumigation, roasting, natural fermentation, treatment with lime and chopping. Processing procedures involving the formation of certain shapes, bundling and special drying may also have an impact on the quality of the medicinal plant materials.
   (e) **Processing facilities:** Facilities should preferably be located in areas that are free from objectionable odours, smoke, dust or other contaminants, and are not subject to flooding. Roadways should not be near vicinity, building ceilings, floors should be clean. Sufficient lighting, ventilation and water supply should be maintained.
2. ***Bulk packaging and labelling:*** immediate packing and labelling is necessary. Packaging material should be clean and stored in dry places. Appropriate labels should be affixed to each batch packing.
3. ***Storage and transportation:*** Conveyances used for transporting bulk medicinal plant materials from the place of production to storage for processing should be cleaned between loads. Bulk transport, such as ship or rail cars, should be cleaned and, where appropriate, well ventilated to remove moisture from medicinal plant materials and to prevent condensation.
4. ***Equipment:*** should be clean and well labelled
5. ***Quality assurance:*** regular auditing visits to cultivation or collection sites and processing facilities by expert representatives of producers and buyers and through inspection by national and/or local regulatory authorities.
6. ***Documentation:*** SOP should be prepared for each stage.
7. ***Personnel (growers, collectors, producers, handlers, processors):*** same as GAP

Section 5: Other Relevant

Issues

5.1 Ethical and legal considerations: Must be carried out in accordance with legal and environmental requirements and with the ethical codes or norms of the community and country in which the activities take place. The provisions of the Convention on Biological Diversity must be respected.

- ***Intellectual property rights and benefits-sharing:*** Agreements on the return of immediate and/or long-term benefits and compensation for the use of source medicinal plant materials must be discussed and concluded, in writing, prior to collection or cultivation.
- ***Threatened and endangered species:*** Medicinal plants that are protected by national and international laws, such as those listed in national "red" lists, may be collected only by relevant permission according to national and/or international laws.

5.2 Research needs

A national and/or regional inventory of medicinal plants may facilitate the identification of medicinal plants used by communities (including endangered species), outline their distribution and assess their abundance. It can also be used as a tool in tackling questions concerning intellectual property rights issues. Member States are encouraged to establish such inventories.

Research is greatly needed to improve the agronomy of cultivated medicinal plants, promote the exchange of information on agricultural production and investigate the social and environmental impact of medicinal plant cultivation and collection.

Data sheets and monographs should be developed on medicinal plants that take into account the particular situation of regions and countries. Such information materials can be useful instruments for promoting technical advancement. General as well as specific education and training materials should be developed for local growers and collectors of medicinal plants.

1.2.2 Organic Farming

Biodynamic agriculture is a holistic, ecological, and ethical approach to farming which focuses exclusively on organic farming. It avoids use of inorganic and synthetic chemicals, pesticides and fertilizers. It favors traditional farming with use of modern technology.

Organic farming is an agricultural system that uses fertilizers of organic origin such as compost manure, green manure, and bone meal and places emphasis on techniques such as crop rotation and companion planting.

Integrated Pest Management is important aspect of organic farming which involves:

- *Cultural method or traditional methods like clean cultivation without giving chance to spread pest, crop rotation and plowing, variation in time of planting, proper use of fertilizers and irrigation, use of resistant varieties, intercropping, pruning*
- *Mechanical, physical control or biological control like use of pheromones and hormones; use of attractants, repellants and sterilants*
- *Use of biopesticides like fungi (Beauveria, entomophthora), bacteria (Bacillus thuringiensis), Virus (Nuclear polyhedrosis Virus),*
- *Use of botanical pesticides like neem, pyrethrin*

The principal methods of organic farming include

- **Crop rotation**: It is the practice of growing different types of crops in the same area in sequenced seasons. Different crops need different nutrients. Depletion in soil nutrition is observed due to growing of same crops in the same place for many years due to use of only one type of nutrient by crops. But rotation of crops can balance soil nutrition by reducing soil erosion and increasing soil fertility and crop yield.
- **Use of green manures**: Green manure comprises cover crops which are grown only for production of green manures. These crops in green condition are allowed to incorporate in soil by ploughing to improve soil nutrition and fertility.
- **Use of compost**: Composting of waste is an aerobic (in the presence of air) method of decomposing solid wastes. The process involves decomposition of organic waste into humus known as compost which is a good fertiliser for plants. Vermi-compost is excretions produced by live earthworms in soil provided with sufficient biomass. Use of bio fertilizers (example: *Rhizobium*, *Azotobacter*, Blue green algae, Azolla , *Mycorrhizae* etc) and kitchen waste are also promising in improvement of soil fertility.
- **Mechanical control:** It employs manual labor along with different devices for collection and destruction of pests.
- **Biological pest control**: Biological control is a method of controlling pests such as insects, mites, weeds and plant diseases using other organisms. It relies on predation, parasitism, herbivorism, or other natural mechanisms like use of herbivores and pathogens, but typically also involves an active human management role. It requires thorough understanding of effective organisms. There are three basic types of biological pest control strategies:
    - Importation: use of natural enemy of a pest
    - Augmentation: breeding and release of locally-occurring natural enemies
    - Conservation: use of measures to increase natural enemies

Due to popularity of medicinal plants for primary health care and prevention of diseases, natural resources of these plants are destroyed by human being. But sound knowledge of Cultivation technology has resulted in gradual depletion of raw material from wild sources. Cultivation of medicinal plants requires knowledge, skills, and technologies used to grow intensively produced plants for human food and non-food uses and for personal or social needs. Actual work involves plant propagation and cultivation with the aim of improving plant growth, yields, quality, nutritional value, and resistance to insects, diseases, and environmental stresses. Wild medicinal plant collection damages natural environment due to extinction of a species and many times it is difficult to collect correct plant from remote areas like mountains, forests etc. So cultivation of medicinal plants allows preservation of endangered medicinal plants and thus natural resources improves quality and quantity as well as yield of drugs and builds up national economy.

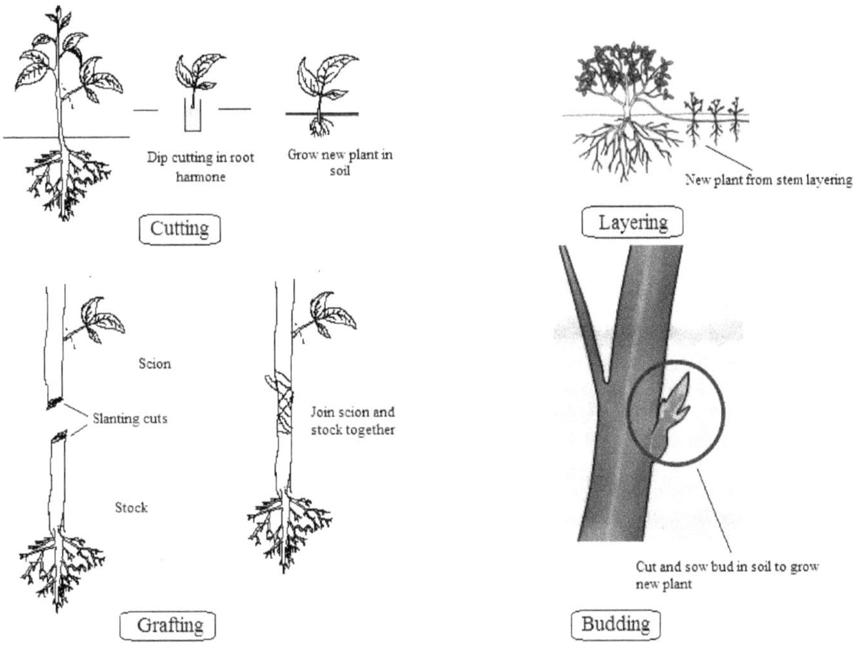

Fig. 1.1 Different Asexual (vegetative) propagation methods

Following are Methods of propagation

Method	Sexual (seed) propagation	Asexual (vegetative) propagation (Fig. 1.1)		
Material of propagation	Seeds are sowed by broadcasting (scattering of extremely small seeds) or dibbling (sowing of large size seeds into holes) method	**Natural**: Bulbs (garlic), tubers (aconite), offsets (aloe), corms (saffron), rhizomes (ginger), roots, suckers (banana), stolons (licorice)	**Artificial**: Cuttings (rose, brahmi), layering (lemon), grafting (mango), budding (hibiscus)	**Tissue culture**: Laboratory developed cultures of plants (Example: Banana)
Advantages	Cheap method of raising Seedlings which are long-lived, sturdy and suitable for plants which cannot be propagated by asexual method	Uniformity in yield and other characters, fast in growth, seedless, nutrients improved or disease resistant varieties can be obtained		
Disadvantages	Time consuming and costly as to grow seed-lings first and then actual plant, poor uniformity in yield of seedlings,	Poor adaptability to climatic changes and hence short lived		

1.2.3 Pest and Pest Management in Medicinal Plants

Pest is an undesirable animal or plant species. The overall losses due to pest infestation tune to millions of rupees every year. The control of pests thus, assumes primary importance in the context of cultivation of medicinal and aromatic plants. Pest control in the recent years has become a major problem in our homes, gardens and agriculture. The insect population of the universe is increased to such an extent that governmental agencies and public health offices are constantly struggling to keep barest of this potential danger to crop plant. The different types of pests infesting the medicinal plants are: fungi, virus, Insects, Weeds, Non insect pests

Fungi: Many fungi affect plants differently. Here few examples are discussed

- Aschochyta atropea: Formation of grayish white irregular spots which further cause necrosis of leaves, called leaf necrosis
- Cercospora atropea: Round to angular brown spots with chestnut coloured margins on both sides of leaves, called leaf spot.
- Phytophthora nicotinae: Dropping of young leaves and branches, yellowing of older leaves and drying of whole apical portion, called phytophthora root rot. (disease most occur on belladonna and some other plants)

Viruses: Many different viruses are also the cause of the some disease occurring on plants. They are mosaic causing necrosis of leaves, petioles and stem on different solanaceous plants. Tobacco mosaic virus, Cucumber mosaic virus, Tobacco ring spot virus affects Digitalis. Cucumber mosaic virus (one of the strain) affects hyocymus, rauwolfia, tobacco, datura, vinca and eucalyptus. Other viruses are Yellow vein mosaic, graft transmissible virus, distortion mosaic etc.

Insects: It is found that Total no. of insect species are equivalent to **Total** number of species of all other forms of life put together. Throughout world, about 1 million insect species have been reported. All insects are belongs to Arthropods of animal kingdom. These arthropods are roughly divided into two morphological groups, according to their Mouthparts. Their effects involve biting, chewing, piercing and sucking. Various insect pests which attack medicinal plants are: Agrotis spes., Heliothis armigera, Odoutotames obesus, Flea beetle, Empoasca pteridis etc.

- Mentha: Phytomyza atricornis
- Rauwolfia: Diaphonia nilgirica, Indomia cretacerus, Plantia viridicolis
- Dill: Papillio machon, Hyadaphis coriavdri
- belladona leaves: Gonocephalum spc., Agrotis flammatra
- Others, which cause damages, are caterpillar, lepidopterus larve, weevil, aphids, pyrilla, locusts, spinder, ticks, mites etc.

Weeds: A weed is undesirable plant. Weeds are considered as dreadful pests because losses due to them estimated to be more than those occurring due to pests and disease combination together. Weed leads to loss of Nutrients, Water, Light and space. Increase in cost of labour and equipment. Low product quality, Enhanced chances for attacks of bacteria, fungi and insects, Some weeds also cause allergies:

- Hay fever by Rag weed, Medican tea, Yellow dock, Parthenium
- Dermatitis by Poison ivy, Western poison oak, Poison sumac
- Others, Fatal effect by Corn cokle (cyanogenetic glycoside), Poisonous: Datura, menispermous spc.

Non-Insect Pests: They are grouped into two categories. Vertebrates like monkeys, rats, birds, rabbits and hares, squirrels, antelopes, deer, pigs. Ievertebrates like nematodes, crabs, snails, mites and symphylids.

Methods of Pest Control

Mechanical Method	It employs manual labor along with different devices for collection and destruction of pests. A proper approach is made for collection and destruction of Eggs, Larvae, Pupae, and Adults of insects. The better way for protection from rodents like rat is construction of concrete warehouses. Warehouses should have metal reinforcement corners on window frames. The method adopted for trapping flying insect is flavored attractant placed in funnel shaped container, which are mixed with saw dust. The insect can easily get an entry in the trap, but find very hard to come out. The mouse and rat traps are also used. The simple techniques used are: Hand picking, Pruning, Burning, Trapping of pests. ***Advantage*** • Skilled labours are not required • Cost required is very less • There are no any side effects ***Limitations*** • Time and labour requirement is high • Applicable only on small scale • Requires repeated application
Physical Method	Reduction of pest population by using device which affect them physically or alter their physical environment. Manipulation of temperature, humidity, light is used for this purpose. This includes following types: • Sun drying:. • Disinfection of gowdouns by heating [50-70^{0}C] • Burning • Refrigeration/Cold storage • Moisture: [less than 10 %] • Use of light • Use of Ionizing radiation to sterile • Use of Ultrasonic sound • Hot water
Cultural/*Agricultural Method*	It covers advanced plant breeding techniques capable of inducing genetic manipulations resulting in production of pest-resistance species. It has achieved much success in producing hybrid varieties, which are resistance to fungal and bacterial attack, as compared to limited success with insect. The systemic insecticides have been developed which are absorbed through the root and reach to leaves by which all the foliage portion becomes distasteful for insects. Another aspect is agricultural control is ploughing, which should be sufficiently deep so as to eradicate weeds as well as early stages of insects. If a plant is found out to be favored by insects as

Contd...

	major source of food, the land under cultivation of such plant should be subjected to crop rotation. Another method for checking supply of food to insects is by changing the environment which is in many cases, may leads to obstruction in their life cycle. Proper drainage source serve this purpose to a greater extent. ***Advantages*** • Economic • Safe ***Disadvantages*** • Effective for single pest only • Few visible results observed • Not effective at epidemic condition • Detailed knowledge of biology of pest is required
Chemical Method	Chemical control is done by with help of Pesticides. Pesticides are chemicals derived from synthetic and natural sources effective in small concentration against pest. Because of toxic effect of all such chemicals used as pesticides their use is regulated by the **Insecticides** act, in India; Federal insecticide, fungicide and rodenticide act, in US; The agriculture (poisonous substances) regulation, in UK. Various forms of preparation of pesticides used:Spray or wetable powders, Powders, Granulates, Self-emulsifying concentrates, Solution in mineral oil fractions, Fumigants. Chemical Pesticides may be classified according to the type of organism against which they are effective, as follows ***Fungicides:*** they are used to prevent or control the plant disease caused by phytopathogenic fungi and most widely used as seed or soil fungicidal disinfectant. They can be of different types based on their use as follows: *Disinfectants for seeds:* These fungicides give prior protection to seeds against fungal disease causing pathogens which are admixed with the seed in the form of their spores, hyphae and scieratia. Dithiocarbamates, Organo-phosphorous compounds, Pyridine derivatives, Carboxins etc. *Disinfectants for soil:* There are some fungicides, which can be useful for the disinfection of the soil and thereby kill the phyto-pathogenic bacteria, which cause fungal infection through soil. However this is more difficult and expensive. *Leaf fungicides:* These are fungicides, which are used for the protection of the leaves and fruits. Bordeaux mixture, Copper oxy chlorides, Colloidal sulphur, Barium sulphate, Thiurams and dithiocarbamates, Nitro compounds like dichloro nitro aniline etc ***Herbicides:*** They are the weed killers, which are used for destroying the unwanted plants or to prevent their growth. Example- Carbamates, Urea derivatives, Growth promoters, Quaternary ammonium compounds, Di-and triazines. They are of several types that differ in their mode of action as: Total herbicides, Selective herbicides, Water weed killers, Harvesting aids ***Insecticides:*** Major insect controlling agents are insecticides, insect repellents, insect attractant and insect sterilizing agents. The insecticides can be of three types like Respiratory toxin or food toxin or contact toxins. Beside these they can be classified by the mode of action as general cell toxins (protein precipitants), enzyme toxins (phosphoric acid ester and N- alkyl carbamates) and nerve toxins (Example-chlorinated hydrocarbons). The insecticides used for the protection of the medicinal plants can be of two types based on the site of their action those which do not penetrate into the plant and systematic insecticides. ***Acaricides*:** They are substances that are used to control the infestation caused by the mites, especially spider mites. These mites belong to the arthropod and multiply very

Contd...

	rapidly. They cause rapid damage to the foliage of culti-vated plants. These insects acquire resistance to the chemicals because of their rapid multiplication and therefore new acaricides have to be developed. Examples: Phosphoric and thiophos-phoric acid esters, Carba-midic esters, Chlorinated aromatics with or without sulphur in the molecule ***Nematodes*:** For the control of the phyto-pathogenic thread worms i.e. nematodes living free in the soil and also occurring in the plants. The agents, which are responsible for the control of the nematodes, are Halogenated hydrocarbons, Carbamidic and thiocarbamidic acid derivatives and Thio-phosphoric acid esters ***Rodenticides*:** Rodents are the mammals such as the rats, mouse and rabbit, which have sharp gnawing incisor teeth. The fecal pellets and hairs from the fur of the rats and mice characterize this contamination. The pesticides acts against rodent are called rodenticides. Examples: Warfarin, Arsenic trioxide, Thallium sulfate ***Advantages*** • Highly effective method • Get quick results • Useful at variable climatic conditions • Wide range for selection of chemicals • Economic method ***Disadvantages*** • Repeated application of chemicals is required • Non target species like natural enemies of insect get affected. • Resurgence of minor pest • Residue in food • Direct hazard to the applicator • Resistance in insect
Biological Control Biopesticides/ Bioinsecticides	See details as follows

1.2.4 Biopesticides/Bioinsecticides

This method uses biochemicals, microorganisms or plant mediated pest control. If the method is properly designed it may emerge as an effective, safe, and economical method of pest control.

Biochemical pesticides: It include substances that interfere with mating, such as insect sex pheromones (Examples- 7, 8-epoxy-2-methyloctadecane from gypsy-moth), as well as various scented plant extracts that attract insect pests to traps.

Plant derived Biopesticides/Bioinsecticides: The reason for using new natural pesticides is that these are active at highly acceptable levels, biodegradable and do not leave toxic residues while the commonly used phosphorous and chlorinated insecticides contaminate the environment. [Table 1.2.]

Microbial pesticides: It consists of a microorganism (Example- a bacterium, fungus, virus or protozoan) as the active ingredient. Microbial pesticides can control many different kinds of pests, although each separate active ingredient is relatively specific for its target pest[s]. For example, there are fungi that control certain weeds and other fungi that kill specific insects. The most widely used microbial pesticides are subspecies and strains of *Bacillus thuringiensis,* or

Bt. Each strain of this bacterium produces a different mix of proteins and specifically kills one or a few related species of insect larvae.

Predators: Organisms which feed on other insects having body size greater or equal to the insect is called predators. This includes,

- Lady bird beetle: This insect feeds on aphids.
- *Chrysoperia carnea*: The larvae of this insect feed on all soft bodied insects like aphids, jassids, white flies, mealy bug, etc.
- *Cryptolaemus montrouzieri*: This insect feeds on mealy bugs on grapes.

Parasites: Those insects whose larvae feed internally or externally on the body of other insect is called parasites. This includes,

- Egg parasite: Trichogramma chilonis parasites egg of Helicoverpa armigera.
- Larval parasite: Bracon hibitor parasites larvae of H.armigera.
- Pupal parasite: Goniopthalmus halli parasites pupae of H.armigera.
- Adult parasite: Epiricania melanoleuca parasites adults of sugarcane pyrilla.
- Egg larval parasite: Copidosoma kohleri parasities egg of potato tuber moth and comes out at larval stage by killing the pest.

Pathogens: Microorganisms like bacteria, virusus, fungi, protozoa and nematodes develop diseases to the pest and thus help in killing pest. [Table 1.3]

Table 1.1 Different Classes of Pesticides based on the Chemical Composition

<table>
<tr><th>Class</th><th>Examples</th><th>Action on plants</th><th>Action on animals</th></tr>
<tr><td>Chlorinated hydrocarbons</td><td>Aldrin, Benzene hexachloride (BHC), Chlordane, DDT, Dieldrine, Endrin, Heptachlor, Lindane , Methoxychlor</td><td rowspan="3">➢ Inhibition of photosynthesis
➢ Inhibition of oxidative phosphorylation</td><td rowspan="3">➢ Inhibition of Ach esterase
➢ Neurotoxication</td></tr>
<tr><td>Chlorinated phenoxyalkanoic acid</td><td>2, 4- D (2, 4- dichlorophenoxy acetic acid), 2, 4, 5- T</td></tr>
<tr><td>Organophosphorous</td><td>Carbaphenathion, Malathion, Parathion, Demeton, Ethion</td></tr>
<tr><td>Carbonate insecticides</td><td>Carbaryl</td><td rowspan="5">➢ Hormone analogue
➢ Inhibition of chlorophyll synthesis
➢ Inhibition of pentothenate synthesis</td><td rowspan="5">➢ Inhibition of neuromuscular junction</td></tr>
<tr><td>Dithiocarbamate fungicides</td><td>Ferbamn, Nabam, Thiram, Zineb, Ziram</td></tr>
<tr><td>Inorganic pesticides</td><td>Alumminium phosphate, Calcium arsenate, Lead arsenate</td></tr>
<tr><td>Miscellaneous</td><td>Brompproplylate, Chloropicrin, Ethylene dibromide, Ethylene oxide, Methyl bromide</td></tr>
<tr><td>Pesticides of plant origin:</td><td>Nicotine, Pyrethrum, pyrethroids, Rotenoids</td></tr>
</table>

Table 1.2 Examples of Plant derived Biopesticide/Bio-insecticides

Pyrethrum (African daisy)	Biological source: dried flower heads of *Chrysanthemum cinerariifolium* and *Chrysanthemum coccineum* of family Asteraceae. It contains oleoresin mixture of six compounds: Pyrethrin-I and II, Cinerin-I and II, Jasmoline-I and II *Mode of action*: It is contact poison which affects on CNS through sodium channel and causes paralysis
Sabadilla lily	*Biological source:* seeds of *Schoenocaulon officinale* of family Liliaceae. It contains vetratridine, sabadine alkaloids. *Mode of action:* It is contact poison and affects on CNS through sodium channel and causes paralysis
Castor oil	*Biological source:* seeds of *Ricinus communis* of family Euphorbiaceae. It contains toxic protein ricin. *Mode of action:* Impairs chain elongation in protein synthesis, causing cell death and tissue damage
Ryania	*Biological source:* Roots of *Ryania specios* of family Salicaceae. It contains diterpene alkaloid- ryanodine *Mode of action:* Affects CVS, CNS by inhibiting calcium release proteins
Derris (tuba) root	*Biological source:* Root and rhizomes of *Derris elliptica* of family Fabaceae. The main active principle is iso-flavonoid rotenone. *Mode of action:* It is inhibitor of respiratory chain and affects by inhibiting electron transport and thus exhibits feeding deterrent activity.
Neem	*Biological source:* Whole plant of *Azadhiracta indica* of family Meliaceae. It contains triterpenoid- azadirachtin *Mode of action:* Anti-feedent, antifungal, nematicidal, affects hormones of insects
Nux vomica	*Biological source:* Seeds of *Strychnous nux-vomica* of family Loganiaceae. It contains indole alkaloids –Strychnine and Brucine. *Mode of action:* Rodenticide by strong convulsant action
Red squill	*Biological source:* Bulbs of *Urginia maritima* of family Liliaceae. It contains cardioactive sterols- proscillaridin, scillroside, scillarenin *Mode of action:* It causes emesis, blocks cardiovascular and central nervous system.
Tobacco	*Biological source:* Whole plant of *Nicotiana tabacum* of family Solanaceae. It contains alkaloid- Nicotine *Mode of action:* It predominantly affects respiratory system but also acts as a slight contact and stomach poison.
Custard apple	*Biological source:* Seeds of *Annona squamosa* of family Annonaceae. It contains alkaloid, essential oils and glycosides. *Mode of action:* It is cytotoxic and causes electron transport inhibition.
Essential oil	There are many well known essential oils (like ocimum, lemon grass, citronella, clove, thyme, mint, cinnamon, rosemary etc) which have insecticide or insect repellent properties. Insecticide linalool (present in ocimum, coriander, cinnamon, lavender and birch oil) has been demonstrated to act on the nervous system. Eugenol (Present in clove, cinnamon, tulsi oil) mimics octopamine action by increasing intracellular calcium levels to act as insecticide. Eugenol and its derivatives, safrole and its derivatives are found potent toxic and repellent to *Periplaneta americana (American cockroach)*. Mustard oil from *Brassica nigra* contains allyl isothiocyanate which is antifungal.

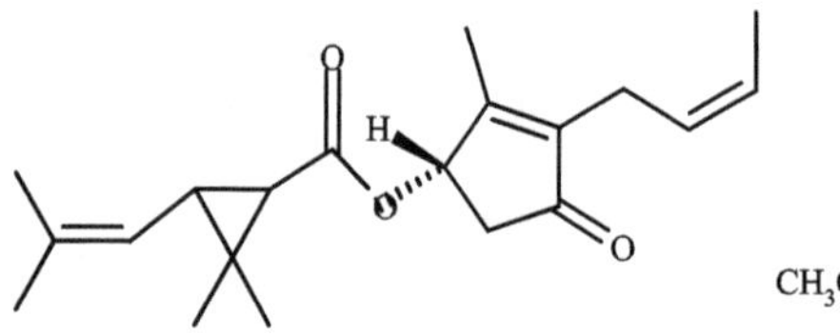

Cinerin I

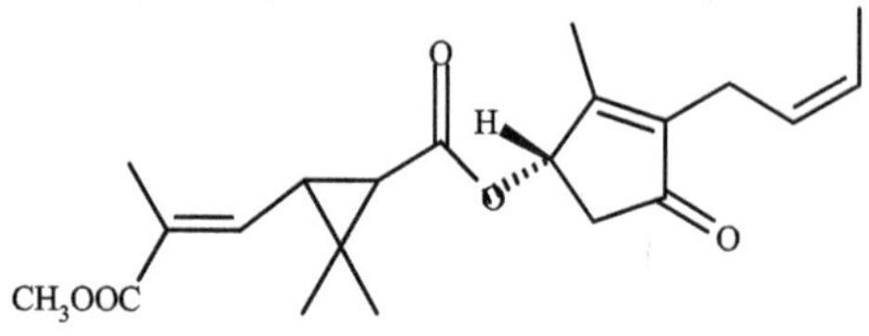

Cinerin II

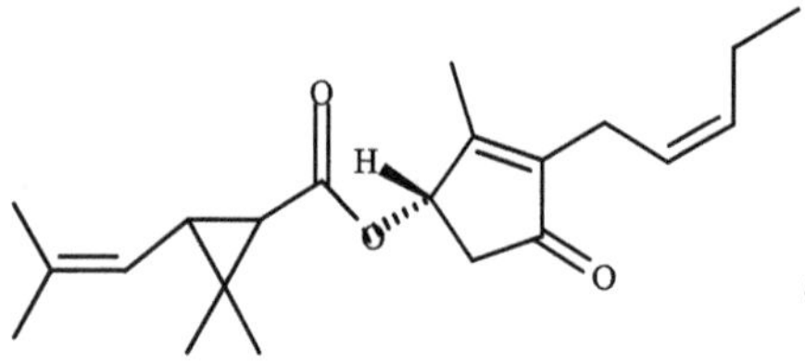

Jasmolin I

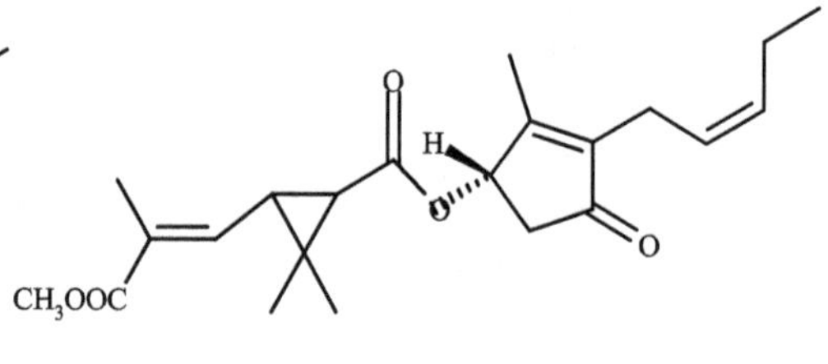

Jasmolin II

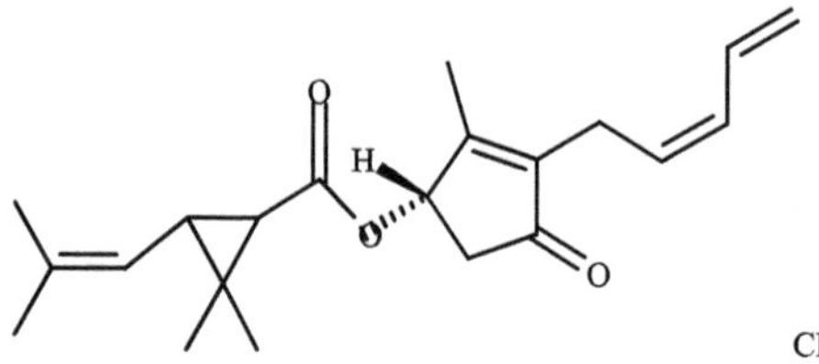

Pyrethrin I

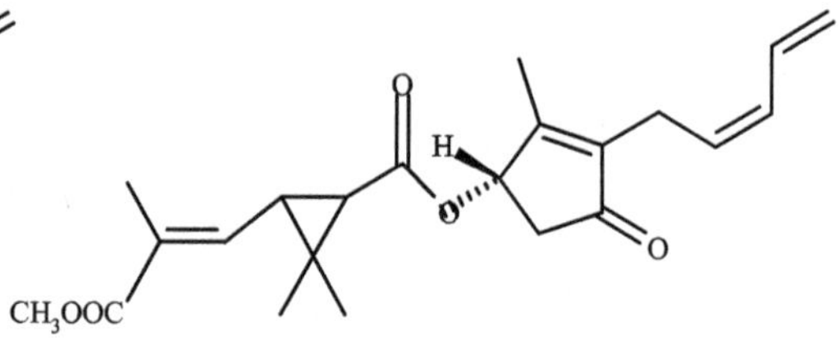

Pyrethrin II

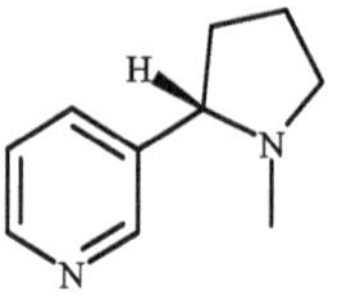

Nicotine

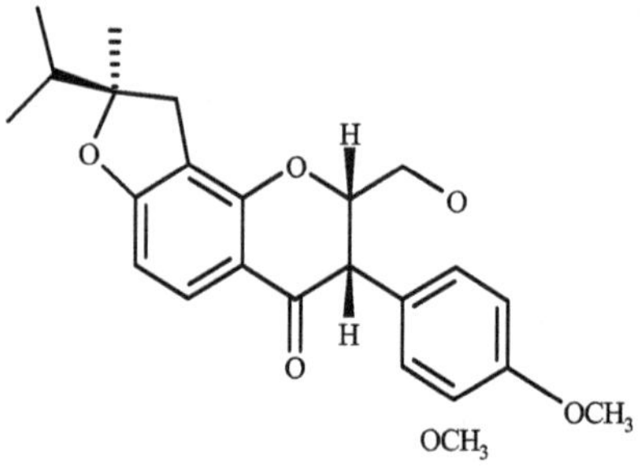

Rotenone

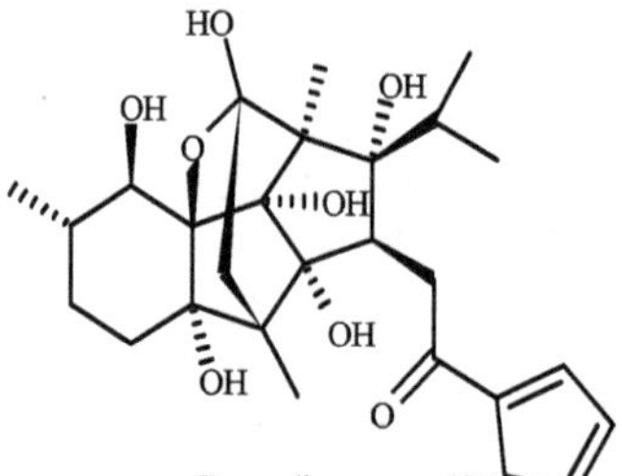

Ryanodine

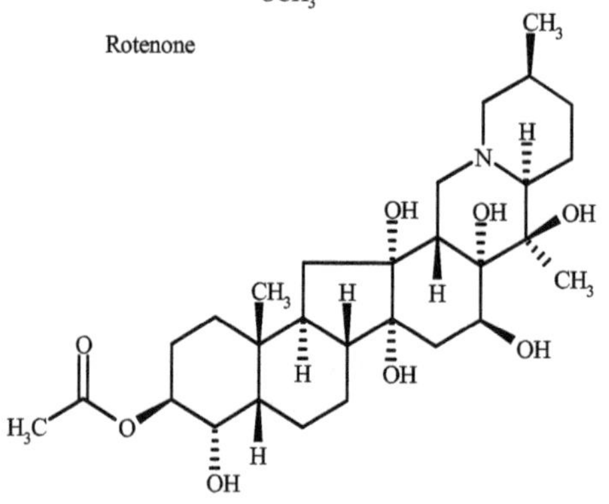

Fig. 1.2 Chemistry of natural pesticides

Table 1.3: Examples of Pathogen derived Biopesticide/Bio-insecticides

Control Agent	Mode of Action	Examples	Control Agent
Bacteria	Produce toxins that are detrimental to certain insect pests when ingested	Bacillus thuringiensis (BT)	Lepidopterans
		Bacillus popilliae	Japanese beetle
		Agrobacterium radiobacter	Crown gall disease
Viruses	Kills insects when ingested. Insect's feeding behavior is disrupted thus it starves and dies.	Baculoviruese: Nuclear polyhedrosis virus (NPV)	Lepidopteran and Hymenopteran
		Baculoviruses: Granulosis virus (GV)	Lepidopteran
		Baculoviruese: Group C	Arthropods
		Entomopo	
Fungi	Controls insects by growing on them secreting enzymes that weaken the insect's outer coat, and then getting inside the insect and continuing to grow, eventually killing the infected pest	Entomophaga praxibulli	Grasshoppers
		Zoophthora radicans	Aphids
		Neozygites floridana	Cassava green mite
Protozoa	Kills insects when ingested. Insect's feeding behavior is disrupted thus it starves and dies.	Nosema	Grasshoppers
		Vairimorpha	Lepidoptera
		Malamoeba	Locusts
Nematode	They kill their target organisms by entering natural body openings or by penetrating the insect cuticle directly.	Heterorhabditis bacteriophora	Black vine weevil, Japanese beetles
		Phasmarhabditis hermaphrodita	Various slugs and snails

1.3 Indian Systems of Medicine

1.3.1 Basic principles involved in Ayurveda, Siddha, Unani and Homeopathy

1.3.1.1 Ayurveda System

It is about 5000 year old system of medicine native to India. It is holistic system of medicine which considers whole body while treating disease and not just a diseased part of body. Ayurveda has thousands year's evidence based history so it can be just complete system rather alternative system or complementary system. Ayurveda is a Sanskrit word which means (*Ayur*- life and *veda* – to gain knowledge or science) science of life. Ayurveda deals with different types of plants, minerals and animal products. Charak samhita by Charak includes the principle components or theory of Ayurveda. Sushrut samhita edited by Sushrut is about the surgical treatments in Ayurveda.

It is assumed that Sushruta was born in the Eastern part of India near Bihar (which was famous for sacred schools and universities at that time). Sushruta was a physician by occupation. In Mahabharata, he is represented as a son of Rishi Visvamitra.

His Samhita, divided into six volumes, compromises all aspects of general medicine. However, due to an extraordinary accuracy and detail of surgery in his work, he is also considered as the father of surgery.

These six volumes contain 184 chapters describing 1120 illness, 700 medical plants, 64 drugs prepared from minerals, and 57 from animal sources. It also discusses different surgical techniques suitable for different body parts along with 14 different types of bandages. Mostly, the Samhita focuses on surgery and midwifery, but it also deals with topics such as genetics, mental illness, embryology, anatomy, geriatric illness, and diabetes.

It has 300 surgical procedures and it classifies surgery into five subheadings such as

- Aharya (extraction of solid bodies),
- Bhedya (excising),
- Chhedya (incising),
- Eshya (probing),
- Lekhya (scarifying),
- Sivya (suturing),
- Vedhya (puncturing), and
- Visravaniya (evacuating fluids).

It describes more than 300 kinds of operations that call for 42 different surgical processes and 121 different types of instruments. For the purpose of anesthesia, he advised the use of wine with the incense of cannabis and this is the oldest form of anesthesia used with no world record before that. The instruments used for surgeries were constructed after the shape of beasts and birds and named after them like the crocodile forceps and hawk's bill forceps.

The Sushruta Samhita is best known for its approach and discussions of surgery. It was one of the first in human history to suggest that a student of surgery should learn about human body and its organs by dissecting a dead body. It describes haemorrhoidectomy, amputations, plastic, rhinoplastic, ophthalmic, lithotomic and obstetrical procedures.

Theory and principles: Ayurveda involves following fundamental principles:

Pancha Mahabhuta	*Prithvi* (earth) *Apa* (water) *Tej* (fire) *Vayu* (air) *Akash* (sky)
Panchshil theory	*Rasa* : Therapeutically active substances *Guna* : Quality *Virya* : Active principle and potency *Vipaka* : The end product of digestion *Prabhava* : Actual effect of drug on body.
Sapta Dhatu theory	*Rasa* (Plasma) *Raktam* (Blood) *Mansa* (Muscles) *Meda* (Fat) *Asthi* (Bone) *Majja* (Bone marrow and nerves) *Shukra* (Reproductive fluid or Semen)
Tridosha theory	*Vatta* = *Vayu* + *akash* = respiration and mobility *Pitta* = *Agni* = digestion and metabolism *Kapha* = *Prithvi* + *apa* = lubrication of joints and stability.
Triguna	*Satva* (good) *Raja* (aggressive) *Toma* (dullness)
Ama	A Sanskrit word meaning "uncooked" or "undigested" is used to refer to the concept of anything that exists in a state of incomplete transformation.

Diagnosis: The non-equilibrium between any of above principles causes to person suffers from diseases. Mental, physical, social and spiritual welfare of human beings is considered by Ayurveda to cure the disease cause. Observation of body color, tongue, nail, eyes, pulse and investigation of blood, urine and fecal matter is criteria of diagnosing actual cause of disease.

Treatment: Panchkarma is an important treatment in Ayurveda which includes Snehan (massage), Swedan (steam), Vaman (vomit), Virechan (expulsion) and Basti (medicated enemas). The medicines are given in the form of powder (churna, bhasma), liquid (asava, arishta and taila), semisolid (leha or paka) and tablets (gutika, vati). Treatment of ayurveda involves use of drugs obtained from plant, animal and mineral sources. Ayurveda also focuses on exercise, yoga, and meditation. One type of prescription is a Sattvic diet.

Dosage forms of Ayurveda are powders (churna), bhasma (metal oxides), asava and arishtha (alcohol containing liquids), quath (extracts), gutika (pills), lep (ointment) or taila (Medicated oils).

There are eight branches of Ayurveda:

1. Kayachikitsa (internal medicine)
2. Kumarbhritya (pediatrics)
3. Trachchikitsa (psychology medicine)
4. Shalakya Tantra [ear, nose and throat]
5. Shalya Tantra (surgery)
6. Agada tantra (toxicology)
7. Rasayana tantra (geriatrics)
8. Vajikaran tantra [gynecology]

1.3.1.2 Siddha System

Sidha system of medicine is one of the oldest medical systems known to mankind even before ayurvedic system which was flourished in Vedic culture, Dravidian culture and Indus Valley Civilization. Tamil traditional medicine is origin of Siddha system and hence most of literature of this system is given in Tamil Language. 18 "Siddhas" (Spiritual persons) developed this system so it is called as Sidha. Sage Agathiyar is considered the guru of all Sidhas.

According to Palm Leaf manuscript, it is believed that it was first described by Lord Shiva to his wife Parvathy and then to their son Lord Muruga. Then he passed this knowledge to his disciple sage Agasthya. Agasthya educated 18 Siddhars. Human beings got this knowledge from 18 Siddhars. Siddhars have to get Siddhi means attainment of supernatural powers.

Theory and principles: Generally the basic principles of Siddha and Ayurveda medicine are almost similar. But siddha system explains in detail about various basic treatments of diseases while surgery like modern treatments are practiced and written in detail in Ayurveda. Like Ayurveda, Siddha medicine also, classifies physiological components of the human beings as vata (air), pitta (fire) and kapha (earth and water). Siddha system is based on 96 principles and out of these Triguna theory, i.e., vatta, pitta and kapha is more prominent. Under normal conditions, the ratio between Vatta, Pitta, and Kapha is 4:2:1, respectively.

Siddha deals with thousands of herbs, animal, mineral and metals. Siddha system believes that health is perfect state of physical, mental, social, moral and spiritual component. It is based on Andapinda Thathuvam means relationship between universe and human body. Siddhas are called as Vaithiyars.

Diagnosis: A Siddha physician studies eight important things of body i.e. nadi (pulse), varna (colour), na (tongue), mala (faeces) kan (eyes), swara (voice), sparisam (touch), and neer (urine).

Guna	Personalities	Complications
Vata	Stout, black, cold and inactive healthy	Increased *Vata* shows arrogant behaviour, paralysis, heart attack.
Pitta	Lean, whitish complexion and perfectionist	Increased *Pitta* shows graying of hair, anemia and instability.
Kapha	Well built, good complexion and well behaved	Increased *Kapha* causes jaundice, heart attack.

Treatment: Siddha medicines are divided into three categories: Thavaram (Herbal), Thadu (inorganic) and Janganam (animal). Internal as well as external medicines are divided into 32 categories each separately. Pressure or massage techniques are also part of treatment and called as Thokkanam. There are 108 varma points for pressure techniques.

Treatment is classified into three categories:

- **Devamaruthuvum (Divine method):** The medicines prepared from metals and minerals come under this topic. The speciality of these medicines is a very small dose brings quick recovery even from chronic ailments. These are highly potent. Most of these medcines has no expiry date that is they can be preserved life-long. In this method use of metals and minerals medicines like parpam, chendooram, guru, kuligai made of mercury, sulphur and pashanams recommended.
- **Manuda maruthuvum (Rational method):** In this method herbal medicines like churanam, kudineer, vadagam are used. They are herbal medicines which have short definite life span. Dose may vary accordingly. They comprise of 34 types – 22 Internal medicines and 12 External medicines
- **Internal medicines :**Charu (juice), Surasam (boiling the extracted juice), Kudineer (decoction), Karkam (Raw materials prepared into paste) etc.
- **External applications :**Vedhu (Steam- therapy), Pattru (Pasting procesed raw drugs on diseased part), Ottradam (Formentation), Kattu (Like Bandaging)
- **Asura maruthuvum (surgical method):** use of surgical method, incision, excisions, use of heat or leech

Treatment in this system emphasizes preparation of fresh medicine. It is then prepared and administered with some Pathya (some restriction). Example- Day time sleeping is not allowed or some food material is restricted like chicken, mango, coconut, mustard, groundnut, almond, tobacco etc. Medicine can be kashayam (extract), churnam (powder), tailams (medicated oil), gulligai (pills), chenduram (metal), bhasmam (calcination product) and or ghritam (medicated ghee).

1.3.1.3 Unani System

This system is also called as Unani-tibb or Yunani Medicine. Arab and Persian physicians such as Rhazes, Avicenna (Ibn Sena), Al-Zahrawi, and Ibn Nafis developed this system.

Book: Ibn Sina's the Canon of Medicine. First book, "On General Means of Treatment" describes that treatments are done in three ways: "one of them is regimen and nutrition; the second, application of drugs; and the third, manual treatment, i.e., surgery". The second book gives rather detailed pharmacological and pharmacotherapeutic characteristic of 811 drugs, among which those of vegetable kingdom constitute 594 (73.7%), of animal kingdom 118 (14.5%) and of mineral origin 99 (12.2%).

Theory and principles: Unani medicine involves concept of the four humours (akhlat) i.e. Phlegm (Balgham), Blood (Dam), Yellow bile (Safra) and Black bile (Sauda). These "humors" and a open air blood sedimentation test exhibits close relation where a dark clot at the bottom resembles black bile, a layer of unclotted erythrocytes resembles blood, a layer of white blood cells resembles phlegm and a layer of clear yellow serum resembles yellow bile. Abnormality in humor leads to disease condition in body.

Diagnosis: The human body is considered to be made up of seven components i.e. 1. Elements (Arkan) 2. Temperament (Mijaz). 3. Humors (Aklat) 4. Organs (Aaza) 5. Faculties (Quwa) 6. Spirits (Arwah). 7. Functions (Afaal) which have direct bearing on the health status of a person and considered by the physician for diagnosis and treatment.

In diagnosis Unani Physican (Hakim) asks a detail history and decides treatment.

Treatment: After diagnosing the disease, treatment involves either to eliminate cause (Izalae sabab), normalize humors (Tadeele akhlat) or to normalise tissues or organs (Tadeele aza). Method of treatment involves modification of essential pre-requisites of health (Ilaj- Bil-Tadbeer) or Panchkarma like in Ayurveda (Ilaj-Bil-Tadbeer) or pharmacotherapy (Ilaj bil advia) or surgery (Ilaj-Bil-Yad).

- Regimental therapy (Ilajbil tadbeer) – Use of exercise, climate change, massage, venesection, leaching, cupping, diet therapy etc.
- Pharmacotherapy (Ilajbil dava) – use of plant, animal and mineral origin drugs, either alone or in combination.
- Surgery (Ilajbil Yad) – Surgical intervention in treatment

As far as possible Unani medicine therapy attempts to use simple physical means to cure a disease. Some of the techniques used in Ilaj bil- Tadbir (Regimental therapy) include Hijamah (Cupping), Fasd (Venesection), Tareeq (Sweating), Idrar-e-Baul (Diuresis), Hamam (Turkish Bath), Dalak (Massage), Kai (Cauterization), Ishal (Purging), Qai (Vomiting), Riyazat (Exercise) and Taleeq (Leeching).

Unani dosage forms are-

- Solid dosage forms [Example: (Habb (pills), quers (tablet), safoof (powder)]
- Liquid dosage forms [Joshnda (decoction), Khisanda (Infusion), Arq (Distillate), Sharbat (Syrup), Qutur (Drops)]
- Semi-solid dosage forms [Huqna (enema) and tila (liniment)].

1.3.1.4 Homeopathy System

Homeo means similar and Pathos means suffering so homeopathy is the "system of similar suffering". German physician Samuel Hahnemann first stated the basic principle of homeopathy in 1796, known as the "law of similars" (let like be cured by like.")

This system was developed by Dr Samuel Hahnemann in Germany. Dr Samuel had written a book *The Curative Powers of Drugs and Some Examinations of Previous Principles* which was based on his study of effect of *cinchona* on his own body where he actually found "law of similars" which indicates similarity between drug and disease.

Theory and principle: Homeopathy emphasises the root cause of the disease and the nature's law of its cure that is 'like cures like'. Thus, homeopathy deals with the following seven principles which are outlined below:

- ***Individualisation*** : No two individuals in the world are alike, i.e. the disease affecting two individuals cannot be similar though they may share common symptoms. So the medicines used to cure the same disease in different individuals are different.

- ***Principle of similiar***: Use of the medicine will produce similar symptoms of disease in an healthy individual. For example, watery eyes and burning nose caused by an onion hence an attack of hay fever with watering eyes and a burning nose can be cured homeopathic remedy made from onion.
- ***Principle of simplex***: Only one single simple medicine at one time and no combination is allowed.
- ***Minimum dose*** : Minimum medicine at a time
- ***Law of proving***: Medicine should have the capacity to produce disease state in a healthy individual.
- ***Law of dynamisation***: Medicine should preserve the normal state of healthy body.
- ***Vital force:*** Medicine should have the capacity to arouse sufficient energy to maintain a healthy body.

Diagnosis: It involves knowing of complete hereditary history as well as observation of moods, habits, skin, eyes, tongue, blood, urine etc of patients.

Treatment:

Not considering imponderabilia, the source materials for homeopathic medicines may consist of the following:

- **plant material such** as: roots, stems, leaves, flowers, bark, pollen, lichen, moss, ferns and algae;
- **microorganisms** such as: fungi, bacteria, viruses and plant parasites;
- **animal materials** such as: whole animals, animal organs, tissues, secretions, cell lines, toxins, nosodes, blood products;
- **human materials such** as: tissues, secretions, cell lines and endogenous molecules such as hormones;
- **minerals and chemicals.**

When the symptoms picture matches with the drug picture, the physician always attempts to identify a single medicine. Homeopathic preparation involves "dynamisation" or "potentiation", whereby a substance is diluted with alcohol or distilled water and then vigorously shaken in a process called "succussion". Three logarithmic potency scales are in regular use in homeopathy for dilution. Hahnemann created the "centesimal" or "C scale", diluting a substance by a factor of 100 at each stage. Inert substance like sugars, typically lactose, is used to prepare homeopathic pills and then a drop of liquid homeopathic preparation is placed on pills. Hahnemann began to test what effects substances produced in humans, a procedure that would later become known as "homeopathic proving".

Imponderabilia: Homeopathic medicines prepared from energy, emanating from natural and physical reactions. It means “not weighable”, i.e. which have no perceptible weights. They are energy forms such as sunlight (Sol), magnetic fields (Magnetis Polus Australis), radiation (X-ray).

Mother solution (also called solution): the most concentrated solution prepared from a substance of mineral or chemical origin by dissolving it in alcohol or purified water. It may also be prepared by exposing alcohol or purified water to an energy source (see Imponderabilia).

Mother tincture (also called tincture): The initial homeopathic preparation made from source material that can be further potentized (also called "liquid stock"), sometimes used as homeopathic medicines, is regarded as the most concentrated form of a finished homeopathic medicine. Mother tinctures are obtained classically by maceration or percolation (sometimes also by digestion, infusion, decoction or fermentation) techniques from source materials according to a procedure prescribed by a recognized homeopathic pharmacopoeia. Sometimes a mother tincture corresponds to the first decimal dilution, "1D" or "1X" (10-1), mostly when dry plant material is used as starting material.

Nosodes: Homeopathic medicines prepared from disease products from humans or animals; from pathogenic organisms or their metabolic products; or from decomposition products of animal organs.

Sarcodes: Homeopathic medicines made from healthy animal tissues or secretions. In Greek, sarcode means fleshly.

Potency: The denominated degree of serial trituration or dilution and succession that is reached for each homeopathic medicine. The degrees of dilution or potencies are normally indicated by the letters D, DH or X for successive 1 to 10 (decimal) dilutions, the letters C, CH or K or CK for successive 1 to 100 (centesimal) dilutions while Q or LM denote successive 1 to 50 000 (Hahnemannian quinquagintamillesimal) dilutions.

Dilution by 1 to 10 denotes 1 part processed with 9 parts of diluent (Hahnemannian decimal), dilution by 1 to 100, 1 part processed with 99 parts (Hahnemannian or Korsakovian centesimal), and so on.

The number preceding the letters (Example- D, C or LM) normally indicate the number of dilution steps employed.

As a consequence of different views in various approaches in homeotherapy and because the notion of these terms may depend on the nature of the starting materials, the terms "high potency" and "low potency" cannot be defined unambiguously.

Potentization (also called dinamization): The combined process of serial dilution and succussion or trituration at each step in the manufacture of homeopathic medicines from stocks. (According to the tenet of homeopathy, potentization represents the process by which the activity of a homeopathic medicine is developed.)

The potentisation steps in a potency row can be performed in different dilution ratios:

D or X: 1:10

C or CH: 1:100

LM 1:50,000.

So, for example, D4 means potentised four times in the ratio 1:10. The higher the number of potency the lower the concentration.

1.3.2 Preparation and Standardization of Ayurvedic Formulations

1.3.2.1 Bhasma

Bhasma is a calcinated preparation in which the gem or metal is converted into ash. *Example- Suvarnabhasma, Pravalbhasma, Lauhbhasma, Shankhbhasma.* Bhasmikaran is a process by which a substance which is otherwise bioincompatible is made biocompatible by certain samskaras or processes. The objectives of samskara are elimination of harmful matters from the drug, modification of undesirable physical properties of the drug, conversion of some of the characteristics of the drug and enhancement of the therapeutic action. Various steps involved in the preparation of bhasma(or bhasmikaran) are: 1. Sho-dhan- Purification, 2. Maran - Powdering, 3. Chalan- Stirring, 4. Dhavan - Washing, 5. Galan- Filtering, 6. Putan- Heating, 7. Mardan- Triturating, 8. Bhavan- Coating with herbal extract, 9. Amrutikaran - Detoxification and 10. Sandharan - Preservation.

Selection of these steps depends on the specific metal. Sometimes there is an overlapping of the steps Example- maran is achieved by puttan. The bhasmas' used in Ayurveda for treatment of various diseases for the past several centuries is the oldest form of nano-technology. Nano particles are 1 crore times smaller than a hair and due to its small size, the basic characteristics also get changed. Due to change in electrical, thermal, magnetic, optical, chemical and biological characteri-stics, the particles can be used for various products.

Steps involved in the preparation of bhasma (or bhasmikaran) are:

- ✓ Shodhan –Purification
- ✓ Maran - Powdering
- ✓ Chalan- Stirring
- ✓ Dhavan - Washing
- ✓ Galan- Filtering
- ✓ Putan- Heating
- ✓ Mardan- Triturating
- ✓ Bhavan- Coating with herbal extract
- ✓ Amrutikaran - Detoxification and
- ✓ Sandharan- Preservation
- ✓ specified metal, mineral, and animal product (*Kasaya*)
- ✓ cakes are made (*Cakrikas*) and dried under the sunlight
- ✓ mud tray and closed with another tray and the clay smeared with cloth of seven consecutive layers
- ✓ Dig a pit of appropriate size. Half of the pit is filled with dried cow dung cakes
- ✓ Put tray. Pack with the cow dung cake. Fire is lit from all sides and in the middle of the pit
- ✓ Cool at room temperature. Remove tray, break seal, podwer the chakrikas.

Preparation

1. ***Shodhana:*** In *Ayurveda* the very first stage of metal purification is called *Shodhana* to eliminates harmful matter, modifies or converts undesirable properties to desirable enhanced therapeutic actions. Shodhana is of two types, *Samanya shodhana* and *Vishesh shodhana.* In *Samanya Shodhana,* the sheets of metals are heated till red hot and are successively dipped into liquids like oil, buttermilk, cow's urine etc. The procedure is repeated seven times. In *Vishesh Shodhana* For some metals a specific process is described for shodhan Example- for purification of Jasad, the molten mass is poured in cow's milk 21 times.

2. ***Marana:*** Maran literally means killing where metal lose its metallic characteristics and physical nature. Here the purified drug is grounded with the specified metal, mineral and animal product (*Kasaya*) for a specified period of time to from small cakes (*Cakrikas*) which are further dried under the sunlight. The dried cakes are placed in a single layer in a mud tray and closed with another tray and the clay smeared with cloth of seven consecutive layers. This tray is then placed into the half filled pit with dried cow dung cakes and the pit is again packed with the cow dung cake. Fire is lit from all sides and in the middle of the pit. After specified burning, it is allowed to cool at room temperature. The clay tray is removed, and the seal is broken. The contents are taken out and finely powdered.

3. ***Chalan:*** Process of stirring with iron rod or plant stick during heating the metal is known as chalan. Iron serves as catalyst and the phytoconstituents of plant stick may be enhancing the therapeutic effect. For example, stick of Neem is used for chalan process of Jasad bhasma, which is used topically for ophthalmic diseases.

4. **Dhavan**: This means several time washing of product with water to remove the excess amounts of agents used in shodhan or maran stage.

5. **Galan:** It means sifting of the product either through a fine cloth or through sieves of suitable mesh so as to separate residual material larger in size.

6. **Puttan:** The term puttan means ignition. This is key process in manufacturing the bhasma which involves heating the product in a special shallow earthen pot called as Sharav in a faster and uniform format. The classification of putta is primarily done on the basic nature of the process and is as under: 1. Chandra-putta 2. Dhanyarashiputta 3. Surya-putta 4. Bhugarbhaputta 5. Agniptuta.

Characteristics: The final Bhasma should be free from metallic luster. Bhasma when rubbed between fingers should be so fine so as to get easily into the lines or crevices of finger. In water Bhasma should float on the surface.

1.3.2.2 Asava and Arishta

Asava and *arishtas* are the self generated fermented alcoholic liquid preparations. Fermentation is brought about by the addition of *dhataki* (*Woodfordia fruticosa*) flowers. Fermented alcohol facilitates the extraction of active constituents in the drug and also acts as a preservative. Both *Asava* and *arishtas* contain up to 12% of alcohol and hence are also called medicinal wines. *Arishtas* are prepared with decoctions of herbs in boiling water while *asavas* are prepared by direct use of fresh herbal juices.

Aristha Preapartion	Asava Preapartion
Clean, dry and powder the crude drug and prepare the decoction in potable water. The wooden pots should be fumigated with pimply *churna* and also smeared with ghee before addition of parent material or sugar.	Boil the required quantity of potable water; add sugar, *jaggery* or honey, cool and transferr to the wooden vessel.previously fumigated with pimply *churna* and also smeared with ghee
Then add pure sugar (cane sugar), honey or jaggery (very old), according to the preparation, to the decoction.	Then, add finely powdered drug mentioned in the formula.
Now add *dravas*, other powder ingredients and *dhatakipushpa,* if mentioned.	Now add *dravas*, other powder ingredients and *dhatakipushpa,* if mentioned.
Place the vessels in the basement (underground cellar) all under a heap of paddy to ensure constant atmospheric temperature during the whole process of fermentation. After the specified period, generally from 7-10 days, remove the pot and decant the fluid. After 2-3 days when the fine particle of sediment is settled down, the arishta is bottled.	Place the vessels in the basement (underground cellar) all under a heap of paddy to ensure constant atmospheric temperature during the whole process of fermentation. After the specified period, generally from 7-10 days, remove the pot and decant the fluid. After 2-3 days when the fine particle of sediment is settled down, the Asava is bottled.

Arishta Preparation: Clean, dry and powder the crude drug and prepare the decoction in potable water. Filter and the prepared decoction and transfer to the wooden pots. The wooden pots should be fumigated with pimply *churna* and also smeared with ghee before addition of parent material or sugar. Then add pure sugar (cane sugar), honey or jaggery (very old), according to the preparation, to the decoction. Now add *dravas*, other powder ingredients and *dhatakipushpa,* if mentioned. Close the vessel with the lid and seal the edges with the clay smeared cloth of seven consecutive layers. Place the vessels in the basement (underground cellar) all under a heap of paddy to ensure constant atmospheric temperature during the whole process of fermentation. After the specified period, generally from 7-10 days, remove the pot and decant the fluid. After 2-3 days when the fine particle of sediment is settled down, the arishta is bottled. **Example:** *Ashokarishta, Dharakshrishta, Dashmularishta.* Arishta can be stored for any length of time in a well stoppered glass bottle.

Characteristics: The filtered final arishta should not contain any particle of sediment. The taste should not be sour. The preparation should have the characteristic odour of fermented liquid. If any growth of mould is observed, reject immediately. Mix equal quantity of water and aristha before consumption.

Asava Preparation: For the preparation of *asava*, boil the required quantity of potable water; add sugar, *jaggery* or honey, cool and transferr to the wooden vessel. Then, add finely powdered drug mentioned in the formula. Cover the container with a lid and the edges are sealed with seven consecutive layers of clay smeared cloth. The vessel is kept in the basement for the specified period of time, after which the pot is removed and the liquid is decanted or filtered. **Example:** *Kumariasava, Chonclanasavo, Lauhasava. Asava* can be stored for any length of time in a well stoppered glass bottle.

Characteristics: The filtered final Asava should not contain any particle of sediment. The taste should not be sour. The preparation should have the characteristic odour of fermented liquid. If any growth of mould is observed, reject immediately. Mix equal quantity of water and Asava before consumption.

Table 1.4 Examples of few Asavas and Aristhas

Name	Uses
Abhayarishta	Carminative and appetizer. Indicated in piles, anemia, colitis, cardiac, lesions, spleen and other intestinal disorders, Also removes constipation.
Arjunaristha	Tonic and cardiac stimulant. used in diseases of heart and respiratory disorders.
Ashokarishta	Alterative, stimulant and astringent. Used in leucorrhoea, haematuria, menorrhagia and other female complaints
Balarishta	Antirheumatic and diuretic. Indicated in hemiplegia, rheumatic pains.
Chandanasava	Diuretic and urinary antiseptic .Used in gonorrhoea, spermatorrhoea and other urinary diseases.
Dashmoolarishta	Bitter tonic,Alterative and stimulant, Useful in cough, menonervous diseases, consumption, anemia, jaundice, piles and as a parental tonic.
Drakshava	Stimulant antipyretic, diuretic, it is invigorating and nourishing. Used in phthisis, insomnia, loss of appetite, cough, general debility and premature sanity.
Kalmeghasava	Expectorant, Laxative, stimulant. Used in chronic respiratory disorder, flatulence and other disease of alimentary system.
Kumariasava	Alterative tonic and haematinic. Used in anemia, enlargement of the liver, endocrinal, deficiency, tympanites, cough, asthma and constipation.
Kutajarishta	Astringent, stimulant, and antiperiodic. Used in dysentery, diarrhea, fever and sprue.
Punarnavarishta	Diuretic, alterative and haematinic Indicated in beriberi, Edema, abdominal disorders and liver complains
Vidangasava	Carminative, anthelmintic. Used in paralysis, Paraplegia, lock jaw and in destroying worms.

1.3.2.3 Leha (Avaleha/Paka)

Leha also called as *avalehaor paka*, is a semisolid Ayurvedic preparation consisting of *kasayas*, or powder drugs alongwith*jaggery*, sugar or Khanda-sari and ghee or oil or liquid. Example-*Vasavaleha, Dhrakshavaleha, Musalipaka, Suvarnleha.*

Preparation: Dissolve *jaggery*, sugar or sugar-candy in the liquid and strain to remove the foreign particles. Boil this solution over a moderate fire. When *paka* becomes thready (*Tantuvat*), or when it sinks in water without getting easily dissolved, it should be removed from the fire. Then add fine powders of drugs with continuous stirring to form a homogenous mixture. Add ghee or oil, if mentioned while the preparation is hot and mix well. Add Honey, if mentioned when the preparation becomes cool and mix well until the *paka* is obtained.

Characteristicsp: *Leha* should neither be hard nor be a thick fluid. *Leha* should roll between the fingers. *Leha* should be kept in glass and porcelain jars. Normally *leha* should be used within 1 year.

1.3.2.4 Churna

Churna is a solid Ayurvedic preparation of fine powder of the drug/s which is often taken with some *anupan* such as milk, ghee or honey. Finer the powder the better it's therapeutic effect.

Preparation : Clean, dry, powder and sieve through cloth, the drugs mentioned in the formula. This can be also done by a disintegrator or mechanical sifter. When there is more than one drug, each drug should be separately powdered, sieved and weighed. As some of the drugs contain more fibrous material than the others, it should be treated by a special process as mentioned in the formula. Finally, mix all the powders well together. If salt, sugar, camphor is mentioned, then it should be powdered and added separately at the end.

Characteristics: Powder should be fine at least of 80 mesh size. It should be kept in an air tight container. It should be used within 6 months.

1.3.2.5 Gutika/Vati

This is a solid Ayurvedic formulation in the form of small tablets of drugs of plant, animal or mineral origin. Example- *Astaksarigutika, agnitundivati*

Preparation: Dry and powder the mentioned drugs separately. Reduce the mineral to bhasma or sindura unless otherwise mentioned. If required, prepare *kajjali* of some drugs. The processed *kajjali* is put in *kalba* and ground to a soft paste with the prescribed liquid. When more than one fluid is mentioned, use them in succession while grinding. When the mass does not stick to the fingers then mold into the *vati*, add sugandhadravas like *kasturi*, *kapoor* with continuous grinding. Now roll the pills and dry under sun or shed. Pills should be kept in an air tight container.

Characteristics: It should not lose its original taste, colour, smell and form. It should be used within 24 months in case of plants and indefinite period for minerals.

Shelf life of Ayurvedic drugs

Sr.No	Dosage form	Shelf life or date of expiry with effect from the date of manufacture
(i)	Anjana	
	a) Anjana made from Kasthaushadhi	1 year
	b) Anjana made from Kasthaushadhi along withRasa/Uprasa/ Bhasma	2 years
	c) Anjana made only from rasa/Uprasa/Bhasma	3 years
(ii)	Arka	1 year
(iii)	Asava Arista	10 years
(iv)	Avaleha, Khanda, Paka, Guda	3 years
(v)	Chuma, KwathaChuma, LepaChuma, DantaManjan, (Chuma)	2 years
(vi)	Dhoopan	2 years
(vii)	Dravaka, Lavana, Kshara	5 years
(viii)	Ghrita	2 years
(ix)	Guggulu	5 years
(x)	Gutika/Vati	
	(i) Gutika or Vati containing Kasthaushadhi along withRasa / Uprasa/ Bhasma/ Guggulu (including LepaGutikaand GhanVati)	5 years
	(ii) Gutika or Vati containing only Kasthaushadhi (including LepaGutika and GhanVati)	3 years

Contd...

Sr.No	Dosage form	Shelf life or date of expiry with effect from the date of manufacture
	(iii) Gutika / Vati containing only Ras / Uprasa / Bhasmaexcept Naga, Vanga and TamraBhasma	10 years
(xi)	Kama/ Nasabindu	2 years
(xii)	KupipakvaRasayana	10 years
(xiii)	Malahar	3 years
(xiv)	Mandura-Lauha	10 years
(xv)	Naga Bhasma, Vanga Bhasma and TamraBhasma	5 years
(xvi)	Netrabindu	1 years
(xvii)	Parpati	10 years
(xviii)	Pishti and Bhasma except Naga, Vanga and TamraBhasma	10 years
(xix)	PravahiKwatha	3 years
(xx)	Rasayoga	
	(i) Rasayoga Containing only Rasa / Uprasa / Bhasma except Naga, Vanga and TamraBhasma	10 years
	(ii) Rasayoga Containing Rasa / Uprasa/ Bhasma along with Kasthaushadhi/Guggulu	5 years
(xxi)	Sattva (derived from medicinal plant)	2 years
(xxii)	Sharkar / Panak/Sharbat	3 years
(xxiii)	Shvetaparpati	2 years
(xxiv)	Taila	3 years
(xxv)	Varti	2 years

Subjective Questions

1. How to authetify herbal materials?
2. How to process herbal raw material?
3. What is biodynamic agriculture?
4. What is biopesticide?
5. How to manage pest in medicinal plant?
6. What are basic principles involved in Ayurveda or Sidhha or Chinese medicine system?
7. How to prepare and evaluate Ghutika or Bhasma or Lehya
8. What is difference between Asava and Aristha?
9. How agriculture and cultural or mechanical and Physical methods of pest control are replted?
10. What is IPM?
11. What are plant pesticides?
12. What are different mills used to pulverize crude drugs? Give example based on type of crude drugs?

13. Give suitable examples of different storage containers used for crude drugs.
14. What is shelf life of Leha and Bhasma?
15. What is shelf life of Gutika and taila?

Multiple Choice Questions (MCQs)/Objective Questions

1. According to WHO, the terminology used to represent crude plant materials such as leaves, flowers, fruits, seed, stem, wood, bark, rhizome or other plant parts which may be entire or fragmented or powdered is called as

   a. Shrub c. Tree

   b. Herb d. All of the above

2. The study or practice of the medicinal or therapeutic use of plants especially as a form of alternative medicine is known as ....

   a. Herbalism c. Paraherbalism

   b. Herbal medicine d. Both a and b

3. Alternative and pseudoscientific practices of using unrefined plant or animal extracts as unproven medicines called as ....

   a. Herbalism c. Paraherbalism

   b. Herbal medicine d. Both a and b

4. Any medicinal product exclusively containing one or more herbal substances as active ingredients/ one or more herbal preparations or a combination of two is known as ....

   a. Herbal medicine c. Dietary food

   b. Herbal product d. Herbal drug

5. Which one of the following formulation is NOT herbal drug preparation?

   a. Tincture c. Extract

   b. Infusion d. Talc

6. Which one of the following serves as intermediate in the process of producing finished herbal products or herbal dosage forms for therapeutic use ....

   a. Herbal medicine c. Herbal material

   b. Herbal preparation d. Both a and b

7. The word herb is derived from ....word "Herba"

   a. Italian c. Latin

   b. Spanish d. Greek

8. Sources of herbs are ....

   a. Animals c. Marine

   b. Insects d. Plants

9. Quality, safety and efficacy of a herbal drug material depends on largely ....
   a. Correct identification of herb
   b. Authentication of herb
   c. Cultivation technique
   d. Both a and b

10. The process of quality assurance that ensures the correct plant species and plant parts used as raw materials for herbal medicines is called as ....
    a. Identification
    b. Authentication
    c. Quality control
    d. None

11. Which one of the following is NOT quantitative microscopy?
    a. Lycopodium spore method for percentage purity
    b. Pallisade ratio
    c. Stomata index
    d. None

12. According to WHO, Upper limit for number of *E.coli* per gram of crude drug material is ...
    a. 10
    b. 10^4
    c. 10^2
    d. 9

13. Aflatoxin contamination is determined by ....
    a. TLC using standard Aflatoxins (B_1,B_2,G_1,G_2) mixture
    b. HPLC using standard Aflatoxins (B_1,B_2,G_1,G_2) mixture
    c. Microbial plate culture
    d. None of the above

14. Which one of the following methodin primary processing is used for enzymatic degradation of toxic ingredients of crude herbal materials?
    a. Sweating
    b. Aging
    c. Heating
    d. Drying

15. For which drug, aging technique is utilized for neutralization of toxic ingredients before utilization as herbal medicine?
    a. Rhubarb
    b. Cascara
    c. Datura
    d. None

16. Primary processing is an important step in herbal drug processing because of ....
    a. Increases secondary metabolite levels of drug
    b. Enhances cost effectiveness
    c. Neutralizes toxic ingredients and reduces side effects of drug
    d. All of the above

17. The process in which herbal drug material is kept in boiling water for short period of time without being fully cooked to increase storage life of crude drug is known as .....
    a. Sweating
    b. Aging
    c. Blanching
    d. Steaming
18. Before decoction or infusion, which primary process is implemented commonly?
    a. Blanching
    b. Steaming
    c. Stir frying
    d. Bleaching
19. In which method, boiling water is poured over the herb or herbal material to produce a dilute liquid preparation?
    a. Decoction
    b. Infusion
    c. Maceration
    d. Percolation
20. Tincture is typically made up of .....
    a. 1 part herbal material and 5-10 parts of solvent
    b. 2 parts of herbal material and 5-10 parts of solvent
    c. 3 parts of herbal material and 5-10 parts of solvent
    d. 4 parts of herbal material and 5-10 parts of solvent
21. Which one of the following is responsible for water holding capacity of soil?
    a. Clay
    b. Fine soil particles
    c. Humus
    d. Tree plantation
22. In organic farming, which two factors plays very important role for the desired growth of plants?
    a. Rain fall
    b. Organic matter
    c. Water holding capacity of soil
    d. Both b and c
23. Which one of the following micro organisms is NOT responsible for nitrogen fixation?
    a. E.coli
    b. Azospirillium
    c. Azolla
    d. Bijericcia
24. The quality, safety and efficacy of a medicinal herb highly depends on......
    a. Cultivation technique
    b. Collection technique
    c. Appropriate harvesting
    d. All of the above
25. Phytopthora root rot disease in belladonna occurs due to microorganism......
    a. Ascochyta atropae.
    b. Cercospora atropae.
    c. Phytopthoranicotianae
    d. Phytopthoraerythrosceptica
26. Leaf necrosis in medicinal plants is caused by.........
    a. Cercospora atropae
    b. Ascochyta atropae
    c. Pythium spinosum
    d. One

27. Cucumber mosaic virus is observed on which Medicinal plants?
    a. Digitalis.
    b. Hyoscyamus.
    c. Datura
    d. Both a and b
28. All insect pests belongs to phylum ....
    a. Anthropoda
    b. Vertebrate
    c. Invertebrate
    d. None
29. Which weed is responsible for allergic response hay fever?
    a. Parathenium.
    b. Mexican tea.
    c. Yellow dock
    d. All
30. Which one of the following weed belongs to poisonous category?
    a. Menispermus species.
    b. Datura.
    c. Both a and b
    d. None
31. Which one of the following is NOT invertebrate pest?
    a. Crabs
    b. Snails
    c. Rats
    d. Mites
32. Which one of the following is not mechanical method of pest control?
    a. Hand picking
    b. Pruning
    c. Burning
    d. pesticides
33. Sex pheromone 7,8 – epoxy – 2 methyloctadecane, a biological pest control is obtained from.........
    a. Screw worms
    b. Lady bug
    c. Gypsy moth
    d. None of the above
34. Which one of the secondary metabolite acts as rodenticide?
    a. Strychnine
    b. Quinine
    c. Atropine
    d. Warfarin
35. Which one of the following is NOT Herbicide?
    a. 2,4 – dichlorophenoxy acetic acid
    b. Calcium arsenate
    c. Sulphuric acid
    d. DDT
36. Organophosphorous compounds and carbamates exert pesticidal activity on animals by...
    a. Neurotoxication
    b. Inhibition of neuromuscular junction
    c. Inhibition of acetyl cholinesterase
    d. None
37. On which date, Bioincecticides were registered under insecticides Act 1968 by Central Insecticide Board, Ministry of Agriculture, New Delhi?
    a. 26/03/1995
    b. 26/03/1996
    c. 26/06/1998
    d. 26/06/1999

38. *Agrobacterium tumefaceins* was registered as biopesticide under insecticide act 1968 in
    a. 2002
    b. 2003
    c. 2004
    d. 2005
39. Carbamates acts as weedicide by ....
    a. Inhibition of pentothenate synthesis
    b. Inhibition of oxidative phosphorylation
    c. Inhibition of chlorophyll synthesis
    d. None
40. The insecticidal principles in pyrethrum are located in which part of pyrethrum plant?
    a. In oleoresin secretion of leaves
    b. In oleoresin secretion of floral parts
    c. In oleoresin secretion of stem
    d. None
41. Asava is prepared by ....
    a. Soaking drug in water before decoction
    b. Drug is coarsely powdered and added to water
    c. Both a and b
    d. None of the above
42. In Arishta preparation, the ratio of crude drug to water is generally ......
    a. 1:4
    b. 1:16
    c. Both a and b
    d. None
43. In Arishta preparation, sugar is jaggery is added to........
    a. Concentrated decoction as last part of process
    b. Dilute solution of coarse powdered drug
    c. Before decoction of crude drug
    d. None
44. Amongst Asava and Arishta, which preparation contains high amount of water?
    a. Asava
    b. Arishta
    c. Both a and b
    d. None
45. Which method is used for standardization of Asava and Arishta preparation?
    a. Water content determination
    b. Microbial content determination
    c. Alcohol content determination
    d. Both a and b

46. Which one of the following ingredient is used as binding agent in Gutika preparation?
    a. Jaggery
    b. Sugar
    c. corn floor
    d. gum
47. Which parameters are investigated for standardization of Gutika preparation?
    a. Disintegration time
    b. Solubility
    c. Dissolution time
    d. Both a and c
48. Which one of the ingredient is used as flavouring agent as well as carminative in Gutika?
    a. Coriander
    b. Dill
    c. caraway
    d. Fennel
49. Churna is Ayurvedic formulation prepared from.......
    a. Fresh herbs in powdered form
    b. Dried herbs in powdered form
    c. Both a and b
    d. None
50. Which excipients are used in Churna preparation?
    a. Jaggery
    b. Sugar
    c. fennel
    d. None of the above
51. Which phytochemical parameters are investigated during standardization of Churna preparation?
    a. Ash value
    b. Foreign particle determination
    c. Moisture content determination
    d. All of the above
52. Which parameter is critical for shelf life of Churna preparation?
    a. Ash value
    b. Moisture content
    c. Solubility
    d. Both a and b
53. Lehya is ....Ayurvedic dosage form
    a. Solid
    b. Liquid
    c. Semi-solid
    d. Powdered
54. Which ingredients are used for preparation of Lehya?
    a. Kashaya or churna
    b. Madhu
    c. Ghrita
    d. All of the above
55. What is the role of Ghrita in Lehya preparation?
    a. Laxative
    b. Lipophillic agent
    c. Hydrophobic agent
    d. Preservative

56. Which parameter is used for standardization of lehya preparation?
    - a. Ash value
    - b. Saponification value
    - c. Moisture content
    - d. All of the above

57. In Bhasma preparation, the step in which purified metals are amalgamated with mercury and purified sulphur to form black, lusterless, fine smooth mass is called as
    - a. Bhavana
    - b. Kupipaka
    - c. Kajjali
    - d. Marana

58. The presence of luster in finally prepared bhasma indicates ....
    - a. Incomplete Shodhana process
    - b. Incomplete Marana Process
    - c. Incomplete bhavana process
    - d. None

59. The particle size of swarnabhasma is generally...............
    - a. 100 – 120 nm
    - b. 56 – 57 nm
    - c. 200 – 250 nm
    - d. 150 – 200 nm

60. Which step in bhasma preparation removes toxicity of metals?
    - a. Shodhana
    - b. Marana
    - c. Bhavana
    - d. All

Answer Key

1. b	2. d	3. c	4. b	5. d	6. b	7. c	8. d	9. d	10.b
11. d	12. b	13. a	14. b	15. b	16. d	17. c	18. a	19. b	20. a
21. c	22. d	23.a	24. d	25. d	26. a	27. d	28. a	29. c	30. c
31. d	32. d	33. c	34. a	35. c	36. c	37. d	38. c	39. c	40. b
41. b	42. c	43. a	44. a	45. c	46. a	47. d	48. d	49. b	50. c
51. d	52. b	53. c	54. d	55. b	56. b	57. c	58. a	59. b	60. b

Unit 2

2.1 Nutraceuticals

2.1.1 General Aspects, Scope, Market Growth, Types, Regulations, Classifications of Products Available in the Market

2.1.2 Health Benefits and Role of Nutraceuticals in Ailments

2.1.2.1 Diabetes

2.1.2.2 Cardiovascular diseases

2.1.2.3 Cancer

2.1.2.4 Irritable bowel syndrome (IBS) and various Gastro intestinal diseases

2.1.3 Study of Herbs as Health Food

2.2 Herbal-Drug and Herb-Food Interactions

2.2.1 General Introduction to Interaction and Classification

2.2.1.1 Classification/Types of Interactions

2.2.2 Study of Few Herbal Drugs and their Possible Side Effects and Interactions

2.1 Nutraceuticals

2.1.1 General Aspects, Scope, Market Growth, Types, Regulations, Classifications of Products Available in the Market

General aspects

Nutraceutical is word coined by Dr. Stephen in 1989, a combination of the words "nutrition" and "pharmaceutical", is a food or food product that reportedly provides health and medical benefits, including the prevention and treatment of disease. It is defined as food stuff (as a fortified food or a dietary supplement) that provides health benefits. Nutraceuticals are non-specific biological therapies used to promote wellness, prevent malignant processes and control symptoms. Nutraceutical foods are not subject to the same testing and regulations as pharmaceutical drugs. As per the Food Safety Standard Act, 2006 (Chapter 4, Section 22) it has been recommended that Food should be classified as follows:

- Novel foods
- Genetically modified food
- Irradiated food
- Organic foods
- Foods for special dietary use
- Functional foods
- Nutraceuticals
- Health Supplements

This makes it very clear that Nutraceuticals are a part of the food segment and it should not be considered as a form of pharmaceutical or drug formulation.

Scope of Nutraceuticals

- ➢ Awareness that prevention is better than cure
- ➢ People especially of younger generation are becoming progressively more health-conscious
- ➢ Gradual shift toward natural ingredients
- ➢ Unnourished population
- ➢ Increased work stress, busy schedule and Agricultural pollution unable to provide proper nutrition
- ➢ High cost of health care with the expensive disease-treatment approach
- ➢ Chronic diseases without effective medicines

So there is great demand of alternative beneficial products like dietary supplement, functional food and nutraceuticals by people as well as researchers to explore therapeutic values.

Nutraceuticals have numerous health and nutritional benefits which helps in immunity enhancement, reduction of disease risk and also have anti-ageing effect.

But, unrealistic claims, poor packaging and labeling, poor stability and poor taste masking are few of challenges in the field of nutraceuticals.

Market Growth of Nutraceutical

Globally, the US and Japan are the most developed markets for nutraceuticals, due to the consumer acceptability achieved in these regions. India, China and Brazil are developing nations which show huge potential for the nutraceuticals market, India and China have emerged as a key sourcing destination for natural ingredients. The global market for Nutraceuticals is projected to reach US$ 250 billion by 2018, driven primarily by the growing affinity among the general populace towards adopting a healthy lifestyle. Nutraceutical foods were the largest market segment in 2007, worth $39.9 billion. This is expected to increase $56.7 billion in 2013. Nutraceutical supplements have the second largest market share, generating $39.0 billion in 2007. This segment should reach $48.8 billion in 2013. The nutraceutical beverages segment represents the fastest growing segment and is expected to have the largest share of the market by 2013. This segment was worth $38.4 billion in 2007 and is expected to increase to and $71.3 billion in 2013.

Types of products available in market

Functional Food

- Probiotics Fortified Food
- Omega Fatty Acid Fortified Food
- Branded Ionized Salt
- Branded Wheat Flour Market
- Other Functional Food

Functional Beverages

- Fruit & Vegetable Juices and Drinks
- Dairy & Dairy Alternative Drinks
- Noncarbonated Drinks
- Other

Dietary Supplements

- Proteins & Peptides
- Vitamins & Minerals
- Herbals
- Other

Personal Care and pharmaceuticals

Major Key players:

- ➢ GlaxoSmithKline: Horlicks, Boost, and Viva.
- ➢ Britania: Nutraceutical biscuits and juices

- Parle: Nutraceutical biscuits and juices
- Kellogg: Vitamin and mineral fortifies breakfast options
- Amway: Nutrilite
- Baidyanath: Chyawanprash
- Nestle: ActiPlus
- Danone: Yakult
- Coca-Cola: Minute Maid juices
- PepsiCo: Tropicana juices
- Abott: Pediasure, Ensure or Glucerna

Segments wise Key players in India

- **Functional/ fortified foods**: Cargill, Britannia, Kelloggs, Nestle, PepsiCo, Heinz, Baggrys, GlaxoSmithKline Consumer Healthcare, Patanjali, Mother Dairy, General Mills, Ruchi Soya
- **Functional beverages**: Redbull, Coca-cola, PepsiCo, Goldwin Healthcare, GlaxoSmithKline, Hector Beverages
- **Dietary supplements**: Amway, Dabur, Herbalife International, Danone, Novartis

Regulations

Different countries have different Nutraceutical terminologies and their regulations which are as follows

Country	Body Known as	Body Governed by	Definition covers
Canada	Natural health products in 2004	FDA	Vitamins, mineral, homeopathic, Chinese medicine, amino acids, essential fatty acids
EU	Food supplements in 2002	Food safety authority	Concentrated sources of nutrients, substances with nutritional or physiological effects
Russia	Biologically active food in 1997	Ministry of health and social development	Vitamins, amino acids, dietary fibers, para-pharmaceuticals (bioflavonoid, polysaccharides)
USA	Dietary supplement in 1994	FDA	Vitamins, minerals, botanicals, amino acids, extract
Australia	Complementary medicines in 1991	Department of health and ageing	Herbal medicines, vitamins, minerals, nutritional supplements.
Japan	Foods for specific health use in 1991	Japan health and nutrition food association	Functional foods that can have three functions: nutrition, sensory satisfaction, physiological improvement
India	Foods for special dietary use in 2005	Food safety and standards act passes in 2006 yet to be implemented	Vitamins, minerals, botanicals, extracts
China	Health Food	State Food and Drug Administration (SFDA) in 2003	Any finished product or raw material intended for people to eat or drink, as well as any product that has traditionally served as both food and medication, with the exception of products used solely for medical purposes.

Classification

Generally nutraceutical are grouped as follows:

- Substances with established nutritional functions, such as vitamins, minerals, amino acids and fatty acids, also defined nutrients;
- Herbs or botanical products as concentrates and extracts, often called herbals; and
- Reagents derived from other sources (Example-. pyruvate, chondroitin sulphate, steroid hormone precursors) serving specific functions, such as sports nutrition, weight-loss supplements and meal replacements, also indicated as dietary supplements

Nutraceuticals can be classified on the basis of their nomenclature which is as follows:

Dietary supplements	Vitamins, minerals, herbs or other botanicals, amino acids, and substances such as enzymes, organ tissues, and metabolites.
Functional foods	It can be any ordinary food that has components or ingredients added to give it a specific medical or physiological benefit, other than a purely nutritional effect
Medical foods	It covers probiotics, antioxidants manufactured in liquids, tablets, capsule form
Farmaceuticals	It is a melding of the words farm and pharmaceuticals. It refers to medically valuable compounds produced from modified agricultural crops or animals (usually through biotechnology).

Nutraceuticals can be classified on the basis of their market which is as follows:

Dietary supplements	Vitamins, minerals, extracts, protein supplements, ayurvedic supplements (Chyawanprash, honey), powders
Functional foods	Fortified food, prebiotics, probiotics, iodinated food, gluten free food,
Functional Beverages	Energy drinks, nutritional drinks, fortified juices, sport drinks

Nutraceuticals are commonly classified on the basis of ingredients which is as follows

Minerals	Over twenty dietary minerals are necessary for human being and each have its specific role in maintain health ➢ Calcium: maintaining bone strength important in nerve, muscle and glandular functions. ➢ Iron: Metabolism and energy production. ➢ Magnesium: for nerve and muscle function ➢ Phosphorous: Part of genetic material. ➢ Chromium: With insulin helps to convert carbohydrates and fats into energy. ➢ Cobalt: Essential component of vitamin B12 ➢ Copper: Part of hemoglobin and collagen production ➢ Iodine: Essential for proper functioning of the thyroid. ➢ Zinc: Essential for immune function, would healing, blood clotting ➢ Selenium: Essential for fertility and sperm motility

Contd...

Vitamins	Vitamin is an organic compound required by an organism as a vital nutrient in limited amounts and cannot be synthesized in sufficient quantities by an organism, and must be obtained from the diet. Dietary supplements, often containing vitamins, are used to ensure that adequate amounts of nutrients are obtained on a daily basis, if optimal amounts of the nutrients cannot be obtained through a varied diet. ➢ Vitamin A: Antioxidant, essential, for growth and development and in the treatment of certain skin disorders. ➢ Vitamin E: Antioxidant, helps form blood cells, muscles, lung and nerve tissue, boosts the immune system. ➢ Vitamin K: Essential for blood clotting. ➢ Vitamin C: Antioxidant, for healthy bones, gums, teeth and skin, in wound healing, prevent common cold and attenuate its symptoms. ➢ Vitamin B_1 (Thiamine), B_2 (Riboflavin), B_3 (Niacin), B_5 (Panthothenic acid), B_6 (Pyridoxol), B_7 (Biotin): energy production, essential in nerve functions, healthy eyes, skin. ➢ Vitamin B_9 (Folic acid): Produce the genetic materials of cells, in pregnancy for preventing birth defects, RBCs formation, protects against heart disease. ➢ Vitamin B12 (Cobalamine): Proper functioning of nervous system
Antioxidants	Antioxidants are widely used in dietary supplements and have been investigated for the prevention of diseases such as cancer, coronary heart disease and even altitude sickness. An antioxidant is a molecule that inhibits the oxidation of other molecules. Oxidation is a chemical reaction that transfers electrons or hydrogen from a substance to an oxidizing agent. Oxidation reactions can produce free radicals. In turn, these radicals can start chain reactions. When the chain reaction occurs in a cell, it can cause damage or death to the cell. Antioxidants terminate these chain reactions by removing free radical intermediates, and inhibit other oxidation reactions. They do this by being oxidized themselves, so antioxidants are often reducing agents such as thiols, ascorbic acid, or polyphenols, vitamins, minerals.
PUFA	Polyunsaturated fatty acids (PUFAs) are fatty acids that contain more than one double bond in their backbone. This class includes many important compounds, such as essential fatty acids. Essential fatty acids, or EFAs, are fatty acids that humans and other animals must ingest because the body requires them for good health but cannot synthesize them. The term "essential fatty acid" refers to fatty acids required for biological processes, and not those that only act as fuel. Only two EFAs are known for humans: alpha-linolenic acid (an omega-3 fatty acid) and linoleic acid (an omega-6 fatty acid). Other fatty acids that are only "conditionally essential" include gamma-linolenic acid (an omega-6 fatty acid), lauric acid (a saturated fatty acid), and palmitoleic acid (a monounsaturated fatty acid). Essential fatty acids play a part in many metabolic processes, and there is evidence to suggest that low levels of essential fatty acids, or the wrong balance of types among the essential fatty acids, may be a factor in a number of illnesses, including osteoporosis Moreover, PUFAs play an important physiological role in the body mainly in the synthesis of eicosanoids or "local hormones" (prostaglandins, prostacyclins, thromboxanes, and leukotrienes). Hence, the deficiency of fatty acids and lipids significantly affects vascular fragility, reduces immune functions, interferes with clotting process, and increases the chance of forming atherosclerosis.

Contd...

Prebiotics	Prebiotics (Oligofructose, galacto-oligsachharides, lactulose) are non-digestible food ingredients that stimulate the growth and/or activity of bacteria in the digestive system in ways claimed to be beneficial to health. Traditional dietary sources of prebiotics include soybeans, inulin sources, raw oats, unrefined wheat, unrefined barley, and yacon. Some of the oligosaccharides that naturally occur in breast milk are believed to play an important role in the development of a healthy immune system in infants.
Probiotics	Probiotic are Live microorganisms which when administered in adequate amounts confer a health benefit on the host. Lactic acid bacteria (LAB) and bifidobacteria are the most common types of microbes used as probiotics; but certain yeasts and bacilli may also be used. Probiotics are commonly consumed as part of fermented foods with specially added active live cultures; such as in yogurt, soy yogurt, or as dietary supplements. Probiotics generally include the following categories of bacteria: Lactobacilli such as *L. acidophilus, L.casei, L.delbrueckii subsp. bulgaricus, L.brevis, L.cellobiosus.* Gram-positive cocci such as *Lactococcus lactis, Streptococcus salivarius* subsp. *Thermophilus, Enterococcus faecium* Bifidobacteria such as *B.bifidun, B.adolescentis, B.infantis, B.longum, B. thermophilum.*
Fibers	Dietary fiber (roughage or ruffage) is the indigestible portion of plant foods having two main components: soluble (may be prebiotic and/or viscous) fiber that is readily fermented in the colon into gases and physiologically active byproducts, and insoluble fiber (may be metabolically inert and provide bulking or metabolically fermented in the large intestine as a prebiotic fiber). Bulking fibers absorb water as they move through the digestive system, easing defecation. Fermentable insoluble fibers mildly promote regularity, although not to the extent that bulking fibers do, but they can be readily fermented in the colon into gases and physiologically active byproducts.
Health drinks	Health drinks are either just water fortified with some kind of flavor or teas, milk, juices enriched with healthy ingredients. Dairy drinks (19%), general health drinks (13.4%), ready-to-drink (RTD) tea and coffee (11.2%) and sports and energy drinks (10.%) are famous types of health drinks. Claims like "rich "or "free" needs scientific evidences.
Phytochemicals	Polyphenols useful to prevent and control arterial diseases. Flavonoids useful to block the Angiotensin converting enzyme inhibitors (ACE) and strengthen the tiny capillaries that carry oxygen and essential nutrients to all cells. Glucosamine and chondroitin sulfate obtained from fish and animals are used against osteoarthritis and regulate gene expression and synthesis of NO and PGE2.

2.1.2 Health Benefits and Role of Nutraceuticals in Ailments

2.1.2.1 Diabetes

Diabetes mellitus (DM), commonly known as just diabetes, is a group of metabolic disorders characterized by a high blood sugar level over a prolonged period of time. Serious long-term complications include cardiovascular disease, stroke, chronic kidney disease, foot ulcers, damage to the nerves, damage to the eyes and cognitive impairment. There are three main types of diabetes mellitus:

- ***Type 1 diabetes*** results from failure of the pancreas to produce enough insulin due to loss of beta cells. This form was previously referred to as "insulin-dependent diabetes mellitus"

(IDDM) or "juvenile diabetes". The loss of beta cells is caused by an autoimmune response. The cause of this autoimmune response is unknown.

- ***Type 2 diabetes*** begins with insulin resistance, a condition in which cells fail to respond to insulin properly. As the disease progresses, a lack of insulin may also develop. This form was previously referred to as "non insulin-dependent diabetes mellitus" (NIDDM) or "adult-onset diabetes". The most common cause is a combination of excessive body weight and insufficient exercise.
- ***Gestational diabetes*** is the third main form, and occurs when pregnant women without a previous history of diabetes develop high blood sugar levels.

In recent years a wide range of herbal dietary supplements and herbal medicines have scientifically proven to benefit type 2 diabetes mellitus in preclinical studies, however, few have been proven to do so in properly designed randomized clinical trials.

Phytochemicals	Soy contains the largest concentration of isoflavones, a class of phytoestrogens. Phytoestrogens are structurally similar to estradiol and mimic its effects. Soy and phytoestrogens have received increasing attention due to the health benefits associated with their consumption. In animal studies, soy and phytoestrogens are effective at reducing adipose tissue and improving glucose uptake. Isoflavones, are phytoestrogens which have structural/functional similarities to human estrogen. Soy isoflavones have been studied most and their consumption have been associated with lower incidence and mortality rate of type II diabetes, heart disease, osteoporosis and certain cancers.
Fatty acids	Omega-3 fatty acids supplementation in type 2 diabetes has a favorable impact in lowering triglycerides and VLDL-cholesterol, and reducing blood pressure and inflammatory markers. Omega-3 fatty acids have been suggested to reduce glucose tolerance in patients predisposed to diabetes. For the synthesis of a long chain *omega*–3 fatty acids, insulin is required; the heart may thus be particularly susceptible to their depletion in diabetes. Ethyl esters of omega–3 fatty acids may be potential beneficial in diabetic patients. Lipoic acid is an antioxidant which is used for the treatment of diabetic neuropathy and seems to be effective as a long-term dietary supplement for protection of diabetics from complications.
Dietary fibers	Dietary fibers from psyllium have been used extensively both as pharmacological supplements, food ingredients, in processed food to aid weight reduction, for glucose control in diabetic patients and to reduce lipid levels in hyperlipidemia. Soluble dietary fiber is associated with lower postprandial glucose levels and increased insulin sensitivity in diabetic and healthy subjects, effects that are generally attributed to the viscous and/or gelling properties of soluble fiber.
Minerals	Chromium is a trace element that may be deficient in persons with diabetes. It has been suggested that chromium supplements may increase insulin sensitivity and improve glucose tolerance in patients with type 2 diabetes. Prospective epidemiology links magnesium -rich diets to decreased risk for diabetes, with an inverse correlation between magnesium intake and fasting insulin levels, suggesting an improvement in insulin sensitivity.

2.1.2.2 Cardiovascular diseases

Worldwide, the prevalence of CVD and the researches in this area is increasing. CVD is a term which is used for disorders of the heart and blood vessels and includes coronary heart disease (heart attack), peripheral vascular diseases, cerebrovascular disease (stroke), hypertension, deep vein thrombosis, pulmonary embolism, rheumatic heart disease, heart failure, and so on.

CVDs are the major cause of death globally: more people die annually from CVDs than from any other cause. Most cardiovascular diseases can be prevented by addressing behavioural risk factors such as tobacco use, unhealthy diet and obesity, physical inactivity and harmful use of alcohol using population-wide strategies.

Heart attacks and strokes are usually acute events and are mainly caused by a blockage that prevents blood from flowing to the heart or brain. The most common reason for this is a build-up of fatty deposits on the inner walls of the blood vessels that supply the heart or brain.

Nutraceuticals in the form of vitamins, minerals, antioxidants, dietary fibers and omega-3 polyunsaturated fatty acids (*omega*–3 PUFAs) together with physical exercise are recommended for prevention and treatment of CVD. The molecules such as polyphenols alter cellular metabolism and signaling, which is believed to reduce arterial disease.

Phytochemicals	Phytosterols compete with dietary cholesterol by blocking the uptake as well as facilitating its excretion from the body. Hence, they have the potential to reduce the morbidity and mortality of CVD. Phytosterols occur in most plant species and although green and yellow vegetables contain significant amounts of sterols, their seeds concentrate them. Flavonoids are widely distributed in vegetables, onion, endives, cruciferous, grapefruits, apples, cherries, pomegranate, berries, black grapes, and red wine, and are available as flavones, flavanones and flavonols, playing a major role in prevention and curing the CVD. Flavonoids block the angiotensin-converting enzyme, block the cyclooxygenase enzymes that break down prostaglandins, and prevent platelet aggregation. They also protect the vascular system that carries oxygen and nutrients to cells. Anthocyanins, tannins (proanthocyanidins), tetrahydro-β-carbolines, stilbenes, dietary indoleamines, serotonin and melatonin, in plant foods are hypothesized to impose health benefits. Orange juice containing pulp is rich in flavonoids. Hesperidin is a flavanone glycoside which is classified as a citrus bioflavonoid. Citrus sinensis and tangelos are the richest dietary sources of hesperidin. The peel and membranous parts of lemons and oranges have the highest hesperidin concentrations. Hesperidin is used for the treatment of venous insufficiency and hemorrhoids. Flavonoid intake was significantly inversely associated with mortality from coronary heart disease and the incidence of myocardial infarction. Flavonoids in regularly consumed foods may reduce the risk of death from coronary heart disease, especially in elderly people. Buckwheat seeds possess phytosterols, flavonoids, flavones, proteins and thiamin-binding proteins, etc., Buckwheat proteins lower blood cholesterol and hypertension. Dietary fibers have also cholesterol-lowering property with beneficial effects in prevention and alleviation of CVD and diabetes.

Contd...

	The rhizome of *Zingiber officinalis* is a common condiment for various foods and beverages. It has a long history of medicinal use and has a positive effect on CVD. Ginger has potent antioxidant and antiinflammatory activities and recently it has been recommended for various diseases including hypertension and palpitation. This plant has a good protective effect on toxicity of synthetic drugs, too.
Fatty acids	Fatty acids of the omega-3 series (*omega*–3 fatty acids) present in fish are dietary components affecting plasma lipids and the CVD, like arrhythmias. Octacosanol, present in whole grains, fruits and leaves of many plants, has lipid lowering property, with no side-effects.

2.1.2.3 Cancer

Cancer has emerged as a major public health problem in developing countries. According to the World Cancer Report the cancer rates are increasing and it would be 15 million new cases in the year 2020 that is, a rise in 50%. A healthy lifestyle and diet can help in prevention of cancer. Carotenoids are a group of phytochemicals responsible for different colors of the foods. They have antioxidant activities and effective on cancer prevention. Recent interest in carotenoids has focused on the role of lycopene in human health, especially in cancer disease.

Phytocehemicals	Plants rich in daidzein, biochanin, isoflavones and genistein, also inhibit prostate cancer cell growth. Because of the unsaturated nature of lycopene it is considered to be a potent antioxidant and a singlet oxygen quencher. Lycopene concentrates in the prostate, testes, skin and adrenal where it protects against cancer. The linkage between carotenoids and prevention of cancer and CAD, heightened the importance of vegetable and fruits in human diet. Lycopene contained vegetables and fruits exert cancer-protective effect via a decrease in oxidative stress and damage to DNA. Lycopene is one of the major carotenoids and is found exclusively in tomatoes, guava, pink grapefruit, water melon and papaya. β-carotene has antioxidant activity and prevents cancer and other diseases. Among the carotenes, β-carotene has the most antioxidant activity. Alpha-carotene possesses 50–54% of the antioxidant activity of β-carotene, whereas epsilon carotene has 42–50% of the antioxidant activity. Chronic inflammation is associated with a high cancer risk. Chronic inflammation is also associated with immune-suppression, which is a risk factor for cancer. Ginseng is an example of an antiinflammatory molecule that targets many of the key players in the inflammation-to-cancer sequence. Nowadays, phytochemicals with cancer-preventive properties have been on high attention. Chemopreventive components in fruits and vegetables, among other beneficial health effect, have potential anticarcinogenic and antimutagenic activities. A broad range of phyto-pharmaceuticals with a claimed hormonal activity, called "phyto-estrogens," is recommended for prevention of prostate and breast cancers. Citrus fruit flavonoids are able to protect against cancer by acting as antioxidants. Soyfoods are a unique dietary source of isoflavones, the polyphenolic phytochemicals exemplified by epigallocatechin gallate from tea, curcumin from curry and soya isoflavones possess cancer chemopreventive properties.Soybean seems to offer protection against breast, uterine, lung, colorectal, and prostate cancers. β-carotene found in yellow, orange, and green leafy vegetables and fruits such as tomatoes, lettuce, oranges, sweet potatoes, broccoli, cantaloupe, carrots, spinach, and winter squash has anticancer activity. Saponins are reported to possess antimutagenic and antitumor activities and might lower the risk of human cancers, by preventing cancer cells from growing. Saponins are phytochemicals which can be found in peas,

Contd...

	soybeans, and some herbs with names indicating foaming properties such as soapberry, soapwort and soapbark. They are also present in tomatoes, potatoes, alfalfa, spinach, and clover. Commercial saponins are extracted mainly from *Yucca schidigera* and *Quillaja saponaria*. Tannins also scavenge harmful free radicals and detoxify carcinogens. Tannins present in grapes, lentils, tea, blackberries, blueberries and cranberries is a proven anticarcinogen is used in alternative medicine and to prevent cancer. Ellagic acid, present in walnuts, pecans, strawberries, cranberries, pomegranates and red raspberry seeds, is an anticancer agent. Pectin is a soluble fiber found in apples has been shown to prevent prostate cancer metastasis by inhibiting the cancer cells from adhering to other cells in the body. Several studies have shown that pectin decreases serum cholesterol levels. Naturally occurring phenolic acid derivatives are reported to possess potential anticancer properties. Phenolic compounds such as curcumin, gallic acids, ferulic and caffeic acid are reported to possess anticancer activity. Glucosinolates and their hydrolysis products, including indoles and isothiocyanates, and high intake of cruciferous vegetables has been associated with lower risk of colorectal and lung cancer. Bio-transformation products of glucosinolates include dithiol thiones, isothiocyanates, and sulforaphane. They block the enzymes that promote tumor growth, particularly in liver, colon, lung, breast, stomach and esophagus. The sulfur compounds, in garlic have been found to boost the immune system and reduce atherogenesis and platelet stickiness and cancer. Sulforaphane rich in broccoli is a potent phase 2 enzyme inducer. It produces D-glucarolactone, a significant inhibitor of breast cancer. Sulforaphane is an antioxidant and stimulator of natural detoxifying enzymes. Sulforaphane has been reported to reduce the risk of breast cancer and prostate cancer. Curcumin is a polyphenol derived from the plant *Curcuma longa*, commonly called turmeric. Curcumin has been reported to possess antioxidative, anticarcinogenic, and antiinflammatory properties.
Vitamins and Minerals	Consumption of fruits and vegetables having cysteine, glutathione, selenium, Vitamin E, Vitamin C, lycopene, and various phytochemicals elevates the levels of antioxidative capacity. However, more investigations are needed to determine their beneficial effects in cancer prevention or treatment.

Several studies have shown the values of alternative and complementary medicine as adjuvant to chemotherapy or radiotherapy. Complimentary therapy may be reliable and useful supportive measure for prostate cancer patients. Majority of the studies have shown a preventive role for nutraceuticals in cancer, however more elaborate studies are needed.

2.1.2.4 Irritable bowel syndrome (IBS) and various Gastro intestinal diseases

Irritable bowel syndrome (IBS) is a gastrointestinal tract dysfunction, affecting the general population, and young people in particular. This syndrome is manifested with abdominal pain, stool pattern alteration, distention, bloating, straining, abdominal discomfort, and urgency. Genetic background and environmental factors are important in the pathogenesis of IBS, but the precise cause of IBS is still unknown.

Probiotics, prebiotics, synbiotics, fibre and herbal medicinal products are, for some aspects, at the same time both current and promising therapeutic approaches for the management of IBS.

One of the pathogenetic pathways of IBD is represented by an imbalanced immune response to microbes, together with an impairment of gut microbiota, in individuals with genetic susceptibility. Probiotics, prebiotics and synbiotics may restore the intestinal microbial balance, thus enhancing gut barrier function and improving local immune response

Stimulant laxatives of plant origin have been commonly used for a long time for the treatment of constipation. The most popular of them are senna, cascara, frangula, aloe and rhubarb, obtained from the dried leaves and pods of some *Cassia* species, the dried barks of Rhamnus purshiana or Rhamnus frangula, the latex contained in the leaves of some *Aloe* species and the dried rhizome of some *Rheum* species respectively.

2.1.3 Study of Herbs as Health Food

Alfa-alfa: *Medicago sativa*, Fabaceae	Phytoestrogens like spinasterol, coumesterol, coumestan; rich proteins content, seeds are rich in PUFA, Carotenes, vitamins from B-group, C, D, E, K	Antioxidant, Hypochlolesteremic
Amla: *Emblica officinalis*, Euphorbiaceae.	Proteins, carbohydrates, tannins, ascorbic acid,phyllembin.	Antioxidant, hair tonic, in diarrhea, in anemia, laxative, jaundice, diuretic
Ashwagandha *Withaniasomnifera*, Solanaceae	Tropane and pyrrolidine alkaloids, steroidal lactones	Immunomodulatory, Antistress, anti-inflammatory
Chicory: *Cinchorium intybus*, Asteraceae	Vitamin A, B-Complex, carotenes, minerals, sesquiterpene lactones, dietary fibers such as inulin and fructo-oligosaccharides,	Roots are coffee substitute, anti-inflammatory, antiparasitic, hepatoprotective
Garlic: *Allium sativum*, Liliaceae	Diallyl disulphide, allin, allicin, polysulphides, volatile oils, proteins, vitamins, lipids, amino acids	Food supplement, treatment of cough, cold, bronchitis, hypertension, cancer, atherosclerosis, antifungal, hypoglycemic.
Ginger: *Zingiber officinale* Zingiberaceae	Volatile oil,starch, zingerol, Zingiberine, shaogol,fat, sesquterpenes,	Stimulants, carminative, stomachic, scistosomiasis, Motion sickness, Mouth washes.
Ginseng: Asian or Korean ginseng (*Panax ginseng*) and American ginseng (*Panax quinquefolius*), Araliaceae	Steroidal saponins, phytosterols	Immunomodulatory, Antistress
Honey: *Apis mellifera*, Apidae.	Glucose, fructose, sucrose, maltose, succinic acid, dextrine, diastase, traces of vitamins & proteins	Demulcent, Expectorant, suspending agent, antiseptic.
Fenugreek/Methi: *Trigonella, foenumgracum* Leguminaceae	Saponins-Trigoneline, phytosterols, mucillagenous hydrocolloids, proteins, lipids, volatile oil.	Hypoglycemic, demulcent, flavoring agent, condiments, emollient in indigestion
Spirulina (type of blue-green algae) *Arthrospira platensis* and *A. maxima.*	It is a biomass of cyanobacteria and rich in protein, vitamins, minerals, and carotenoids	Antioxidant, potent dietary support in malnourishment

2.2 Herbal-Drug and Herb-Food Interactions

2.2.1 General Introduction to Interaction and Classification

Herbs are often administered in combination with therapeutic drugs, raising the potential of herb-drug interactions. Herbal drug interaction means drug or herbs interact with each other and produces harmful or benefit effects. Between herbs and drugs may increase or decrease the pharmacological or toxicological effects of either component. Synergistic therapeutic effects may complicate the dosing of long-term medications. Many times herb-drug an interaction is not necessarily produces a toxic reaction but cause either an increase or decrease in the amount of drug in the blood stream. A decrease in the amount of drug could occur by herb components binding up the drug and preventing it from being absorbed into the blood stream from the gastrointestinal tract, or by stimulating the production and activity of enzymes that metabolize the drug to form inactive products. A decrease in drug dosage by virtue of an interaction could make the drug ineffective; an increase in drug dosage could make it produce adverse effects.

2.2.1.1 Classification/Types of Interactions

Both pharmacokinetic and/or pharma-codynamic mechanisms have been considered to play a role in these interactions, although the underlying mechanisms for the altered drug effects and/or concentrations by concomitant herbal medicines are yet to be determined. Most natural products are a complex mixture of unknown chemical constituents which also varies depending on the part of the plant used (bark, stems, leaves, roots, rhizomes), climate, growing conditions, harvesting, and storage conditions. Combination products composed of multiple natural products complicate matters further. Manufacturing process, Misidentification and no strict quality controls standard are also increasing interactions. Another important limiting factor concerning herbal-drug interactions is the reliability of the existing evidence.

Classification/Types of Interactions	
Types	**Mode of action**
Pharmacodynamic Interaction	Additive, synergistic, antagonistic
Pharmacokinetic interactions	
Absorption interactions	pH, solubility, Chelation, Binding with proteins
Transport and distribution interactions	Competition for plasma protein transport
Metabolism interactions	Enzyme (cytochrome P450 oxidases CYP1A2, CYP2C9, CYP2C19, CYP2D6, CYP2E1 and CYP3A4) inhibition or inductor
Excretion interactions	pH of urine in case of renal excretion and glucuronidation in bile excretion

Examples of Drug Interactions

Pharmacodynamic interaction	Concomitant use of digoxin (cardiotonic) acts well at low levels of potassium (K) and furosemide (Diuretic) favours the loss of K^+. This could lead to hypokalemia (low levels of potassium in the blood), which could increase the toxicity of digoxin.
	Gingko + Anticogulant = Additive

Contd...

Pharmacokinetic interaction	
Absorption interactions	In the case of the antacids, an increase in pH can inhibit the absorption of other drugs such as zalcitabine (absorption can be decreased by 25%), tipranavir (25%) and amprenavir (up to 35%). Gingko decrease absorption of Alprazolam
Metabolism interactions	Grapefruit juice interacts by Enzymatic inhibition with Calcium channel blockers: nifedipine, felodipine, nimodipine, amlodipine, Cyclosporine, tacrolimus
Excretion interactions	Drugs that act as weak bases (Example- Reserpine, Amphetamine, Procaine, Ephedrine, Atropine, Diazepam) are increasingly excreted as the pH of the urine becomes more acidic, and the inverse is true for weak acids (Phenobarbital, Warfarin, Theophylline, Phenytoin).

Examples of Pharmacokinetic interaction

Herb	Drug	Mechanism	Effect
Psyllium, Aloe	Lithium	Psyllium inhibit absorption of lithium	Drug absorption inhibited.
Rhubarb, Aloe	Digoxin, warfarin	Decreases digoxin and warfarin action.	Drug effect decreases.
Black willow	Warfarin carbamazepin	Black willow displaces the highly bound protein like warfarin and carbamazepin.	Increases absorption and excretion of drug.
Liquorice	Corticosteroids	Liqourice Decreases metabolism of corticosteroids.	Increases toxic effect of drug.
Hypercin	Digoxin theophyllin	Hypercin increases metabolism of these drugs.	Drug effect gets reduces.

Examples of Pharamacodynamic interaction

Herb	Drug	Mechanism	Effect
Garlic	Warfarin	Both showing antiplatelate action.	Drug effect gets increases.
Garlic	Saquinavir	Induction of CYP3A4 enzyme.	Drug effect decreases.
Gingko	Aspirin, warfarin, ibuprofen	Antiplatlate action.	Increases bleeding.
Gingko	Omeprazole	Induction of CYP2C19 enzyme	Drug effect decreases.
Ginseng	Phenelzine	Increases drug toxicity	Toxic effect increases.
Ginseng	Digoxin	False elevation of digoxin by unknown mechanism.	No effect.
Green tea	Warfarin	Green tea contains vit. K	Decreases drug effect.
Kava	Alprazolam	Additive CNS depressant effect.	Increases drug effect.
Kava	Levodopa	Kava may antagonize dopamine.	Decreases drug effect.
Noni juice	Warfarine	Noni juice contains vit K	Drug effect decreases.
Papaya	Warfarin	unknown	Increases drug effect.
Peppermint oil	Nifedipine	Increases oral bioavailability	Increases drug effect.
Psyllium	Carbamzepine, lithium	Psyllium decreases absorption.	Decreases drug effect.
Hypercin	Buspirone	Induction of serotonin syndrome.	Increases drug toxicity.

By searching the literatures, it was found that a total of 32 drugs interacting with herbal medicines in humans. These drugs mainly include anticoagulants (warfarin, aspirin and phenprocoumon), sedatives and antidepressants (midazolam, alprazolam and amitriptyline), oral contraceptives, anti-HIV agents (indinavir, ritonavir and saquinavir), cardiovascular drug (digoxin), immunosuppressants (cyclosporine and tacrolimus) and anticancer drugs (imatinib and irinotecan). Most of them are substrates for cytochrome P450s (CYPs) and/or P-glycoprotein (PgP) and many of which have narrow therapeutic indices.

- However, several drugs including acetaminophen, carbamazepine, myco-phenolic acid, and pravastatin did not interact with herbs. Both pharmaco-kinetic (Example-. induction of hepatic CYPs and intestinal PgP) and/or pharmaco-dynamic mechanisms (Example-. synergistic or antagonistic interaction on the same drug target) may be involved in drug-herb interactions, leading of altered drug clearance, response and toxicity.
- Toxicity arising from drug-herb interactions may be minor, moderate, or even fatal, depending on a number of factors associated with the patients, herbs and drugs.
- Predicting drug-herb interactions, timely identification of drugs that interact with herbs and therapeutic drug monitoring may minimize toxic drug-herb interactions. It is likely to predict pharmacokinetic herb-drug interactions by following the pharma-cokinetic principles and using proper models that are used for predicting drug-drug interactions.
- Identification of drugs that interact with herbs can be incorporated into the early stages of drug development. A fourth approach for circumventing toxicity arising from drug-herb interactions is proper design of drugs with minimal potential for herbal interaction.
- So-called "hard drugs" that are not metabolized by CYPs and not transported by PgP are believed not to interact with herbs due to their unique pharmacokinetic properties. More studies are needed and new approached are required to minimize toxicity arising from drug-herb interactions.
- Cases have been published reporting enhanced anticoagulation and bleeding when patients on long-term warfarin therapy also took *Salvia miltiorrhiza* (danshen). *Allium sativum* (garlic) decreased the area under the plasma concentration-time curve (AUC) and maximum plasma concentration of saquinavir, but not ritonavir and paracetamol (acetaminophen), in volunteers.
- A. sativum increased the clotting time and international normalised ratio of warfarin and caused hypoglycaemia when taken with chlorpropamide. *Ginkgo biloba* (ginkgo) caused bleeding when combined with warfarin or aspirin (acetylsalicylic acid), raised blood pressure when combined with a thiazide diuretic and even caused coma when combined with trazodone in patients.
- *Panax ginseng* (ginseng) reduced the blood concentrations of alcohol (ethanol) and warfarin, and induced mania when used concomitantly with phenelzine, but ginseng increased the efficacy of influenza vaccination.
- *Scutellariabaicalensis* ameliorated irinotecan-induced gastro-intestinal toxicity in cancer patients. *Piper methysticum* (kava) increased the 'off' periods in patients with Parkinsonism taking levodopa and induced a semicomatose state when given concomitantly with alprazolam. Kava enhanced the hypnotic effect of alcohol in mice, but this was not observed in humans. *Silybum marianum* (milk thistle) decreased the trough concentrations of indinavir in humans.

- Piperine from black (*Piper nigrum* Linn) and long (*P. longum* Linn) peppers increased the AUC of phenytoin, propranolol and theophylline in healthy volunteers and plasma concentrations of rifamipicin (rifampin) in patients with pulmonary tuber-culosis. *Eleutheroccussenticosus* (*Siberian ginseng*) increased the serum concen-tration of digoxin, but did not alter the pharmacokinetics of dextromethorphan and alprazolam in humans.
- *Hypericum perforatum*(hypericum; St John's wort) decreased the blood concentrations of ciclosporin (cyclosporin), midazolam, tacrolimus, amitriptyline, digoxin, indinavir, warfarin, phenprocoumon and theophylline, but did not alter the pharmacokinetics of carbamazepine, pravastatin, mycophenolate mofetil and dextromethorphan.
- Cases have been reported where decreased ciclosporin concentrations led to organ rejection. Hypericum also caused breakthrough bleeding and unplanned pregnancies when used concomitantly with oral contraceptives. It also caused serotonin syndrome when used in combination with selective serotonin reuptake inhibitors (Example-. sertraline and paroxe-tine).

Examples of Herb-Drug Interactions

Herbal Supplement	Common Uses	Potential Problems	Potential Interactions With
Ephedra *(Ma Huang, Ephedrine, Pseudo-ephedrine)*	To treat asthma, cough, and to induce weight loss	Seizures; Adverse cardiovascular events, hypertension	Cardiac glycosides; General anesthesia; MAO inhibitors; Decongestants, stimulants
Garlic	To decrease cholesterol and blood clot formation	Enhances bleeding	Anticoagulants
Ginger	To relieve nausea	Enhances bleeding; CNS depression; Hypotension; Cardiac Arrhythmia; Hypoglycemia	Anticoagulants; Enhances the effects of barbiturates; Antihypertensives; Cardiac drugs; Hypoglycemic drugs
Ginseng	To increase energy and reduce stress	Enhances bleeding; Tachycardia and hypertension; Mania	Anticoagulants; Stimulants; Antihypertensives; Antidepressants/Phenelzine; Digoxin; Potentiates the effects of corticosteroids and estrogens
Liqcorice	To treat hepatitis and peptic ulcers	Hypertension; Hypokalemia; Edema	Antihypertensives; Potentiates the effects of corticosteroids
St. John's Wort	To treat mild depression, anxiety, seasonal affective disorder	Enhances bleeding; hastens metabolic breakdown of drugs; contra-indicated for organ transplant recipiants	Anticoagulants; Antidepressants; Decreases the effectiveness of cyclosporine, antiviral drugs; Digoxin; Dextrometorphan; Prolongs the effects of general anesthetics; MAO inhibitors

2.2.2 Study of Few Herbal Drugs and their Possible Side Effects and Interactions

St John's wort ***Hypericum perforatum***	***Introduction:*** Hypericum perforatum is a yellow-flowering,perennial herb indigenous to Europe that has been introduced tomany temperate areas of the world and grows wild in manymeadows. The common name comes from its traditional flower-ing and harvesting on 24 June, the birthday of John the Baptist(St. John's Day) ***Chemical constituents:*** Naphthodianthrones (Example-. hypericin and its derivatives), phloroglucinols derivatives (Example-. hyperforin, which inhibits the reuptake of a number of neurotransmitters, including serotonin), and flavonoids. ***Uses***: Treatment of mild-to-moderate depression. As a monotherapy, *Hypericum* has an encouraging safety profile. ***Interaction***: However, relevant and, in some case, life-threatening interactions have been reported, particularly with drugs which are substrate of cytochrome P450 and/or P-glycoprotein. More than 70 % ofall prescription medications are susceptible to SJW-mediated interactions, the consequences of which are decreased oral bio-availability, enhanced systemic clearance, and reduced drug efficacy. Well-documented *Hypericum* interactions include • Induces CYP3A4, thus increasing the metabolism of oral midazolam, alprazolam1 and quazepam, and reducing the bioavailability of these benzodiazepines • Decreases the bioavailability of both nifedipine and verapamil by inducing their metabolism by the cytochrome P450 isoenzyme CYP3A4 in the gut • Serotonin syndrome has been seen with St John's wort alone, and so additive serotonergic effects appear with SSRIs • Reduced plasma drug concentration of antiretroviral (Example-. indinavir, nevirapine) and anticancer (i.e., irinotecan, imatinib) drugs.
Kava kava- *Piper methysticum*	***Introduction:*** Kavakava (Piper methysticum G. Forst.; family Piperaceae) haslong been a traditional beverage consumed among South Pacific islanders to imbue psychotropic, hypnotic, and anxiolytic effects. Since the 1990s, commercial kava extracts formulated as tablets and/or capsules have been marketed as dietary supplements for the alleviation of stress, anxiety, or insomnia ***Chemical constituents:*** Kavalactones- kavain, dihydrokavain, methysticin, dihy-dromethysticin, yangonin, desmethoxyyangonin) ***Uses:***Anxiolytic and sedative properties. ***Interaction***: Several liver failure cases which led to its ban in many countries. • Several kavalactones, the assumed active principles of kava extracts, are potent inhibitors of several enzymes of the CYP 450 system (CYP1A2, 2C9, 2C19, 2D6, 3A4 and 4A9/11). • Potential pharmacokinetic drug interactions with other herbal products or drugs, which are metabolised by the CYP 450 enzymes.

Contd...

Ginkgo biloba	***Introduction:*** Termed living fossils, ginkgo trees (family Ginkgoaceae) have ex-isted since the early Jurassic period 150 million years ago. Thelone species that avoided extinction (Ginkgo biloba L.) is now cul-tivated in Asia, Europe, North America, New Zealand, and Argen-tina. Ginkgo is a popular ornamental tree recognizable by its un-usual fan-shaped leaves that turn bright yellow in autumn. InAsia, the tree has long been held sacred for its therapeutic value ***Chemical constituents:*** Flavonoids (quercetin, kaempferol, and isorhamnetin) and terpenoids (bilobalide and ginkgolides A/B/C/J). It ***Uses:***Improvement of cerebral circulation, memory improvement and antioxidant activity. ***Interaction***: There is some concern that ginkgo leaf extract might increase the risk of bruising and bleeding, and interactions with anticoagulants/antiplatelet drugs. However, Intake of the standardized Ginko extract, together with synthetic drugs appears to be safe as long as daily doses up to 240 mg are consumed
Ginseng: Panax ginseng	***Introduction:*** Of the five major Panax species (family Araliaceae) worldwide,Asian ginseng (Panax ginseng C. A. Meyer) and American ginseng(Panax quinquefolius L.) are the most widely used and extensivelystudied. P. ginseng root has an almost 2000-year history of use intraditional Chinese medicine (TCM) as an adaptogen (a plant thatincreases resistance to stress and fatigue) and a restorative tonic ***Chemical constituents:*** Ginsenosides, a group of triterpene glycosides (steroidal sapo-nins), are unique to Panax species. More than 40 ginsenosideshave been identified in the roots of *P. ginseng and P. quinquefolius*. Ginsenoside nomenclature employs the designation Rx, where "x" represents the retention factor (Rf) value from the sequence of spots (from bottom to top) on thin-layer chromatography plates. ***Uses:*** Immunostimulatory, antithrombotic, antioxidative, anti-inflammatory, and anticancer effects. ***Interaction***: • Ginseng may interact with concomitant medications and alter metabolism and/or drug transport, which may alter the known efficacy and safety of a drug; thus, the role of ginseng may be controversial when taken with other medications. • Ginseng appear to modestly lower blood-glucose levels and may therefore potentiate the blood-glucose-lowering effects of conventional oral antidiabetics. • May reduce the effects of warfarin as ginsengs also contain anti-platelet components, excessive bleeding cannot be ruled out. • Psychoactive effects of ginseng may be additive with those of MAOIs.
Ma-haung: Ephedra gerardiana	***Introduction:*** Ephedra, commonly called as Ma-Haung is dried young stems of *Ephedra gerardiana*, *E. sinica* and *E. equisetina* of family ephedraceae. ***Chemical constituents:*** Ephedrine and pseudoephedrine **Uses:** Asthma, bronchitis, hayfever and colds. It is banned by the FDA in the US due to abuse as a stimulant and slimming aid.. ***Interactions***: • The most notable of these interactions is the potential for hypertensive crises with MAOIs • Ephedrine can raise blood pressure and combined use with caffeine has resulted in hypertensive crises or development of acute psychosis.

Contd...

	• Ephedrine and caffeine may cause catecholamine release and an increase in intracellular calcium release which leads to vasoconstriction. Myocardial ischaemia may occur as a result of this vasoconstriction (in the coronary artery), and this may result in myocardial necrosis and cell death.
Garlic : Allium sativum L.	***Introduction:*** Members of the family Alliaceae have been an important part of the human diet for thousands of years. Allium species, such as garlic (*Allium sativum* L.) and onions (*Allium cepa* L.), are a rich source of sulfur-containing compounds, many of which are volatile and give rise to the characteristic flavor and aroma of these species ***Chemical constituents:*** Organosulfur compounds [allyl thiosulfinates (Example-. allicin), alkyl sulfides (Example-. diallyl sulfide), vinyldithiins, andajoene], steroid saponins, and other phyto-chemicals **Uses:** Treat respiratory infections (such as colds, flu, chronic bronchitis, and nasal and throat catarrh) and cardiovascular disorders (antihypertensive, antithrombotic, lipid-lowering properties), fibrinolytic, antimicrobial, anticancer, expectorant, antidiabetic Ingredient in foods. ***Interactions***: • Garlic may have additive blood pressure-lowering effects with lisinopril, and may • Cause bleeding in those taking warfarin or fluindione. • Antiplatelet effects of garlic may be additive with conventional antiplatelet drugs and NSAIDs, • Garlic may reduce isoniazid levels.
Black pepper/piperine	***Introduction:*** Dried ground black pepper (Piper nigrum L.; family Piperaceae) has been used since antiquity as both a flavoring agent and medicine. In fact, for almost two millennia Piper species (Example-. P.nigrum and P. longum) have been essential components of several Ayurvedic medicine preparations. Black pepper is one ofthe most commonly used spices and may be found on nearly every dinner table in the industrialized world. ***Chemical constituents:*** piperine, andrelated pungent alkaloids known as piperamides ***Uses***: Recognizing piperine's utility as a bioavailability enhancer, manydietary supplement manufacturers incorporate P. nigrum or P.longum extracts into botanical formulations as a means of improving phytochemical efficacy. **Interactions:** • Piperine is its ability todramatically enhance the oral absorption of concomitantly ad-ministered medications. • Drugs affected and the observed percent increase in mean AUC include phenyt-oin (16–133%), rifampicin (69 %), proprano-lol (103%), theophylline (96%), and nevirapine(170%). • Piperine increases the pharmacodynamic effects of hexo-barbital and zoxazolamine in a dose-dependent fashion

Subjective Questions

1. What is Nutraceutical and How to classify it?
2. Write a note on Nutraceuticals useful in Diabetes or cancer or CVS diseases
3. Give health benefits of any five popular nutraceutical herbs

4. With which drugs hypercium found to be more interactive?
5. Give brief account on drugs interacting with gingko.
6. Discuss herb-drug interaction with examples
7. What is difference between Prebiotics and probiotics?
8. How antioxidants are useful in treating or preventing various diseases?
9. What is PUFA?
10. What is difference between Prebiotics and dietary fibers?
11. What is FSSAI?
12. What is IBS?
13. What are types of Drug-drug-food/herb interaction?

Multiple Choice Questions (MCQs)/Objective Questions

1. The present US market for nutraceutical is ....
   a. More than 3 billion US dollars
   b. More than 3 million US dollars
   c. Not estimated
   d. None of the above
2. Which one of the following is an important dietary anticarcinogen?
   a. Tocopherol
   b. Selenium
   c. Ascorbic acid
   d. None of the above
3. Which one of the following is rich source of tocopherol?
   a. Wheat germ oil
   b. Pea nut oil
   c. Sunflower oil
   d. Soyabean oil
4. Poly Unsaturated Fatty Acids belongs to linolenic group ....
   a. Omega - 4 type
   b. Omega -6 type
   c. Omega -3 type
   d. Both b and c
5. Probiotics are ....
   a. Nutraceutical food for gut microbes
   b. Living microorganisms improving gut microbe balance
   c. Both a and b
   d. None
6. *Bifidobacterium* and *Lactobacilli* species are used as ....
   a. Probiotics
   b. Prebiotics
   c. Both a and b
   d. None of the above
7. Chicory is reach in fibrous polysaccharide ....
   a. Inulin
   b. Cellulose
   c. Starch
   d. None of the above

8. Which one of the following is best known prebiotic?
   a. Dextrin
   b. Agave
   c. Inulin
   d. All of
9. Which type of nutraceuticals is beneficial in Irritable bowel syndrome and various intestinal diseases?
   a. Probiotics
   b. PUFA
   c. Dietary fibers
   d. None of the above
10. Recommended daily dose of dietary fibers for adult is ....
    a. 5 gm
    b. 30 gm
    c. 15 gm
    d. 25 gm
11. Parent fatty acid of Omega -3 family is ....
    a. Linoleic acid
    b. Linolenic acid
    c. Oleic acid
    d. Lauric acid
12. Biological source of spirulina is ......
    a. Blue green algae Spirulina platensis, family Oscillatoriaceae
    b. Blue green algae Chlorella, Family Trebouxiophyceae
    c. Blue green algae Spirulina maxima, family Oscillatoriaceae
    d. Both a and c
13. Which one of the following is source of Gamma linolenic acid?
    a. Olive
    b. Almond
    c. Spirulina
    d. All of the above
14. Spirulina exerts anticancer activity by ....
    a. Enhancing nuclear enzyme activity
    b. Enhances DNA repair
    c. Both a and b
    d. None of the above
15. Which compound present in garlic exerts antibiotic activity?
    a. Ajoene
    b. Allicin
    c. S –alllylcysteine
    d. vinyldithiins
16. Which components of Alfalfa exert strong estrogenic activity?
    a. Coumestrol
    b. Ergosterol
    c. Tocopherol
    d. All of the above
17. Fenugreek has health benefits like ....
    a. Lowering of blood sugar
    b. Increase in milk production
    c. Body detox
    d. All of the above

18. Which one of the following medicinal herb is widely used as rejuvenator?
    a. Alfalfa
    b. Fenugreek
    c. Ashwagandha
    d. Chicory
19. What may happen if ephedra is taken with caffeine?
    a. Enhances risk of hypertension
    b. Enhances risk of hypotension
    c. Hyperglycemia
    d. Hypoglycemia
20. If evening primerose oil is consumed with tricyclic antidepressant drugs,
    a. May worsen temporal lobe epilepsy
    b. May improve schizophrenia
    c. lower the seizure threshold?
    d. None of the above
21. If patient is consuming Gingkobiloba when he is already on Aspirin therapy for heart disease, what kind of interaction may happen in such case?
    a. Gingko biloba will not interact with Aspirin
    b. Gingko biloba may exert synergistic effect which lay lead to stroke
    c. Gingko biloba will lower the bioavailability of Aspirin
    d. Gingko biloba will block the aspirin activity
22. KavaKava which originally reduces stress and anxiety should not be consumed with ....to avoid drug herb interaction.
    a. CNS stimulants
    b. Antipsychotic drugs
    c. hypoglycemic drugs
    d. Antiplatelet drugs
23. Ginger should NOT be consumed with ....to avoid side effects
    a. Antiplatelet agents
    b. Calcium channel blockers
    c. Both a and b
    d. None of the above
24. Garlic may potentiate activity of blood pressure reducing agents because
    a. Garlic increases platelet aggregation
    b. Garlic reduces platelet aggregation
    c. Garlic decrease blood pressure
    d. Garlic increase blood pressure
25. Which one of the following herb may interact with the digoxin activity?
    a. Garlic
    b. Ginger
    c. Ginseng
    d. Kava kava
26. During the treatment with hypericum, tyramine containing food must be avoided because
    a. Interaction may cause palpitation and restlessness
    b. Interaction may cause sedative effect
    c. Interaction may lead to seizures
    d. None of the above

27. Serotonin syndrome may arise if st. John's wort is consumed with
    a. Cholinesterase inhibitors
    b. Monoamino oxidase inhibitors
    c. Calcium channel inhibitors
    d. None of the above
28. Co-administration of hypericum with contraceptives may lead to
    a. Failure of contraceptive
    b. Excessive bleeding
    c. Skin rashes
    d. Dry mouth
29. When getting the treatment with warfarin, which herbs must be avoided to avoid adverse invents?
    a. Ginger
    b. Garlic
    c. Gingko biloba
    d. All of the above
30. Which one of the following herb serves as herbal bioavailability enhancer?
    a. Garlic
    b. Pepper
    c. Ginger
    d. All of the above
31. Food or diet with high level of Vitamin K causes
    a. Increase in therapeutic activity of Anticoagulants
    b. Decrease in therapeutic activity of Anticoagulants
    c. Both a and b
    d. None of the above
32. Caffeine increases serum theophylline levels by ....
    a. 40 - 50%
    b. 5 - 10%
    c. 20 – 30%
    d. None of the above
33. Colchicine may impairs absorption of
    a. Vitamin K
    b. Vitamin D
    c. Iron
    d. Vitamin B12
34. Grape fruit juice blocks vital enzyme ....in small intestine which metabolizes drug
    a. CYP450
    b. CYP3A4
    c. CYP2E4
    d. None of the above
35. St. John wort causes ....in the serum level of indinavir which may result in HIV treatment failure
    a. Decrease
    b. Increase
    c. Accumulation
    d. None of the above
36. High protein meal ....bioavailability of drugs like propranolol having high first pass effect
    a. Increases
    b. decreases
    c. Inhibits
    d. None

37. Tannin present in tea impairs absorption of
    a. Zinc
    b. Magnesium
    c. Iron
    d. Calcium
38. Liquorice should NOT be administered with antihypertensive drugs because
    a. Glycyrrhetinic acid inhibits 11 betahydroxysteroid dehydrogenase
    b. Increases cortisol level in kidney
    c. Both a and b
    d. None of the above

Answer Key

1. a	2. b	3. a	4. d	5. c	6. a	7.a	8.c	9. c	10. c
11. c	12. b	13. b	14. d	15. c	16. c	17. b	18. a	19. d	20.c
21. a	22.a	23.b	24. b	25. c	26. b	27. d	28. a	29. b	30. b
31. d	32. b	33. a	34. c	35. d	36. b	37. b	38. a	39. a	40. c

Unit 3

3.1 Herbal Cosmetics

- 3.1.1 Lipids/Fats/Waxes/Non-volatile Oil
- 3.1.2 Gums/Mucilages/Carbohydrates/Polysaccharides
- 3.1.3 Colorants
- 3.1.4 Volatile Oils/Perfumes and Fragances
- 3.1.5 Skin Whitening (Bleaching) Agents
- 3.1.6 Protective Agents or Antioxidants in Products such as Skin Care, Hair Care and Oral Hygiene Products

3.2 Herbal or Natural Excipients

- 3.2.1 Colorants
- 3.2.2 Sweeteners
- 3.2.3 Binders
- 3.2.4 Diluents
- 3.2.5 Viscosity Builders/ Thickening and Gelling Agents
- 3.2.6 Disintegrants
- 3.2.7 Flavors and Perfumes

3.3 Herbal Formulations

- 3.3.1 Conventional Dosage Forms
  - 3.3.1.1 Syrup
  - 3.3.1.2 Mixture
  - 3.3.1.3 Tablet
- 3.3.2 Novel Drug Delivery Systems (NDDSs)

3.1 Herbal Cosmetics

Cosmetics are defined as "items with mild action on the human body for the purpose of cleaning, beautifying, adding to the attractiveness, altering the appearance, or keeping or promoting the skin or hair in good condition" while functional cosmetics, even if falling under the cosmetic definition, are designated as "items fulfilling specific actions like skin whitening, minimizing the appearance of lines in the face and body, protecting from the sun and sun tanning". Cosmeceuticals are cosmetic products having some specific therapeutic effects.

3.1.1 Lipids/Fats/Waxes/Non-volatile Oil

- Fatty acids are important in maintaining the structure and function of the outer layer or epidermis (stratum corneum, SC) which contains glycolipids, intercellular lipids (cement), and a lipid coat of the skin called the natural moisturizing factor. Lipids in intercellular matrix connect the SC, ensuring its cohesiveness, ability to protect the skin from xenobiotics, and forming a barrier against water loss.
- Chronologically aged skin is characterized by an inherent reduction in epidermal lipid content, resulting in dehydration and altered skin barrier function. Epidermal keratinocyte differentiation and desquamation slows with age, leaving skin dry and flaky.
- Dryness of the skin further accumulates into a reduction of elasticity andwrinkles of the skin consequently as evidenced by biomechanical properties ofthe skin. Therefore, application of skin hydrating cosmetics isnot only to hydrate the skin, but their pleiotropic skin benefits ultimately enhanceaesthetic preference of the skin. That is recently known as corneotherapy.

Classification of lipids	
Simple/ Homolipids	Oils, Waxes, Fats [Fatty acid- saturated, unsaturated (MUFA-Omega 3 faaty acids, Omega 6 fatty acids, PUFA-Omega 9 fatty acids],
Compound / Heterolipids	**Phopshplolipids**-Phosphoglycerides, lecithins, cephalins, plasmalogens, linositols, sphingomyleins **Glycolipids**-glycoproteins, glycopeptides, peptidoglycans, glycosides, glycolipids, and lipopolysaccharides
Derived	Carotendois, terpenes, Steroids

- Vegetable oils are used as a emulsifiers in detergents, creams, lotions, ointments, and makeup to acts a skin moisturizing, smoothing and lubrication, anti-eczema, anti-inflammation and arthritis, soothing of sunburn, and the healing of wounds, ulcers, and burns
- The oils incorporate into the cell membranes and regenerate the damaged lipid barrier of epidermis restricting water loss. The unsaturated fatty acids show pronounced healing effects on dermatoses such as atopic skin inflammation and are used in creams, emulsions, cosmetic milks, ointments, hair conditioners, cosmetic masks, lipsticks, bath fluids, nail polishes, etc
- Fatty acids, triglycerides, and glycerol are used as emollient and hydrating components, acts as a waterproof barrier

- Omega-9 fatty acid like ricinoleic acid from castor oil is found to be very useful for skin dryness, acne, and baldness.
- Omega-6 fatty acid like linoleic acid is found to be very useful in eczema, hair loss, reduced wound healing, and circulatory defects.
- Monounsaturated oleic acid, and also the saturated palmitic and stearic acids present in Cocoa butter are very good emollients, moisturizers, and in the treatment of dry skin.
- Polyunsaturated linoleic acid in Sunflower oil is useful for scaly lesions due to essential fatty acid deficiency, or for psoriasis and burns.
- Jojoba waxy oil (seeds of the desert shrub **Simmondsia chinensis**) is very useful in extrinsic skin aging and hair strengthening due to high penetrability and deliverability to deep skin layers through hydration, antioxidant and anti-inflammatory effects. It reduces wrinkles.
- Ceramides like sphingolipids containing linoleic acyl esters are extremely useful in skin rehydration.
- Oil-free moisturizers without vegetable oils use silicone derivatives such as dimethicone and cyclomethicone to retard moisture loss without the greasy feel.
- Vegetable oils commonly used in facial care are Almond, apricot, hazelnut, borage, jojoba, avocado, olive, wheat germ, macadamia, grapeseed
- Vegetable oils commonly used in hair care areAlmond, borage, avocado, cocoa butter, jojoba, sesame, macadamia.

Following are Examples lipid containing plants and animal sources used in cosmetics

Type	Biological source	Family	Chemical composition
			PUFA/MUFA
Plant			
Almond oil	*Prunus dulcis (Mill.)*	Rosaceae	Aldobionic acid, Vit A, E, stearic and palmitic acid,
Apricot oil	*Prunus armeniaca*	Rosaceae	Amygdalin, oleic and linoleic acid, Vit A, C, and Vit E, stearic and palmitic acid,
Avocado oil	*Perseaameriana*	Lauraceae	Oleic acid(65%), linoleic acid(14%), palmitic acid(6%), high content of ω- 3,6,9 fatty acids.
Borage oil	*Borago officinalis*	Boraginaceae	Palmitoleic acid (11%), oleic acid (20%), stearic acid (4.5%), Linolenic acid (38%), nervonic acid(1.5%), eicosenoic acid(5.5%).
Brazil nut oil	*Bertholletiaexcelsa*	Lecythidaceae	Beta sitosterol(54%), monounsaturated fat (24%), polyunsaturated fat(20%), satureted fat(15%).
Canola oil	*Brassica rapa*	Brassicaceae	Arachidic (5%), eicosenoic (5%), lignoceric(8%), oleic(40%), linolenic(8%), linoleic acids.
Cashew oil	*Anacardium occidentale*	Anacardiaceae	Anacardiac acid (71%), saturated fat (7%), unsaturated fat(0.2%), polysaturated fat (7%), monounsaturated fat(23.79%).

Contd….

Type	Biological source	Family	Chemical composition
			PUFA/MUFA
Chia seeds oil	*Salvia hispanica*	Lamiaceae	Omega -3- fatty acids, palmitic acid, linolenic acid.
Cocoa butter oil	*Theobroma cacao*	sterculiaceae	Stearic (34%), palmitic (25%), oleic (37%) acids and small amount of arachidic and linolenic acid.
Coconut oil	*Cocos nucifera*	Palmae	95% saturated fatty acid, caprylic acid, capric acid, myristic acid.
Corn oil	*Zea mays*	Gramineae	Stearic(4.5%), palmitic(13%), oleic(24%), linolenic(62%), linoleic acids(1.5%). Beta-sitosterol, compesterol.
Castor oil	*Ricinus communis*	Euphorbiaceae	Ricinoleic acid, Ricicine, ricin, phytin
Cottonseed oil	*Gossypium harbaceum*	Malvaceae	Glycerides like palmitooleolinoleins (35-40%), palmitodioleins (20%). Stearic(2.7%), palmitic(33%), oleic(29%), arachidic acid(1%).
Evening Primrose Oil	*Oenothera biennis*	Oenothera	Linoleic acid(74%), linolenic acid(10%).sterols.
Flaxseed/Linseed oil	*Linum usitatissimum*	linaceae	Glycerides of Stearic, palmitic, oleic, linolenic, linoleic acids. Squalene and tocopherol, linamarin and 5% of mucilage.
Grape seed oil	*Vitis vinifera*	Vitaceae	Palmitoleic acid (<1%), oleic acid (15.8%), polyunsaturated fatty acid (69.9%), Linolenic acid (69.6%)
Hazelnut oil	*Carylus avellana*	Betulaceae	palmitic, oleic, linolenic, linoleic acids. Arachidonic acid
Hemp seed oil	*Cannabis sativa*	cannabinaceae	Cannabidilic acid and transterahydrocanabinol.
Jojoba oil	*Simmondsiachimensis*	Simmonodsiaceae	Triglycerides, ionomycin, oleosin
Mustard oil	*Brassica nigra*	Brassicaceae	Arachidic(0.5%), behenic(3%), eicosenoic(8%), erusic(60%), lignoceric(18%), oleic(22%), linolenic(7%), linoleic acids.
Macadamia oil	*Macadamia integrifolia*	Proteaceae	Myristic acid(1.6%), Stearic(6.1%), palmitic(13.1%), oleic(51%), linoleic acids(3.7%), Gadoleic acid(3.7%), behenic acid (1.7%).
Olive oil	*Olea europoea*	Oleaceae	Glycerides of Stearic, palmitic, oleic, linolenic, linoleic acids. Arachidonic acid
Palm oil	*Elaeisguineensis*	Arecaceae	Olein, 3-monochloropropanediol MPCD, little amount f linoleic acid.
Peanut oil	*Arachiahypogaea*	Papilionaceae	Fatty acids like Stearic(3.1%), palmitic(8.3%), linolenic(26%), arachidic acid(24%), eicosenoic acid(3.1%).

Contd....

Type	Biological source	Family	Chemical composition
			PUFA/MUFA
Pecan oil	*Carya illinoinesis*	Juglandaceae	Oleic acid(57%), linoleic acid (30%), polyunsaturated fat (21%)
Perilla oil	*Perilla frutescens*	Lamiaceae	Limonene, linalool, alpha-pinene
Rice bran oil	*Oryza sativa*	Gramineae	Oleic (40-50%), linoleic (30-40%), palmitic acid (12-18%)
Safflower oil	*Carthamus tinctorius*	Composites	Glycerides of Stearic (3%), palmitic(6.5%), oleic(13%), linolenic(76%), linoleic acids(90%).
Sesame oil	*Sesamum indicum Linn.*	Pedaliaceae	Sesamolin oleic acid, linoleic acid.
Soybean oil Partially hydrogenated	*Glycine max*	Leguminosae	Saturated fatty acid (14.9), Oleic (42.4), linoleic (2.6), linolenic acid (34.9), palmitic acid, arachidic acid
Soybean oil	*Glycine max*	Leguminosaev	Saturated fatty acid (15.5), Oleic (22.6), linoleic (7), linolenic acid (51), palmitic acid, arachidic acid
Sunflower oil (<60% linolenic acid)	*Carthamus tinctorius*	Compositae	Saturated fatty acid (10.1), Oleic (82.6), linoleic (0.2), linolenic acid(39.8), palmitic acid, arachidic acid
Sunflower oil (>70% oleic acid)	*Carthamus tinctorius*	Compositae	Saturated fatty acid (9.9), Oleic (82.6), linoleic (0.2), linolenic acid (3.6), palmitic acid, arachidic acid
Sunflower (standard)	*Carthamus tinctorius*	Compositae	Saturated fatty acid (10.3), oleic acid(19.5), linolenic acid(0.9), linoleic acid(65.7),
Tomato seed oil	*Solanum lycopersicum*	Solanaceae	High content of linoleic acid (54%), oleic acid(22%), palmitic acid(14%), stearic acid (6%).
Vigna mungo oil	*Vigna mungo*	Fabaceae	Total 1.64 gm of saturated and unsaturated fat in 100 gm contain Oleic, linoleic, linolenic acid, palmitic acid, arachidic acid
Walnut oil	*Juglans regia*	Juglandaceae	Ferulic acid, myricetin, vanillic acid, coumaric acid, syringic acid, sitosterol, ellagitannin.
Wheat germ Oil	*Triticum aestivum*	Gramineae	Saturated fatty acid (4.7%), linoleic acid (44.1%), linolenic acid (10.8%), vit E, unsaponifiable matter.
Animal Sources			
Beeswax	*Apismellifeca*	Apidae	Myricin, melissic acid, cerolein, cero
Cocca butter	*Theobroma cacao*	sterculiaceae	Stearic (34%), palmitic (25%), oleic (37%) acids and small amount of arachidic and linolenic acid.
Shea butter	*Vitellaria paradoxa*	sapotaceae	Five principal of fatty acid Stearic, palmitic, oleic, linoleic and arachidic acids. Phenolic compound catechin.
Lanolin	*Ovis aries*	Bovidae	Complex mixture of ester and polystyrene 33 high molecular weight alcohol and 36 fatty acids. Ester of cholesterol and isocholesterol with oleic, linoleic, caranubic, linopalmatic acid.
Lecithin	*Glycine max (soyabean 33-35%)*	Leguminosae	Sterols, phosphatidyl choline.
Ceramides	*Triticum aestivum (wheat germ)*	Gramineae	Sphingosine and fatty acids.

3.1.2 Gums/Mucilages/Carbohydrates/Polysaccharides

- Polysaccharides are macromolecules based on glycosidically linked combinations of up to 40 different monosaccharides, sometimes substituted by nonsugar groups such as alcohols, organic acids, or sulfates. Those from animals, terrestrial plants, marine macroalgae, and nonphotosynthetic microorganisms are widely exploited by industry as biological agents in various fields including agronomy, medicine, cosmetic, nutrition, and others.
- Gums/Mucilages/ Carbohydrates/Polysaccharides serve a variety of functions, such as thickening, emulsifying (keeping ingredients mixed together), creating protective films or barriers, and making products feel either "drier" or more moist, smoother, or more pleasant overall.Another advantage of Polysaccharides is that they are "high molecular weight," which means they do not easily penetrate the skin and are less likely than traditional alternatives to cause stinging, burning or redness.
- Water-based formulations are thin by nature, and polymers are used to thicken them or turn them into gels. When used to increase thickness in products like shampoos, conditioners, creams, and lotions, for example, the formulas feel more rich, smooth, and creamy. Polysaccharides such as starch, xanthan or guar gum, carrageenan, alginates, polysaccharides, pectin, gelatin, agar, and cellulose derivatives can be used as a thickener in cosmetics. More recent developments include combining hydrophobic and hydrophilic polymers into "copolymers" that stabilize products so that they don't get thin under high heat – for example, sunscreens.
- Hair sprays, lotions, gels, and foamscontaining polysaccharides, including starch and cellulose derivatives, natural gums, andmucilages as hair styling agents.
- Polysaccharidesacts as"carrier" for active ingredients in cosmetics, such as antioxidants and antimicrobials or encapsulation of ingredients such as vitamins and peptides so that they are able to work when applied to hair and skin during use.
- Conditioning Polysaccharidesdeposits, adhere, or absorb into the proteins of the skin and hair. They improve skin feel and hair manageability, reduce static and make the skin and hair softer and smoother.
- Major plant polysaccharides are cellulose, pectins, and β-glucans. Gums/mucilagescan be calssified based on source as follows:
    - marine origin/algal (seaweed) gums: agar, carrageenans, alginic acid, and laminarin;
    - plant origin:
        - shrubs/tree exudates: gum arabic, gum ghatti, gum karaya, gum tragacanth, and khaya and albizia gums;
        - seed gums: guar gum, locust bean gum, starch, amylose, and cellulose;
        - extracts: pectin, larch gum;
        - tuber and roots: potato starch;
    - animal origin: chitin and chitosan, chondroitin sulfate, and hyaluronic acid;
    - microbial origin (bacterial and fungal): xanthan, dextran, curdian, pullulan, zanflo, emulsan, Baker's yeast glycan, schizophyllan, lentinan, krestin, and scleroglucan.

- Glucans if combined with polysaccharides and proteins acts as a tissue matrix proteoglycans which enables to retain water and acts as a film formers, humectants, and skin moisturizers and helps in tissue regeneration and wound healing.
- β-glucan (*Saccharomyces* strains) useful in tissue regeneration which behaves like hyaluronic acid in stimulating collagen synthesis by fibroblasts.
- Carragenans from various red algae are used as emulsifiers in the preparation of creams, gels, pastes, and emulsions.
- Oat β-glucan (*Avena sativa*) is an un-branched polysaccharide that has been claimed to alleviate the signs of aging, protect against UV, activate collagen synthesis, and strengthen the hairs.
- β-glucan and hydrolyzed oat protein is also used to moisturize and soothe irritated skin.
- Gums and mucilages are employed as additives as well as acts as a antioxidant and emollient properties.

3.1.3 Colorants

Generally, plant pigments are classified as chlorophylls, carotenoids, flavonoids, phytochromes, betalains and naphthaquinones. These pigments are of great value in the preparation of cosmetics, foods and drugs in the form of colour additives. As compared to synthetic pigments, natural pigments have lower intensity and require large quantities of raw materials. But due to their low toxicity and no carcinogenic effects, natural pigments are always fascinating to mankind. Example:

Following are Examples of natural colorants		
Source	**Color**	**Chemical structure and Use**
Flavonoid namely, brazilin from sappanwood (*Caesalpinia sappan*, Leguminosae)	Red	Color cosmetics 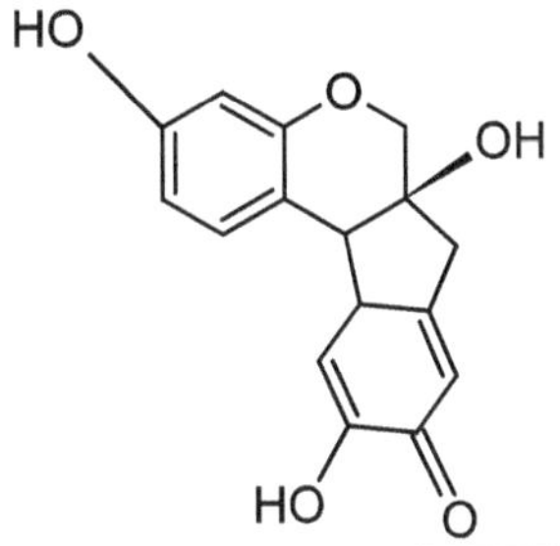 HO OH HO O
Tricyclic anthraquinone Alizarin from Madder (*Rubia tinctorium*) roots	Red	Hair 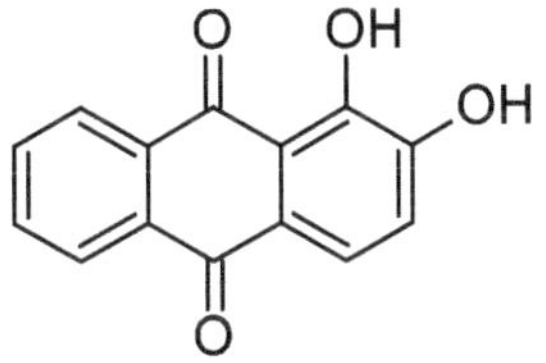 O OH OH O

Contd...

Napthquinone Juglon form walnut (*Juglans nigra*, Juglandaceae) shells and leaves	Brown [C.I. Natural Brown 7 and C.I. 75500]	Hair 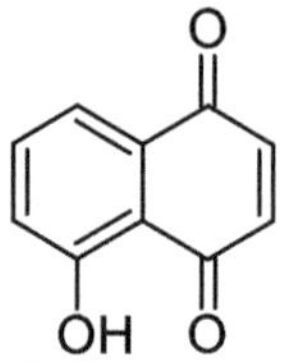
Napthquinone Lawsone from Henna (*Lawsonia inermis*) leaves	Orange yellow	Hair 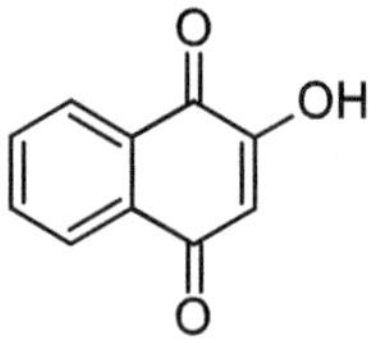
Carmine with the main component carminic acid is an approved food colorant E 120. It is obtained from scales of *Dactylopius coccus* (or cochineals). Carminic acid (C22H20O13) is a red glucosidal hydroxyanthrapurin.	Orange, red	Color cosmetics 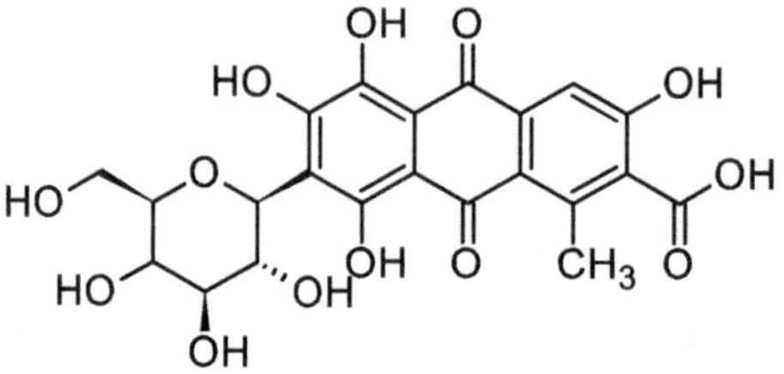
Carotenoid- Bixin from Annatto (*Bixa orellana*) seeds	Orange yellow	Lipstick 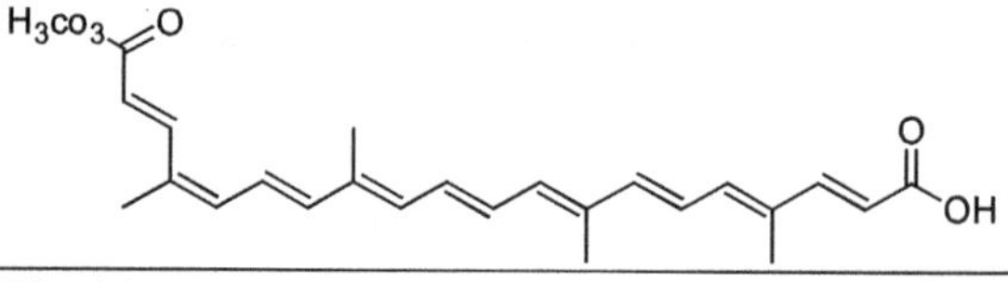
Indigo from *Indigofera tinctoria* and other species leaves	Blue	Lipstick 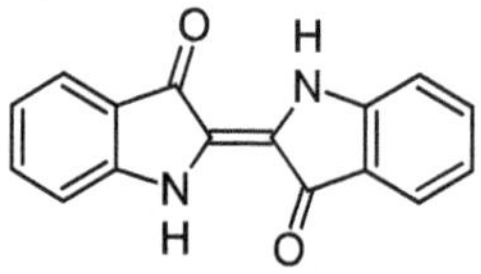
Sesquiterpene Guaiazulene from Guaiacum oil (*Guaiacum officinale*, Zygophyllaceae) and Chammomile (*Matricaria chamomilla*, Asteraceae)	Dark blue	Hair, color cosmetics 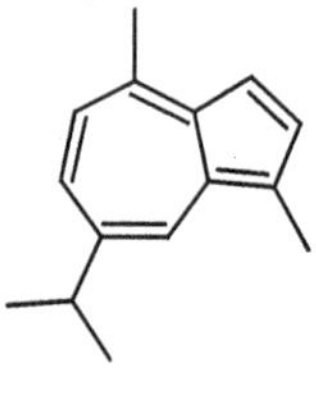
Curcumin a principle Curcuminoids from turmeric (*Curcuma longa*, Zingiberaceae) rhizomes	Ornage, yellow	Color cosmetics 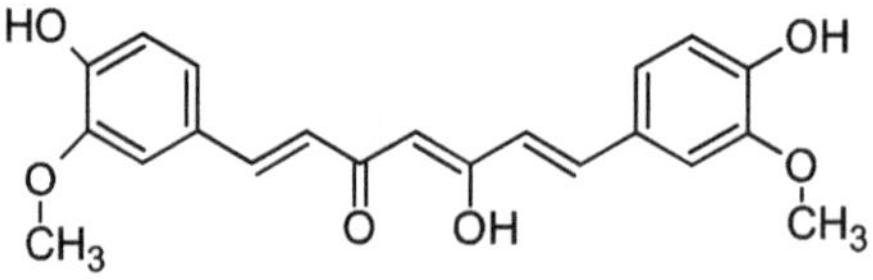

Contd...

Betalains from beet (*Beta vulagris*) roots. **Betalains** are water-soluble nitrogen-containing pigments, which provide red-violet (betacyanins) and the yellow (betaxanthins) colors to some fruits and vegetables	Red–purple betacyanidins and the yellow betaxanthins	Color cosmetics 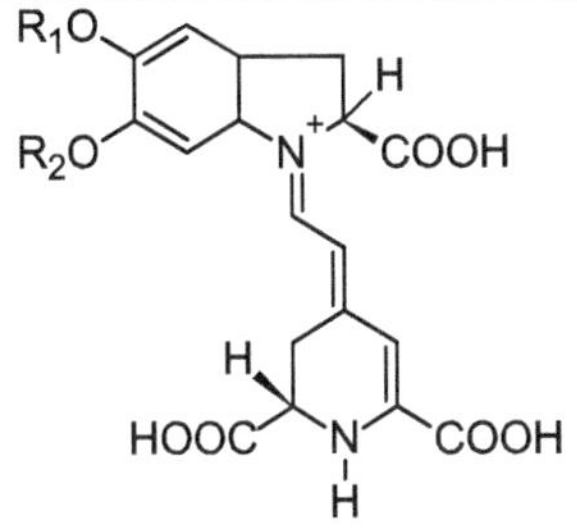 R_1O, R_2O, H, N^+, COOH, H, HOOC, N, COOH, H **Betacyanins** R1= glucosyl or derivatives R2= glucosyl, glucuronyl, derivatives or H H, R, N, H, HOOC, N, COOH, H 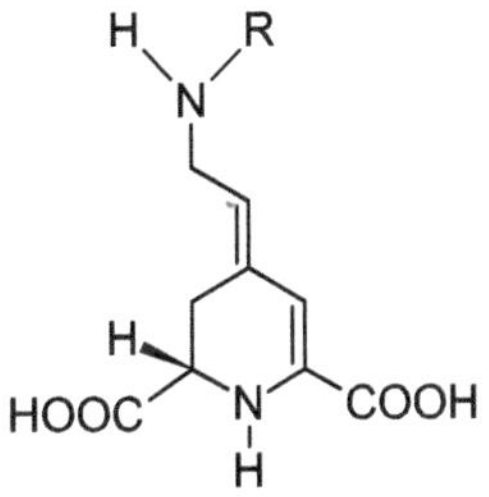 **Betaxanthins** R= amino acid, amine or derivatives
Tannins from barks and leaves of many sources	Yellow, brown, black	Hair
"**Carotenoids**" is a generic term used to designate the majority of pigments naturally found in animal and plant kingdoms. Two classes of carotenoids are found in nature: (a) the carotenes such as β-carotene, which consist of linear hydrocarbons that can be cyclized at one end or both ends of the molecule, and (b) the oxygenated derivatives of carotenes such as **lutein, lycopene, violaxanthin, neoxanthin,** and **zeaxanthin**, known as xanthophylls.	Red, orange, yellow	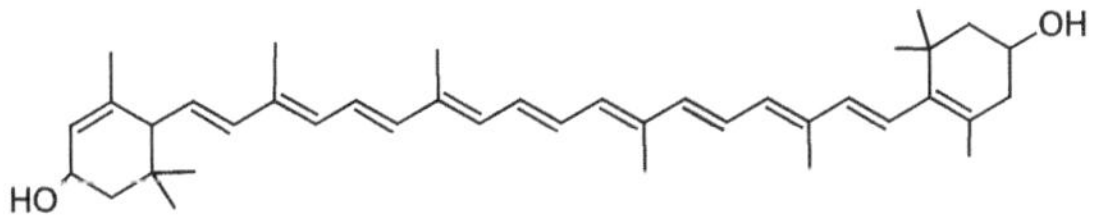 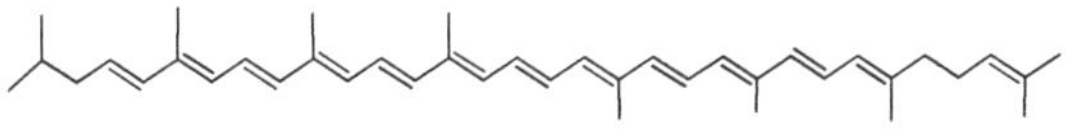 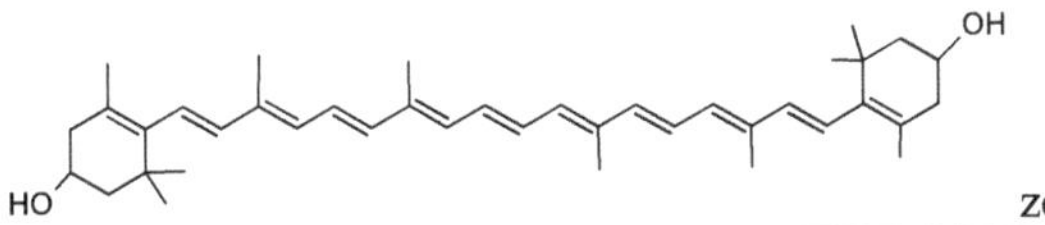 Color cosmetics 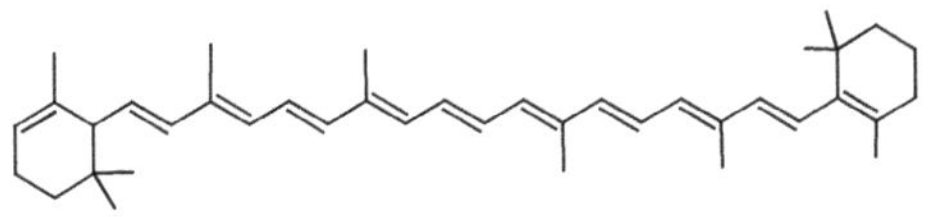 α-carotene 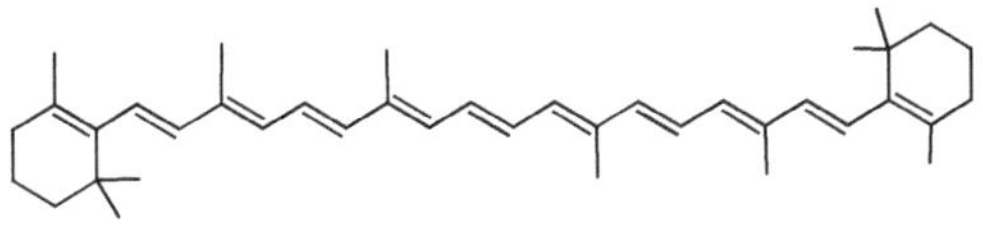 β-carotene 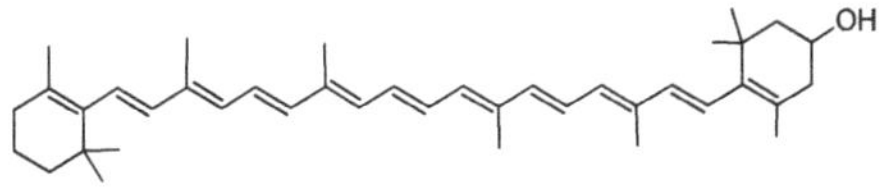 OH β-cryptoxanthin HO, OH lutein lycopene HO, OH zeaxanthin
Anthocyanins Anthocyanins are colored water-soluble pigments belonging to the phenolic group. The pigments are in glycosylated forms.	Orange, red, purple, blue	Color cosmetics Anthocyanins have anti-oxidant, anti-inflammatory, and anti-cancer properties making them useful to protect health in general, but particularly suited to protecting skin from sun damage that contributes to skin aging and cancer.

Contd...

<table>
<tr>
<td>Anthocyanins responsible for the colors, red, purple, and blue, are in fruits and vegetables. Berries, currants, grapes, and some tropical fruits have high anthocyanins content. Red to purplish blue-colored leafy vegetables, grains, roots, and tubers are the edible vegetables that contain a high level of anthocyanins. Anthocyanin is in the form of glycoside while anthocyanidin is known as the aglycone. Anthocyanidins are grouped into 3-hydroxyanthocyanidins, 3-deoxyanthocyanidins, and O-methylated anthocyanidins, while anthocyanins are in the forms of anthocyanidin glycosides and acylated anthocyanins. The most common types of anthocyanidins are cyanidin, delphinidin, pelargonidin, peonidin, petunidin, and malvidin. Acylated anthocyanins are also detected in plants besides the typical anthocyanins. Acylated anthocyanin is further divided into acrylated anthocyanin, coumaroylated anthocyanin, caffeoylated anthocyanin, and malonylated anthocyanin.</td>
<td></td>
<td>
<table>
<tr><th>R1</th><th>R2</th><th>Anthocyanin</th><th>Aglycon</th></tr>
<tr><td>H</td><td>H</td><td>Pelargonin</td><td>Pelargonidin</td></tr>
<tr><td>OH</td><td>H</td><td>Cyanin</td><td>Cyaniding</td></tr>
<tr><td>OCH_3</td><td>H</td><td>Peonin</td><td>Peonidin</td></tr>
<tr><td>OH</td><td>OH</td><td>Delphin</td><td>Delphinidin</td></tr>
<tr><td>OCH_3</td><td>OH</td><td>Petunin</td><td>Petunidin</td></tr>
<tr><td>OCH_3</td><td>OCH_3</td><td>malvin</td><td>Malvidin</td></tr>
</table>
</td>
</tr>
<tr>
<td>Chlorophyll and copper-chlorophyll complex from green plant parts- Piper betel leaves, Eucalyptus leaves.</td>
<td>Bright green</td>
<td>Color cosmetics</td>
</tr>
</table>

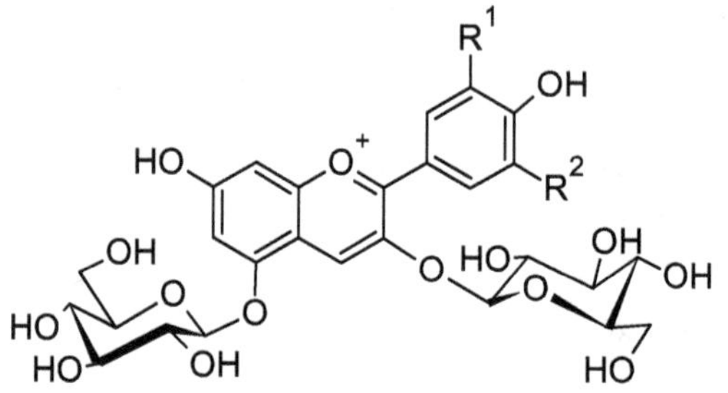

Contd...

Chlorophylls are numerous in types, but all are defined by the presence of a fifth ring beyond the four pyrrole-like rings. Most chlorophylls are classified as chlorins, which are reduced relatives of porphyrins (found in hemoglobin).		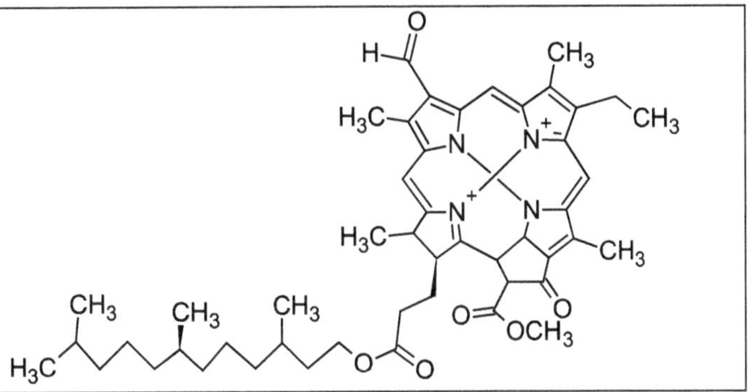

3.1.4 Volatile Oils/Perfumes and Fragances

Volatile oils or essential oils are major part of perfumes as well as flavours. Flavors affect both the sense of taste and smell, whereas fragrances affect only smell. The Fragrance wheel created in 1983 by Michael Edwards is classification method that is widely used in retail and in the fragrance industry.

Various terpenes from mono-terpenoid and sesquiterpenoid class (linear, cyclic, aromatic) with different functional groups (alcohol, aldehyde, ester, ether) are major constituents of natural perfumes. Example: Geraniol (Nerol), linalool, citronellol, citral, pinene, carvone, muskone.

Different perfume sources	
Natural	**Example**
Flowers	Rose, jasmine, osmanthus, plumeria, mimosa, tuberose, narcissus, scented geranium, cassie, ambrette, blossoms of citrus
Wood	Sandalwood, rosewood, agarwood, birch, cedar, juniper, pine
Bark	Cinnamon, cascarilla, sassafras
Fruits	Apples, strawberries, cherries, oranges, lemons, limes
Leaves	Lavender leaf, patchouli, sage, violets, rosemary, citrus leaves
Roots	Vetiver, iris, ginger
Resins	Labdanum, olibanum, myrrh, balsam of peru, benzoin, pine, fir
Animal	Musk, ambergris, civet, hyraceum, castoreum
Synthetic	Synthetic derivatives of benzene, toluene, phenol, naphthalene, cyclopentanone or complete synthetic form of natural perfume chemicals

The *Fragrance wheel* is a relatively new classification method that is widely used in retail and in the fragrance industry. Perfumes are divided as follows:

1. **Floral**
   - Floral
   - Soft Floral
   - Floral Oriental
2. **Oriental**
   - Soft Oriental
   - Oriental
   - Woody Oriental
3. **Fougère**
4. **Woody**
   - Wood
   - Mossy Woods
   - Dry Woods
5. **Fresh**
   - Citrus
   - Green
   - Water

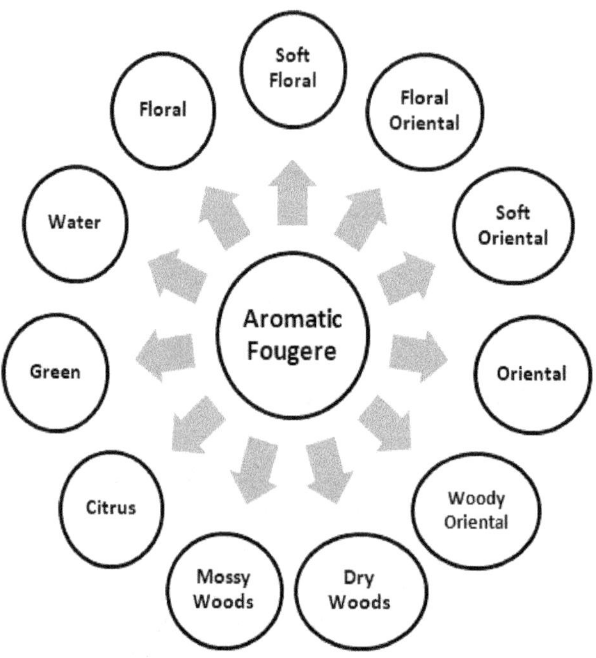

Fig. 3.1 Fragrance wheel

Examples of perfume (volatile oil containing palnts)			
Plant	**Biological source**	**Family**	**Volatile Chemical composition**
Plants			
Agarwood	*Aquilaria malaccencis*	Thymelaeceae	Terpenes, sequiterpenes and oxygenated compound
Ambrette	*Abelmoschus moschatus*	Macalvaceae	Ambrettolide, Farnesol acetate,
Apples	*Malus domestica*	Rosaceae	Vitamin K, B6, Hydroxycinnamic acid, coumarolylquinic acid
Balsam of peru	*Myroxylonbalsamum*	Leguminosae	Styrene, vanillin, coumarin, benzyl alcohol, benzyl cinnamate, cinnamic acid, cinnamyl cinnamate
Benzoin	*Styrax tonkinensis*	Styracaceae	Benzoic acid, cinnamic acid, esters
Birch	*Betula nigra*	Betulaceae	Eugenol, linalool, palmitic acid
Cascarilla	*Croton eluteria*	Euphorbiacea	Cascarillins, lignins, tannins and resins
Cassie	*Acacia farnesiana*	Fabaceae	Essential oil cassie, ellagic acid, naringin, kaempferol
Cedar	*Cedrus deodara*	Pinaceae	Taxifolin, cedeodarin,,ampelopsin, cedrin, cedrinoside, deodarin

Contd...

Plant	Biological source	Family	Volatile Chemical composition
Cherries	*Prunus avium*	Rosaceae	3-caffeoylquinic, p-coumaric acid, catechin
Cinnamon	*Cinnamomum zeylanicum*	Lauraceae	Eugenol, benzaldehyde cuminaldehyde
Citrus	*Citrus species*	Rutaceae	Lipids, vitamins & minerals, flavonoids-limonoids
Fir	*Firs species*	Pinaceae	Camphene, bornyl acetate, santene
Geranium	*Pelargonium graveolens*	Geraniaceae	Geraneol, citronellol
Ginger	*Zingiber officinalis*	Zingiberaceae	Zingiberene, curcumene
Iris	*Iris gemanica*	Iridaceae	Caprylic acid, capric, lauric, tridcanoic palmitic acid
Jasmine	*Jasminum offficinale*	Oleaceae	3-hexanol, linalool, benzyl alcohol
Juniper	*Juniperus communis*	Cupressaseae	A-pinene, camphor, thymol methyl ether
Labdanum	*Cistus ladanifer*	Cistaceae	Tricycline, α-thujene, Sabinene, Terpenilene
Lavender	*Lavendula officinalis*	Labiateae	Esters linalyl acetate linalool, pinene, geraniol, cineol
Lemons	*Citrus limonis*	Rutaceae	Limonene, citral geranyl acetate terpineol.
Limes	*Citrus aurantifolia*	Rutaceae	Vitamin C, citric acid,
Mimosa	*Mimosa pudica*	Fabaceae	Palmitic acid,
Myrrh	*Commiphoramolmol*	Burseraceae	α,β,γ-commiphoric acid, α,β-heerabomyrrholic acid, cuminic aldehyde, eugenol
Narcissus	*Narcissus poeticus*	Amaryllidaceae	β-ocimene, 1,8-cineole, linalool
Olibanum	*Boswellia serrata*	Burseraceae	α-pinene, Sabinene, Limonene, α-Thujene
Oranges	*Citrus species*	Rutaceae	Vitami C, Limonene, citronellal
Osmanthus	*Osmanthus heterophullus*	Oleaceae	Linalool, Terpenoids-Te3, Te5, Te6
Patchouli	*Pogostemoncablin*	Lamiaceae	Germecrene, Patchoulol, Narpatchoulenol
Pine	*Pinus sylvestris*	Pinaceae	Hydrocarbens, terpenoids, phenols, resinous substance, terpentine
Plumeria	*Plumeria rubra*	Apocynaceae	Geraniol, linalool,
Rose	*Rosa alba*	Rosaceae	Geraniol, citronellol, nerol, linalool,
Rosemary	*Rosmarinus officinalis*	Lamiaceae	β-caryophyllene, limonene, α-pinene, 1,8-cineole, carnosol, ursolic acid
Rosewood	*Aniba rosaeodora*	Meliaceae	Linalool,

Contd...

Plant	Biological source	Family	Volatile Chemical composition
Sage	*Salvia officinalis*	Lamiaceae	Thujones, camphor, α-pinene
Sandalwood	*Santalam album*	Santalaceae	α,β-santalol, santene, santenone, teresantol, standalone, santalene
Sassafras	*Sassafras albidum*	Lauraceae	Safrole, camphor, methyleugenol
Strawberries	*Fragaria ananassa*	Rosaceae	Ethyl esters, Palmitic acid,
Tuberose	*Palianthes tuberosa*	Asparagaceae	Methyl benzoate, butyric acid, augenol, nerol, farnesol, geraneol
Vetiver	*Chrysipogon zizanoides*	Poaceae	Citral, geraniol, α and β v
Animal			
Ambergris	*Physeter catoden*	Physeteridae	Ambrene, epicoprostemolcoprostemone
Musk	*Moschus moschiferus*	Cervidae	Musckone, Cholesterine, Albuminoids, Resin
Castoreum	*Caster faber*	Castoridae	Volatile oil, Resin, Castorin, benzyl alcohol, methyl phenol, l-borneol.
Civet	*Viverrazibetha*	Viverridae	Civetone, Indole civetole ethylamine, propylamine.

3.1.5 Skin Whitening (Bleaching) Agents

Skin whitening agents are required to lighten skin in conditions like melasma or postinflammatory hyperpigmentation. They suppress melanin production eiher through competitive inhibition of melanogenesis enzyme tyrosinase or inhibition of the maturation of this enzyme or inhibition of transport of pigment granules (melanosomes) from melanocytes to surrounding keratinocytes. Bearberry, Licorice, Sophora and Peonia plant extracts are found to tyrosinase inhibitors. Following are various plants useful as skin whitening agents:

Tyrosinase inhibition is shown by following natural compounds

Artocarpus lakoocha heartwood	Oxyresveratrol
Astragalus taschkendicus	Askendoside B
Citrus fruit peel	3′,4′,5,6,7,8-hexamethoxy-flavone (nobiletin)
Morus alba Rheum undulatum	1. Oxyresveratrol 2. Hydroxystilbene
Aloe vera	Aloesin; C-glycosylated chromone
Longan seed	Corilagin, gallic acid and ellagic acid or other phenolic/flavonoid glycosides and ellagitannins

Tyrosinase inhibition as well as pigmentation inhibition is shown by following natural compounds:

Source	Compounds (type)
Alpinia galanga and *Curcuma aromatica* medicinal plants	Eugenol and curcuminoids possible active ingredients
Angelica dahurica	Isoimperatorin imperatorin
Artocarpus incisus (best of) 23 heart wood species from Papua New Guinea.	(+)-Dihydromorin, chlorophorin, (+)-norartocarpanone, 4-prenyl-oxyresveratrol, artocarbene, artocarpesin and isoarto-carpesin
Aspergillus fumigatus and *Saccharomyces cerevisiae*	Melanin Degrading Enzymes
Carthamus tinctorius safflower seeds	*N*-feruloylserotonin, *N*-(*p*-coumaroyl)serotonin, and 3) acacetin
Corn bran	Polyamine conjugates, *N,N′*-dicoumaroylputrescine (DCP), *N*-*p*-coumaroyl-*N′*-feruloylputrescine (CFP), and *N,N′*-diferuloyl-putrescine (DFP)
Cucumis sativus	Lutein
Erigeron breviscapus Chinese herb	(2Z,8Z)-matricaria acid methyl ester
Fish, Poultry	Vitamin b3 derivative, niacinamide
Galla Chinensis Radix Clematidis out of 90 Chinese Herbs	Unknown
Gastrodiaelata Blume Orchidaceae	(Synthetic) *p*-hydroxybenzyl alcohol
Glycyrrhiza glabra Licorice extract	Glabrene and 2′,4′,4-tri-hydroxychalcone
Glycyrrhiza uralensis	Glycyrrhlsoflavone and glyasperin C
Grape seed	Oligomeric proanthocyanidins
Grape seed	Proanthocyanidin
Kaempferia pandurata	Chalcone compounds, isopanduratin A and 4-hydroxypanduratin A
Lespedeza cyrtobotrya	Haginin A
Malpighia emarginata Acerola fruit	cyanidin-3-alpha-*O*-rhamnoside. pelargonidin-3-α-*O*-rhamnoside
Morus alba	Mulberroside F (moracin M-6, 3′-di-O-beta-d-glucopyranoside
Piper longum	Piperlonguminine
Pityrosporumovale	Azelaic acid; C9-dicarboxylic acid
Podocarpus macrophyllus	2,3-dihydro-4′,4‴-di-*O*-methylamentoflavone
Polygonum cuspidatum. *Paris polyphylla* *Vitex negundo*	Physcion (anthraquinone + anthraquinone analog) (+)-Lyoniresinol
Punica granatum Pomegranate	Ellagic acid

Contd...

Source	Compounds (type)
Ramulus mori (young twigs of *Morus alba*)	2,3′,4,5′-tetrahydroxy-stilbene (2-oxyresveratrol)
Raspberry	Tiliroside
Rhus Ghinensis; Chinese galls	3 Gallotannins; 2,3,4,6-tetra-*O*-galloyl-d-glucopyranose, 1,2,3,6-tetra-*O*-galloyl-β-d-glucopyranose, and 1,2,3,4,6-penta-*O*-galloyl-β-d-glucopyranose
Rhus succedanea	10′(Z)-heptadecenyl-hydroquinone
Sophora flavescens	Kurarinol, kuraridinol, and trifolirhizin
Sophora japonica and *Spatholobussuberectus* out of 25 Chinese Herbs	High phenolic content, Example-.., gallic acid
Spatholobussuberectus Dunn (Leguminosae) Chinese herb	Butin

3.1.6 Protective Agents or Antioxidants in Products such as Skin Care, Hair Care and Oral Hygiene Products

Free radicals are highly reactive molecules with an odd number of electrons that are generated from oxygen, they can damage various cellular structures, such as DNA, proteins, and cellular membranes. In addition, free radicals may lead to inflammation, which seems to play an additional role in skin aging.

The body possesses endogenous defense mechanisms, such as antioxidative enzymes (*superoxide dismutase, catalase, glutathione peroxidase*) and nonenzymatic antioxidative molecules (*vitamin E, vitamin C, glutathione, ubiquinone*), protecting it from free radicals by reducing and neutralizing them. Some of these antioxidant defense mechanisms can be inhibited by ultraviolet (UV) light. Moreover, as part of the natural aging process endogenous defense mechanisms decrease, while the production of reactive oxygen species increases, resulting in accelerated skin aging.

Hence topical application of antioxidants may neutralize some of the resulting free radicals, and consequently lessen or prevent the signs of aging skin. In addition to their antioxidant activity, most of them possess numerous other biologic properties like wound healing, anti-inflammatory and anticancer. At present, topical antioxidants are marketed to prevent aging and UV-induced skin damage, as well as to treat wrinkles and erythema due to inflammation. For topically administered antioxidants to be effective in preventing skin aging, a couple of considerations should be made when formulating them:

- Product stabilization is crucial. Because antioxidants are very unstable, they may become oxidized and inactive before reaching the target.
- They must be properly absorbed into the skin, reach their target tissue in the active form, and remain there long enough to exert the desired effects.
- In the oral cavity, oxidative stress is associated with gingivitis and other periodontitis. Nevertheless, factors including alcohol consumption, exposure to nicotine, dental procedures, bleaching agents, dental cements, composite fillings and metals used in dentistry also leads to oxidative stress. Periodontal pathogens can induce over production of

ROS and leads to collagen and periodontal tissue breakdown. Recently, it has been affirmed that the onset and development of dental caries is due to imbalances in levels of free radicals, reactive oxygen species, and antioxidants in saliva. Most recently, dental manufacturers and distributors have incorporated antioxidant supplements due to their anti-angiogenic, anti-inflammatory, antiviral, and/or anti-tumor properties into toothpastes, mouth rinses/ mouthwashes, lozenges, fluoride gels and dentifrices, oral sprays, breath fresheners, and other dental products for the control of gingival and periodontal diseases.

- Hair is exposed every day to a range of harmful effects such as sunlight, pollution, cosmetic treatments, grooming practices and cleansing. The UV components of sunlight damage human hair, causing fibre degradation. UV-B attacks the melanin pigments and the protein fractions (keratin) of hair and UV-A produces free radical/reactive oxygen species (ROS) through the interaction of endogenous photosensitizers. UV radiations causes increase in protein and lipid degradation, changes in colour and shine and in adverse consequences for the mechanical properties. Natural antioxidants applications can improve hair mechanical properties and preserve colour and shine of fibres, coats and protects them against UV, reduces lipid peroxidation of the protein degradation and finally improves fiber integrity.

Following are commonly useful antioxidants in Skin cosmetics:	
Vitamin E (tocopherol)	Exerts photoprotective effects, inhibit human macrophage metalloelastase and thus inhibits degradation of elastin, but cuases contact dermatitis
Vitamin C (ascorbic acid)	Potent antioxidant, Ascorbate is required for collagen synthesis and hence reduces production of elastin, topical application cuases stinging and mild irritation
Vitamin B3 (Niacinamide, or nicotinamide)	Antiaging, anti-inflammatory, depigmenting, and immunomodulant,
Coenzyme Q10 (CoQ10)	Suppresses expression of collagenase without any side effect
Idebenone (synthetic analog of coenzyme Q10)	Stronger antioxidant than CoQ10, reduces in skin roughness/dryness, reduction in fine lines/wrinkles, but cuases contact dermatitis
Lycopene	Powerful antioxidant carotenoid, photoprotective, less clinical data available
Green tea polyphenols	Antioxidant, anti-inflammatory, anticarcinogenic, suppress chemo- and photocarcinogenesis
Silymarin polyphenolic flavonoid from milk thistle plant, Silybum marianum	Antioxidant, photoprotective effects
Resveratrol	Antiaging, antioxidant, protects against UVB-mediated cutaneous damage and inhibits UVB-mediated oxidative stress.
Proanthocyanidins from Grape (Vitis vinifera)seed is extract	Stronger scavenger of free radicals than vitamins C and E, Antiaging, antioxidant
Genistein isoflavone from soybeans	Antiaging, antioxidant, photoprotective
Pycnogenol (Phenolic compound)	Antiaging, antioxidant, photoprotective, anti-inflammatory

3.2 Herbal or Natural Excipients

Introduction

A medicine consists of two fundamental parts: the active pharmaceutical ingredient and the excipient. An excipient is a substance formulated alongside the active ingredient of a medication included for the purpose of long-term stabilization, bulking up solid formulations that contain potent active ingredients in small amounts or to confer a therapeutic enhancement on the active ingredient in the final dosage form, such as facilitating drug absorption, reducing viscosity, or enhancing solubility. Pharmaceutical excipients are substances other than the active pharmaceutical ingredient (API) that have been appropriately evaluated for safety and are intentionally included in a drug delivery system.

Natural excipients are generally safe as it is biodegradable, biocompatible and non-toxic – chemically, economic, safe, devoid of side effects and easily availability. But they also possess some disadvantage like Microbial contamination, Batch to batch variation, the uncontrolled rate of hydration, slow process and heavy metal contamination.

Excipients are expected to be inert and should not exert any therapeutic or biological action or modify the biological action of the drug substance but excipients can potentially influence the rate and/or extent of absorption of a drug. As herbal excipients are non toxic and compatible, they have a major role to play in pharmaceutical formulation. Following are few countries/ organisations which regulates excipients:

Sources of natural excipients

Animal	Beeswax, Cochineal, Gelatin, Honey, Lactose, Spermaciti, Lanolin, Musk, Suet.
Vegetable	Kokum butter, Pectin, Starch, Peppermint, Cardamon, Vanilla, Tumeric, Saffron, Guar-gum
Minerals	Bentonite, Kieselghur, Kaolin, Paraffins, Talc, Calamine, Fuller's earth, Asbestos
Marine	Agar, Carrageenans, Alginic acid, Laminarin.

Natural excipients based on phytochemical class

Phytochemical class	Examples
Carbohydrates	Acacia, agar, aliginate, gaur gum, caraggenan, cellulose derivatives, pectin, honey, aloe mucilage, tragacanth
Fixed oil	Almond oil, arachis oil, castor oil, cod liver oil, sesame oil, olive oil, jojoba oil,
Fats	Cocca butter, coconut oil, kokum butter, lard, palm oil, suet
Waxes	Bees wax, wool fat, carnauba wax, spermaceti
Volatil oils	Clove oil, cardamom oil, lemon oil, lavender oil, orange oil, peppermint oil, sandalwood oil, vetiver oil, musk oil
Resins	Asafoetida, ginger and capsicum resin, myrrh, peru balsam tolu balsam, shellac, storax,
Proteins	Casein, gelatin, thaumatin
Enzymes	Diastase, papain, pepsin, pancreatin, rennin
Tannins	Amla, behera, catechu, hirda, tannic acid
Pigments	Chlorophyll, cochineal, annatto, carotene
Polyphenols	Curcumin, gallic acids
Saponins	Soapnut, shikakai, quillaja bark saponins

Classification of Excipients as Per D&C Act [Rule 1945]

Sl. no. & Category	Permitted Excipients	Reference Standard/Grade
A. Additives	Activated Charcoal, Beewax, Cellulose & its derivatives, Soft Paraffin, Carnauba Wax, Beeswax	IP
	Agar, Arachis Oil, Calcium Carbonate	PFA
	Calcium Phosphate Dibasic, Calcium Phosphate Tribasic	IP
	Citric acid & its salts and Tartaric Acid & its salt and Yeast	PFA
	Stearic Acid & its salts and Starch & its derivatives	IP
	Xanthan Gum	USNF
	Zinc oxide, Carbomer, Colloidal Silicon Dioxide, Talc, Sucrose,	IP
B. Preservatives	Acetic acid, Benzoic acid & its salts	PFA
	Butyl paraben, Ethyl paraben	BP
	Methyl Paraben& its salts and Propionic acid & its salts	PFA
	Phenyl mercuric nitrate	IP
	Propyl paraben& its salts and Sorbic acid & its salts	PFA
C. Antioxidants:	Ascorbic acid & its salts &esters, Potassium metabisulphite, Sodium metabisulphite	PFA
	Butylated hydroxyl toluene, Gallic acid esters	PFA
D. Colouring agents:	1. **Natural colours**: Annatto, Carotene, Chlorophyll, Cochineal, Curcumin, Red oxide of Iron, Yellow oxide of Iron (Titanium oxide), Black oxide of Iron 2. **Lakes** – the Aluminium or calcium salts (lakes) of any water soluble colours.	Rule 127 of Drugs and Cosmetics Rules 1945
E. Flavouring agents	As permitted under Fruit Product Order and PFA Act, Rule 163.	
F. Alternate Sweeteners:	Artificial sweeteners may be used for only in proprietary ASU products. Sucralose, Aspartame, Saccharin, Acesulfame K	As in Fruits Product Order

Regulatory Bodies and Regulations for Excipients

Body	Regulation
Japanese pharmacopoeia	31 excipients monograph
USP-NF	41 excipients monograph
World Health Organization	Explained guideline, definition of the pharmaceutical excipients in addition to the quality safety and their required standards
ICH	ICH-Q8(R2) guideline for excipients and its relevancy in drug development
IPEC (The International Pharmaceutical Excipients Council)	Promotes excipients safety and harmonization of regulatory standards and pharmacopoeial monographs
excipients certification scheme (EXCIPACT)	GMP for distributor of excipients
CDSCO (Central Drugs Standard Control Organization), India	Guidance Document IMP/REG/200711 entitled Guidance document on common submission format for import and registration of bulk drug and finished formulation in India. In addition to these guideline, rule 169 of Drug & cosmetic Rule 1945 excipients present permitted excipients in *Ayurvedic* formulation along with their standards permitted in IP, Prevention of Food Adulteration Act 1954 and Bureau of Indian standard act 1986

Different roles of natural excipients with examples

Role	Example
Anti-adherents	Magnesium stearate
Antimicrobials	Curcumin, neem, benzoin, myrrh
Binders	Gums, mucilages like acacia, gelatin, tragacanth, starch
Colorants	Annatto, carotene, chlorophyll, caramel, cochineal
Disintegrants	Starch, cellulose derivatives
Emollient	Glycerin, olive oil,
Emulsifying agent	Acacia, agar, guar-gum, cellulose derivatives,
Fillers and Diluents	Lactose, sucrose, glucose, mannitol, sorbitol, calcium carbonate, and magnesium stearate
Flavorants	Bitter product - mint, cherry or anise Salty product - peach, apricot or liquorice Sour product - raspberry or liquorice Sweet product - vanilla
Glidants	Starch, talc, aerosil
Humectants	Glycerine
Lubricants	Vegetable stearin, magnesium stearate or stearic acid
Lubricants	Coca butter, stearic acid
Polymers	Polysaccharides like: hyaluronic acid , chondroitin sulfate, chitin and chitosan, alginates, and cellulose
Preservatives / Antioxidants	Vitamin A, vitamin E, vitamin C, retinyl palmitate, selenium, cysteine, methionine , Citric acid, sodium citrate
Semisolid bases	Coca butter, bees wax, lanolin, petroleum gelly, paraffin
Suspending agent	Guar gum, gelatin, Aliginate
Sweetners	Licorice, honey, carrot
Thickening agent	Tragacanth, Pectin

3.2.1 Colorants

Source	Color
Flavonoid namely, brazilin fromsappanwood (*Caesalpinia sappan*, Leguminosae)	Red
Tricyclic anthraquinone Alizarin from Madder (*Rubia tinctorium*) roots	Red
NapthquinoneJuglon form walnut (Juglans nigra, Juglandaceae) shells and leaves	Brown [C.I. Natural Brown 7 and C.I. 75500]
NapthquinoneLawsone from Henna (Lawsoniainermis) leaves	Orange yellow
Anthraquinone Carminic from scales of Dactylopius coccus	Orange, red
Carotenoid-Bixin from Annatto (Bixa orellana) seeds	Orange yellow
Indigo from *Indigoferatinctoria* and otherspecies leaves	Blue
Sesquiterpene Guaiazulene from Guaiacum oil (Guaiacumofficinale, Zygophyllaceae)and Chammomile (Matricaria chamomilla, Asteraceae)	Dark blue
Curcumin a principle Curcuminoids from turmeric (Curcuma longa, Zingiberaceae) rhizomes	Ornage, yellow

Contd...

Source	Color
Betalains from beet (*Beta vulagris*) roots. **Betalains** are water-soluble nitrogen-containing pigments, which provide red-violet (betacyanins) and the yellow (betaxanthins) colors to some fruits and vegetables	Red–purple betacyanidins and the yellow betaxanthins
Tannins from Camellia sinensis leaves	Yellow, brown, black
Carotenoids such as lutein, lycopene, violaxanthin, neoxanthin, and zeaxanthin, known as xanthophylls.	Red, orange, yellow
Anthocyanins	Orange, red, purple, blue
Chlorophyll and copper-chlorophyll complex	Bright green

3.2.2 Sweeteners

Natural sweeteners have received much interest due to increasing health concerns over the consumption of sugar as well as problems related to the safety of some nonnutritive artificial sweeteners.In 2018 and 2019, global sucroseconsumption came to 174 million metric tons. Market players operating in the natural sweeteners industry are Evolva Holdings S.A., Cargill, Sunwin Stevia International, Inc., PureCircle, GLG life Tech Corp and Tate & Tyle Plc, Steviocal, Truvia, Procarvit Food Products (India) Pvt Ltd, Herboveda, Madhava Natural Sweeteners, Morita Kagaku Kogyo, Archer Daniels Midland Company, Roquette, Danisco, Sweetener Supply Corporation, Malt Products Corporation, Beijing Ginko Group, Zevia and Clarks UK Ltd.

In the last few years, sugar overconsumption hasbecome pandemic, with serious consequences in public health terms. There is clear evidence for anassociation between eating too much sugar and being at higher risk for dental caries, type II diabetesobesity and cardiovascular diseases, among other non-communicable diseases.

Sweetenerscan be synthetic (Example-.., saccharin, aspartame, sucralose, acesulfame-potassium, cyclamate, alitame, neotame, dulcin), semisynthetic (Example- neohesperidine dihydrochalcone) or natural (Example- rebaudioside and stevioside).

Natural sweeteners encompass wide-ranging compounds like sugars, sugar alcohols, amino acids, proteins, terpenoid glycosides and some polyphenols. Having said that, only those that possessrelevant characteristics, Example- safety, good taste, high stability, good solubility and reasonable cost, are found on the market as widely used sweeteners.

Erythritol is, a sugar alcohol (or polyol), produced from glucose by fermentation with yeast, Moniliellapollinis.Tagatose is hexose monosaccharide, a natural sweetener can be produced commercially from the galactose (lactose is hydrolyzed to glucose and galactose). The galactose is isomerized under alkaline conditions to D-tagatose by calcium hydroxide. The process to produce tagalose powder may involve spray drying.

Examples of natural sweeteners:		
Glycyrrhizin	**General information**	It is triterpene saponin of beta-amyrine type obtained from *Glycyrrhiza glabra* (Licorice) of family Leguminoseae with delayed lingering sweetness
	Production	Prepare water extract of dried powdered roots and separate glycyrrhizic acid by precipitation using sulfuric acid. Then add aqueous ammonia. Wait and precipitate will observe. Re-crystalize with ethanol to yield almost colourless mono-ammonium glycyrrhizinate.
	Toxicology	Due to physiological effects like edema, hypertension large quantity use is not allowed and also it is not approved as a sweetener
	Uses	50-100 times sweetener than sucrose and used as flavouring rather than sweeteners 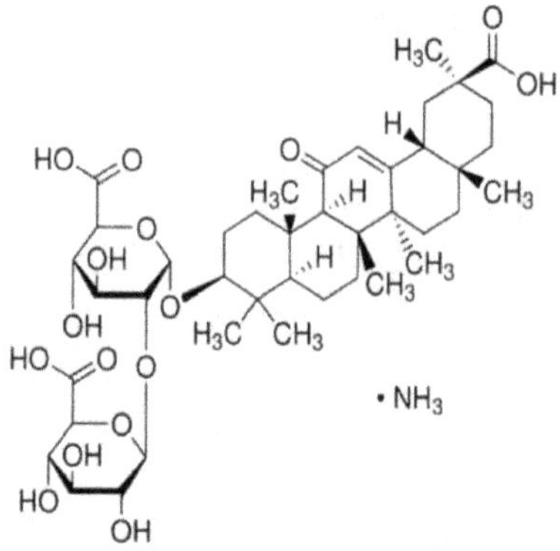 Mono-ammonium glycyrrhizinate.
Neohesperidin dihydrocalcone (NHDC)	**General information**	Semi synthetic sweetener obtained from Naringin present in skin of citrus species i.e. *Citrus aurantium, C. paradise* of family Rutaceae
	Production	Starting material for production of NHDC is naringin. Treat naringin with alkali and produce phloroacetophenone-4-B-Neohesperidoside which is condensed with asovanillin to neohesperidine in chalcone. Hydrogenations under alkaline condition yield neohesperidine dihydrochalcone. as on treatment with KOH, the flavanone ring opens up to yield a chalcone. Catalytic hydrogenation of this chalcone produces neohesperidin. Neohesperidin is industrially use to produce NHDC.
	Toxicology	Menthol-like after -taste limits its applicability. Approval of this sweetener is limited to few countries
	Uses	2000 times sweeter than sucrose; flavouring agent in confectionary product, chewing gum, and beverages. 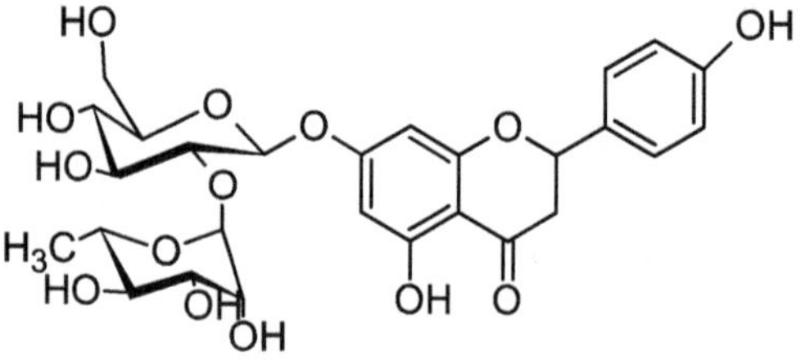 Naringin

Contd....

		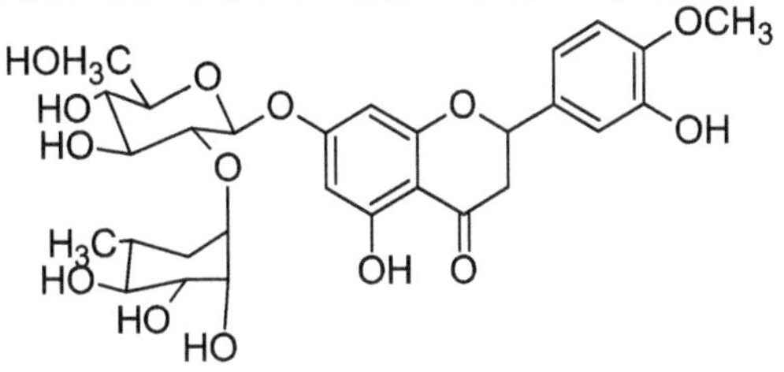 Neo-hesperidin 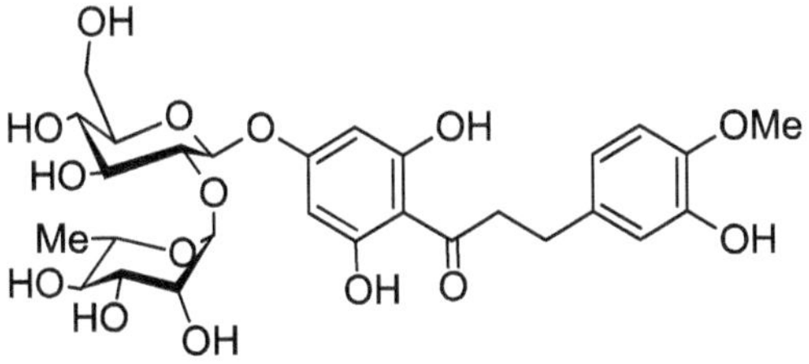 Neohesperidin-dihydrochalcone (NHDC)
Stevioside and Rebaudioside	**General information**	It is Kurene glycoside obtained from leaves of *Stevia rebaudiana*of family compositae.
	Production	Prepare water or hydro alcoholic extract of leaves. Precipitate Stevioside from the extract with methanol. Stevioside can be transformed to rebaudioside by enzymatic action.
	Toxicology	Stevia extract are approved for foods use in several South America and Asia countries
	Uses	300 times sweeter than sucrose. Sweetener for confectionary, soft drinks 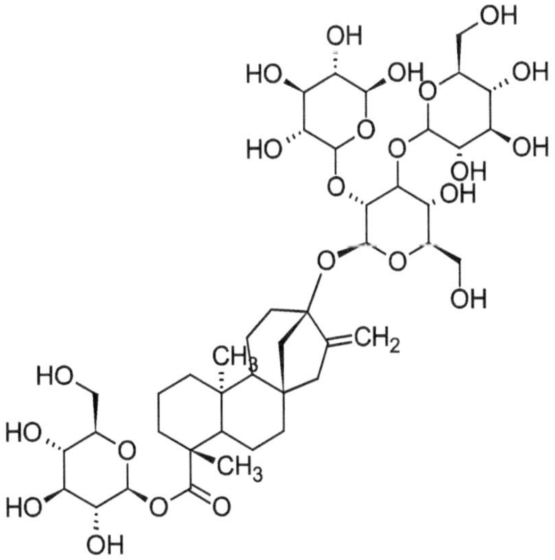 Rebaudioside
	General information	Mixture of structurally related proteins from the arils of the fruits of *Thaumatococcusdaniellii* of family Marantaceae with delayed onset and long persistence sweet taste

Contd….

Thaumatin	**Production**	Prepare water extract of arils of *Thaumatococcus*. Remove solid thaumatin by centrifugation or ultra filtration and purify by ion-exchange chromatography.
	Toxicology	Accepted internationally as a sweetener and food additive in confectionary, Chewing gum, and similar product
	Uses	3500 times sweeter than sucrose flavour enhancer rather than a sweetener 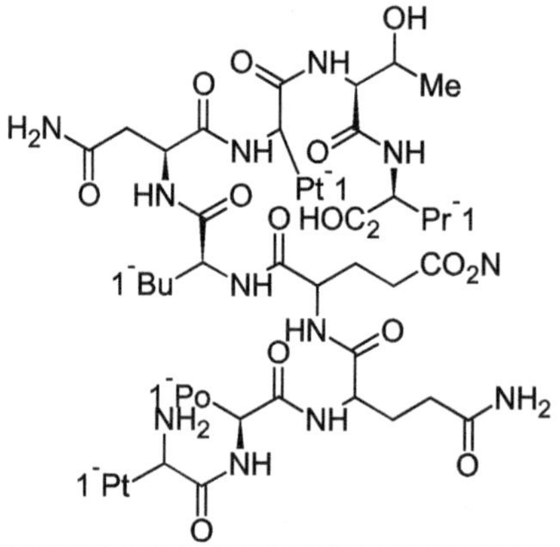
Monellins	**General information**	Sweet polypeptide constituent present in the fruits of tropical plant *Dioscoreophyllumcummisii* of family Menispermaceae
	Production	Monellin is costly to extract from the fruit as the plant is difficult to grow. Alternative production methods like chemical synthesis and expression in micro-organisms are being investigated. For instance, monellin has been expressed successfully in yeast (*Candida utilis*) and synthesised by solid-phase method.
	Toxicology	Affected by conformational changes caused by heat or hydrolytic decomposition, rendering it unsuitable as a normal sweetener.
	Uses	2000 times more sweetner than sucrose
Phyllodulcin	**General information**	It is dihydro-coumarin obtained from *Hydrangea macrophylla* of family hydrangeaceae
	Production	Extract powder with methanol of adjusted pH not less than 8 from normal temperature to about 50°C for 30 min to 6 hr so that hydrangenol is converted into its alkali salt. Then adjust pH to not less than 11 and extract with chloroform to give high-purity phyllodulcin in good yield.
	Toxicology	Delayed onset and lingering after taste, low water solubility
	Uses	400 time sweeter than sucrose 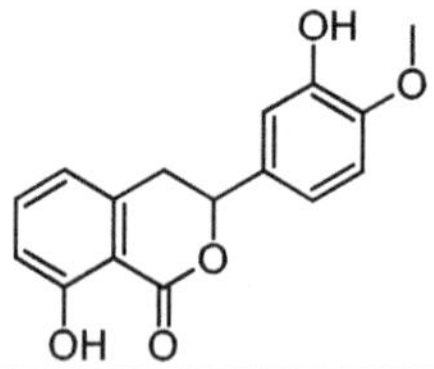

Contd....

Abrusoside	**General information**	It is cycloartane triterpenoid glycoside obtained from *Abrusprecatorius*of family fabaceae
	Production	Extract the plant material with methanol, evaporate and dissolve dry residue in water then partition with diethyl ether. Separate and take water extract to again partition between 1-butanol. Butanol extract containing abrusosides A to D can be purified by the addition of methanol.
	Toxicology	Delayed onset
	Uses	It is 30-100 times sweeter than sucrose 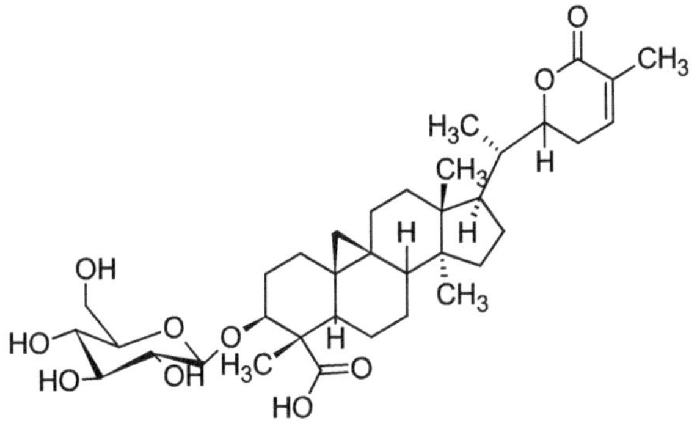
Miscellaneous		
Pentadin	**General information**	A sweet-tasting protein from fruit of Oubli (*Pentadiplandrabrazzeana*Baillon), a climbing shrub growing in some tropical countries of Africa.
	Uses	It is reported to be 500 times sweeter than sucrose on a weight basis, with its sweetness having a slow onset and decline similar to monellin and thaumatin. However, pentadin's sweetness profile is closer to monellin than to thaumatin
Brazzein	**General information**	A sweet-tasting protein from fruit of Oubli (*Pentadiplandrabrazzeana*Baillon), a climbing shrub growing in some tropical countries of Africa.
	Uses	500 to 2000 times sweeter than sucrose. Its sweet perception is more similar to sucrose than that of thaumatin. Unlike other sweet-tasting proteins, it can withstand heat, making it more suitable for industrial food processing
Curculin	**General information**	A sweet protein that was discovered and isolated in 1990 from the fruit of *Curculigo latifolia* of family Hypoxidaceae from Malaysia
	Uses	Cuculin is a taste modifier and 430-2070 times sweeter than sucrose on a weight basis but it is susceptible to heat. It is approved in Japan as a harmless additive.
Miraculin	**General information**	A taste modifier, a glycoprotein extracted from the fruit of *Synsepalumdulcificum.*
	Uses	Miraculin itself is not sweet. It is a readily soluble protein and relatively heat stable, it is a potential sweetener in acidic food. It is approved in Japan as a harmless additive.

3.2.3 Binders

A binder or binding agent is a substance that holds other material/s together by adhesion or cohesion. Binders can be waxes, oils gums, cellulose or protein

Name of Excipients	Source
Gum Ghatti	Anogeissus latifolia (Combretaceae)
Gum acacia	Acacia arabica (Combretaceae)
Khaya gum	Khaya grandifolia (Labiatae)
Albizia gum	Albizia zygia (Leguminoseae)
Cassia tora gum	Cassia tora Linn (Leguminoseae)
Guar gum	*Cyamopsis tetragonoloba (Fabaceae)*
Shatavari mucilage	Asparagus racemosus (Aapocynaceae)
Tamarind seed mucilage	Tamarindus indica (Leguminoseae)
Starch and its derivatives	Arrowroot, cornstarch, katakuri starch, potato starch, sago, wheat flour, almond flour, tapioca and their starch derivatives

3.2.4 Diluents

Diluents are acts as fillers to make up the bulk of solid unit dosage forms when drug itself is inadequate to produce the bulk. Examples: Mannitol, Lactose, Directly compressible Starches, Dextrose, Sorbitol, Microcrystalline cellulose. There are very few examples of diluents of herbal origin.

Saccharine	• ***Source*:** saccharine exudation from the stem of *Fraxinus ornus*, family: Oleaceae. It can be also be obtained chemically by reduction of mannose. • ***Description:*** white, crystalline, odourless, non hygroscopic and sweet powder. The crystals are orthorhombic prisms. The melting point is 166-168 degree C. It is freely soluble in water and insoluble in alcohol. Its specific gravity is 1.52 and optically inactive or slightly levo rotatory. • ***Uses*:** Sweetening agent & 10-19% w/w as a diluents. It doesn't get absorbed by GIT. It is not metabolized and is eliminated by glomerular filtration.
Starches	***Source*:** Starch or amylum is a polymeric carbohydrate consisting of numerous glucose units joined by glycosidic bonds. This polysaccharide is produced by most green plants for energy storage. It is the most common carbohydrate in human diets and is contained in large amounts in staple foods like potatoes, maize / corn (*Zea mays*, Gramineae), rice (*Oryza sativa*, Gramineae) wheat (*Triticum aestivum*, Gramineae) and cassava (*Manihot esculenta*, Euphorbiaceae). ***Modified starches:*** A modified starch is chemically modified to withstand conditions encountered during processing or storage, such as high heat, high shear, low pH, freeze/thaw and cooling. Following are starches with thier E cods: • 1400 Dextrin • 1401 Acid-treated starch • 1402 Alkaline-treated starch • 1403 Bleached starch • 1404 Oxidized starch

Contd....

	• 1405 Starches, enzyme-treated • 1410 Monostarch phosphate • 1412 Distarch phosphate • 1413 Phosphated distarch phosphate • 1414 Acetylated distarch phosphate • 1420 Starch acetate • 1422 Acetylated distarch adipate • 1440 Hydroxypropyl starch • 1442 Hydroxypropyl distarch phosphate • 1443 Hydroxypropyl distarch glycerol • 1450 Starch sodium octenyl succinate • 1451 Acetylated oxidized starch • ***Waxy starches*** are starch without amylase gives more stable paste. • High amylose starch, amylomaize, is gives stable ***gel***. • Sta-Rx 1500 (Staley, USA) is an only ***directly compressible***, partially hydrolysed cornstarch. It is prepared by subjecting cornstarch to physical compression or shear stress in high moisture conditions causing an increase in temperature and a partial gelatinization of some of the starch granules. The end product consists of about 5% free amylose, 15% amylopectin and 80% unmodified starch. • Untreated starch requires heat to thicken or gelatinize. When a starch is pre-cooked, it can then be used to thicken instantly in cold water. This is referred to as a ***pregelatinized*** starch. ***Description:*** Pure starch is a white, tasteless and odorless powder that is insoluble in cold water or alcohol. It consists of two types of molecules: the linear and helical amylose and the branched amylopectin. Depending on the plant, starch generally contains 20 to 25% amylose and 75 to 80% amylopectin by weight. The amylose/amylopectin ratio, molecular weight and molecular fine structure influences the physicochemical properties as well as energy release of different types of starches.
Maltose	• Maltose is a component of malt (germinated cereals- finger millet, foxtail millet, maize (corn), millet, pearl millet, sorghum, Barley, Rice, oats, wheat) a substance obtained in the process of allowing grain to soften in water and germinate. • It is also present in highly variable quantities in partially hydrolysed starch products like maltodextrin, corn syrup and acid-thinned starch.
Sorbitol	• Sorbitol or d-glucitol, a naturally occurring polyol. It is a six carbon sugar alcohol that is is mostly made from potato starch but also found naturally in many fruits, such as berries, cherries, plums, pears, and apples. • Sorbitol is an isomer of mannitol which differs only in the orientation of the hydroxyl group on carbon 2; but differ in sources in nature, melting points and uses. • Due to its sweetness (~60% compared to sucrose) and high-water solubility, sorbitol is largely used as a low-calorie sweetener, a humectant, a texturizer, or a softener. • It is present in a wide range of food products, such as chewing gums, candies, desserts, ice creams, and diabetic foods. In addition, sorbitol is the starting material for the production of pharmaceutical compounds, such as sorbose and ascorbic acid, and it is also used as a vehicle for the suspension of drugs. Furthermore, this polyol is poorly absorbed, or not absorbed at all, in the small intestine. Therefore, it can reach the colon where it can act as a substrate for bacterial fermentation, and for this reason sorbitol could be used as a prebiotic compound.

Contd….

Mannitol	• Mannitol is an isomer of sorbitol, another sugar alcohol; the two differ only in the orientation of the hydroxyl group on carbon 2. While similar, the two sugar alcohols have very different sources in nature, melting points, and uses. • Mannitol is found in a wide variety of natural products, including almost all plants, it can be directly extracted from natural products, rather than chemical or biological syntheses. In fact, in China, isolation from seaweed is the most common form of mannitol production. Mannitol concentrations of plant exudates can range from 20% in seaweeds to 90% in the plane tree. It is a constituent of saw palmetto (Serenoa).

3.2.5 Viscosity Builders/ Thickening and Gelling Agents

Viscosity builders also called as a thickening agent or thickener, are substances which can increase the viscosity of a liquid without substantially changing its other properties. Some thickening agents are **gelling agents (gellants)** forming a gel.

Following are Examples of Viscosity builders/ Thickening and Gelling agents	
Starch and its derivatives	Arrowroot, cornstarch, katakuri starch, potato starch, sago, wheat flour, almond flour, tapioca and their starch derivatives
Vegetable gums	Alginin, guar gum, locust bean gum, and xanthan gum., Gum Tragacanth
Polysaccharides	Agar, carboxymethyl cellulose, pectin and carrageenan, Aloe mucilage
Following are Examples of Polysaccharides used as Viscosity builders/ Thickening and Gelling agents	
Alginic acid , sodium alginate, potassium alginate, ammonium alginate , calcium alginate	Polysaccharides from brown algae
Agar	Polysaccharide obtained from red algae
Carrageenan	A polysaccharide obtained from red seaweeds
Pectin	A polysaccharide obtained from apple or citrus-fruit
Locust bean gum	A natural gum polysaccharide from the seeds of the carob tree

Examples of plant gums used as binders, Disintegrants, Viscosity builders/ Thickening and or Gelling agents

Gum	Biological source	Family	Structure	Pharmaceutical Application
Albizia gum	*Albizia zygia (DC.) J.F.Macbr.*	Fabaceae	Galactose Mannose Arabinose Glucuronic acid 4-0-_-methyl analogue	Tablet binder Emulsifier Coating materials in compression-coated tablets
Almond Gum	*Prunus dulcis (Mill.) D.A.Webb*	Rosaceae	Aldobionic acid L-arabinose L-galactose D-mannose	Emulsifying Thickening Suspending Adhesive Stabilizing "Drug release Uncoated tablet dosage form

Contd....

Gum	Biological source	Family	Structure	Pharmaceutical Application
Bhara gum	*Terminalia bellirica (Gaertn.) Roxb.*	Combretaceae	ß-sitosterol Gallic acid Ellagic acid Ethyl gallate Galloyl glucose Chebulaginic acid	Sustained release Microcapsules employing bhara gum release of famotidine
Cashew gum	*Anacardium occidentale L.*	Anacardiaceae	Galactose Arabinose Rhamnose Glucose Glucuronic acid L-arabinose L-rhamnose D-galactose Glucuronic acid	Suspending agent "Disintegration time "Polymer ratio drug release to a greater extent
Cordia gum	*Cordia myxa L.*	Boraginaceae	Galactose (27%) Rhamnose (21%) Mannose (17%) Xylose (11%) Glucose (10%) Arabinose (9.5%) and uronic acids (5%)	Oral sustained release matrix tablets
Grewia gum	*Grewia mollisJuss.*	Malvaceae	Glucose Rhamnose Galacturonic acid	Controlled release dosage forms Suspending agent Binding property
Guar gum	*Cyamopsis tetragonoloba (L.) Taub.*	Fabaceae	Galactose Mannose	Sustained release Controlled drug delivery Suspending agent
Gum acacia	*Acacia nilotica (L.) Delile*	Fabaceae	1,3-linked _-dgalactopyranosyl	Binder Suspending agent Emulsifying agent Demulcent Emollient
Gum Damar	*ShoreajavanicaKoord. and Valeton*	Dipterocarpaceae	40% a Alpha resin (resin that dissolves in alcohol) 22% Beta-resin 23% Dammarol acid 2.5% Water	Sustained release

Contd….

Gum	Biological source	Family	Structure	Pharmaceutical Application
Gum ghatti	*Anogeissus latifolia (Roxb.*	Combretaceae	_-1-3-linked D galactose units with some ß1-6-linked D-galactose units	Binder Emulsifier Suspending agent
Hakea Gum	*Hakea gibbosa Cav.*	Proteaceae	Glucuronic acid Galactose Arabinose Mannose Xylose which is 12: 43: 32: 5: 8.	Sustained release Binding agent
Honey Locust Gum	*Gleditsia triacanthos L.*	Fabaceae	Galactomannans. ratio of mannose to galactose in tara gumis 3:1	Controlled release carrier
Karaya gum	*Firmiana simplex (L.) W.Wight*	Malvaceae	_-d-galacturonic acid _-l-rhamnose	Suspending agent Emulsifying agent Dental adhesive Sustaining agent Mucoadhesive Buccoadhesive
Khaya gum	*Khaya grandifoliola C.DC.*	Meliaceae	Protein Sugar Phenol 61% Galactose 14% Arabinose 7% Rhamnose, 8% Glucose 5% Glucuronic acid <2% other sugar residues	Binding agent Drug targeting Controlled release
Konjac Glucomannan.	*Amorphophallus konjac K.Koch*	Araceae	D-glucose D-mannose in the ratio 1: 1.6	Gelling properties
Locust bean gum (carob gum)	*Ceratonia siliqua L.*	Fabaceae	D-galacto-Dmannoglycan pentane Proteins Cellulose	Super disintegrant Controlled drug delivery Drug targeting to the colon Super disintegrants Mucoadhesive
Mango Gum	*Mangifera indica L.*	Anacardiaceae		Binding agent Sustained release Disintegrating

Contd....

Gum	Biological source	Family	Structure	Pharmaceutical Application
Moringa oleifera Gum	*Moringa oleifera Lam.*	Moringaceae	Arabinose Galactose Glucuronic acid in the preparation of 10:7:2 Rhamnose	Gelling property Binding property Release retardant property Disintegrating property Emulsifying property
Neem Gum	*Azadirachta indica A.Juss.*	Meliaceae	Mannose Glucosamine Arabinose Galactose Fucose Xylose Glucose	Binding property Sustained release "Matrix tablet
Okra gum	*Abelmoschus esculentus (L.) Moench*	Malvaceae	Galactose Galacturonic acid Rhamnose Glucose Mmannose Arabinose Xylose	Controlled release tablet Sustained-release tablets Suspending agent
Olibanum Gum	*Boswellia serrata Roxb. ex Colebr.*	Burseraceae	5–9% Oil content 13–17% Resin acids, 20–30% Polysaccharides 40–60% boswellic acid	Sustained release Binding agent
Tamarind gum	*Tamarindus indica L.*	Fabaceae	Glucosyl: Xylosyl: Galactosyl 3:2:1	Matrix tablets Biodegradable carrier for colon specific release
Terminalia catappa gum	*Terminalia catappa L.*	Combretaceae		Oral sustained release tablets
Terminalia Gum	*Terminalia randii Baker f.*	Combretaceae		Binding agent "Strength friability
Tragacanth gum	*Astragalus brachycalyx Fisch. ex Boiss., A. gummiferLabill.*	Fabaceae	Pectinaceous Arabino galactans Xylogalacturonans	Sustain release Suspending agent Emulsifying agent

Examples of plant mucilages used as binders, Disintegrants, Viscosity builders/ Thickening and or Gelling agents

Mucilage	Biological source	Family	Structure	Pharmaceutical Application
Aloe Mucilage	*Aloe vera (L.) Burm.f.*	Xanthorrhoeaceae	Arabinan, Arabinorhamnogalactan, Galactan, Galactogalacturan, Glucogalactomannan, Galactoglucoarabinomannan, Glucuronic acid, Polysaccharides	A controlled delivery system
Asario Mucilage	*Lepidium sativum L.*	Brassicaceae	Polysaccharides, Gelatinous type of material	Suspending agent Emulsifying agent
Cassia tora Mucilage	*Senna tora (L.) Roxb.*	Fabaceae	Cinnamaldehyde, Tannins, Mannitol, Coumarins, Essential oils, (aldehydes, eugenol, pinene), Sugars, Resins	Binding Property "Hardness Disintegration Suspending agent
Cocculus Mucilage	*Cocculus hirsutus (L.) W.Theob.*	Menispermaceae	Polysaccharides, Gelatinous type of material	Gelling property Anti-inflammatory
Cordia Mucilage	*Cordia dichotoma G.Forst.*	Boraginaceae	L-rhamnose, D-galactose, D-galacturonic acid, D-glucuronic acid	Binding agent Emulsifying
Dendrophthoe Mucilage	*Dendrophthoe falcata (L.f.) Ettingsh.*	Loranthaceae	L-rhamnose, D-galactose, D-galacturonic acid, D-glucuronic acid	Binder
Fenugreek Mucilage	*Trigonella foenum-graecum L.*	Fabaceae	Mannose, Galactose, Xylose	Better release retardant
Hibiscus rosa-sinensis	*Hibiscus rosa-sinensis L.*	Malvaceae	L-rhamnose, D-galactose, D-galacturonic acid, D-glucuronic acid	Sustained release Binding agent Release-retarding agent
Mimosa mucilage	*Mimosa pudica L.*	Fabaceae	D-xylose, D-glucuronic acid	Disintegrating property
Ocimum Mucilage	*Ocimumamericanum L*	Lamiaceae	Xylose, Arabinose, Rhamnose, Galacturonic acids	Disintegrating property
Phoenix Mucilage	*Phoenix dactylifera L.*	Arecaceae	Carbohydrates 44–88%, Fructose, Sucrose, Mannose, Glucose, Maltose, Pectin (0.5–3.9%), Starch, Cellulose	Binding properties

3.2.6 Disintegrants

- Disintegrants facilitate breakup or disintegration after administration
- Superdisintegrants are improved disintegrant efficacy resulting in decreased quantity levels when compared to traditional disintegrants
- Chemical modification of starch, cellulose, and povidone brought about the development of more efficient disintegrants, capable of good disintegration action at much lower concentrations in the tablet formulations and are referred to as superdisintegrants.

Gums	Agar, Gellan gum, Tragacanth, Alginate
Starch and its derivatives	Sodium starch glycolate, partially pregelatinized starch
Cellulose derivatives	Croscarmellose sodium, microcrystalline cellulose, low-substituted hydroxypropyl cellulose

3.2.7 Flavors and Perfumes

Flavors

Flavorants are not intended to be consumed, which are added to food in order to impart or modify odour and/or taste, are called flavorings or flavourings. It denotes the combined chemical sensations of taste and smell, the same terms are used in the fragrance and flavors industry to refer to edible chemicals and extracts that alter the flavor of food and food products through the sense of smell. Taste Masking flavour examples depending on taste are Salt - Butterscotch, maple; Bitter - Wild cherry, walnut, chocolate-mint, licorice; Sweet - Fruit, berry, vanilla; Acid - Citrus.

Peppermint oil	Obtained by steam distilation of the fresh flowring tops of the plant, *Mentha piperita* Family-Labiatae	Menthol, pulegone menthone, menthofuram, Jasmone, methyl isovalerate, Methyl acetate, Limonene, Isopulegone, Cineol , Pinene, Camphene
Cinnamon oil	Dried inner bark of the shoots of coppiced trees of *Cinnamomum zeylanicum,* Family- Lauraceae	Eugenol, benzaldehyde cuminaldehyde, Cinnamaldehyde, Phellandrene, Pinene, Cymene, Caryophyllene, Starch, Mucilage, Mannitol
Lemom peel oil	Ripe fruits of *Citrus limonis*, Family-Rutaceae	Hesperidin, Pectin, Limonene, citral geranyl acetate terpeneol
Orange peel oil	Dried or fresh outer part of *Citrus aurantium*, Family-Rutaceae	Pectin, Aurantiamarin and aurantianic acid, Hesperidin, Isohesperidin, Neohesperidin, Vit-C, Limonene, Citral
Cardamom oil	Dried ripe fruits of *Elettaria cardamomum,* Family-Zingiberaceae	Terpinil acetate, Alpha-terpeniol, borneol, Cineol, Terpinen, Fixed oil, Starch and protein
Cummin oil	Dried ripe fruits of *Cuminum cyminum* Family-Umbelliferae	Cuminaldehyde, alpha-pinene, beta-pinene, Phellendrene, Cuminic alcohol, Hydro-cuminine
Anise oil	Dried ripe fruits of *Pimpinella anisum,* Family-Umbelliferae	Anethol, methyl chavicol,
Caraway oil	Dried ripe fruits of Carum carvi, Family-Umbelliferae	Carvone, carvacrol, Dihydrocarvone, Caravacrol,

Perfumes

Perfume is a mixture of fragrant essential oils or aroma compounds, fixatives and solvents, usually in liquid form, used to give agreeable scent to human body, food or objects. These are extracted from different raw materials- animals, plants marine sources. The extraction of raw material can be essential oils, absolutes, concretes, or butters. Perfumes vary from each supplier based on when and where they are harvested, how they are processed, and extraction method resulting in different organic compounds, each adding a different note to the overall scen

Plant	Biological source	Family	Volatile Chemical composition
Plants			
Agarwood	*Aquilaria malaccencis*	Thymelaeceae	Terpenes, sequiterpenes and oxygenated compound
Ambrette	*Abelmoschus moschatus*	Macalvaceae	Ambrettolide, Farnesol acetate,
Apples	*Malus domestica*	Rosaceae	Vitamin K, B6, Hydroxycinnamic acid, coumarolylquinic acid
Balsam of peru	*Myroxylonbalsamum*	Leguminosae	Styrene, vanillin, coumarin, benzyl alcohol, benzyl cinnamate, cinnamic acid, cinnamyl cinnamate
Benzoin	*Styrax tonkinensis*	Styracaceae	Benzoic acid, cinnamic acid, esters
Birch	*Betula nigra*	Betulaceae	Eugenol, linalool, palmitic acid
Cascarilla	*Croton eluteria*	Euphorbiacea	Cascarillins, lignins, tannins and resins
Cassie	*Acacia farnesiana*	Fabaceae	Essential oil cassie, ellagic acid, naringin, kaempferol
Cedar	*Cedrus deodara*	Pinaceae	Taxifolin, cedeodarin,,ampelopsin, cedrin, cedrinoside, deodarin
Cherries	*Prunus avium*	Rosaceae	3-caffeoylquinic, p-coumaric acid, catechin
Cinnamon	*Cinnamomum zeylanicum*	Lauraceae	Eugenol, benzaldehyde cuminaldehyde
Citrus	*Citrus species*	Rutaceae	Lipids, vitamins & minerals, flavonoids-limonoids
Fir	*Firs species*	Pinaceae	Camphene, bornyl acetate, santene
Geranium	*Pelargonium graveolens*	Geraniaceae	Geraneol, citronellol
Ginger	*Zingiber officinalis*	Zingiberaceae	Zingiberene, curcumene
Iris	*Iris gemanica*	Iridaceae	Caprylic acid, capric, lauric, tridcanoic palmitic acid
Jasmine	*Jasminum offficinale*	Oleaceae	3-hexanol, linalool, benzyl alcohol
Juniper	*Juniperus communis*	Cupressaseae	A-pinene, camphor, thymol methyl ether

Contd....

Plant	Biological source	Family	Volatile Chemical composition
Labdanum	*Cistus ladanifer*	Cistaceae	Tricycline, α-thujene, Sabinene, Terpenilene
Lavender	*Lavendula officinalis*	Labiateae	Esters linalyl acetate linalool, pinene, geraniol, cineol
Lemons	*Citrus limonis*	Rutaceae	Limonene, citral geranyl acetate terpineol.
Limes	*Citrus aurantifolia*	Rutaceae	Vitamin C, citric acid,
Mimosa	*Mimosa pudica*	Fabaceae	Palmitic acid,
Myrrh	*Commiphoramolmol*	Burseraceae	α,β,γ-commiphoric acid, α,β-heerabomyrrholic acid, cuminic aldehyde, eugenol
Narcissus	*Narcissus poeticus*	Amaryllidaceae	β-ocimene, 1,8-cineole, linalool
Olibanum	*Boswellia serrata*	Burseraceae	α-pinene, Sabinene, Limonene, α-Thujene
Oranges	*Citrus species*	Rutaceae	Vitami C, Limonene, citronellal
Osmanthus	*Osmanthus heterophullus*	Oleaceae	Linalool, Terpenoids-Te3, Te5, Te6
Patchouli	*Pogostemoncablin*	Lamiaceae	Germecrene, Patchoulol, Narpatchoulenol
Pine	*Pinus sylvestris*	Pinaceae	Hydrocarbens, terpenoids, phenols, resinous substance, terpentine
Plumeria	*Plumeria rubra*	Apocynaceae	Geraniol, linalool,
Rose	*Rosa alba*	Rosaceae	Geraniol, citronellol, nerol, linalool,
Rosemary	*Rosmarinus officinalis*	Lamiaceae	β-caryophyllene, limonene, α-pinene, 1,8-cineole, carnosol, ursolic acid
Rosewood	*Anibarosaeodora*	Meliaceae	Linalool,
Sage	*Salvia officinalis*	Lamiaceae	Thujones, camphor, α-pinene
Sandalwood	*Santalam album*	Santalaceae	α,β-santalol, santene, santenone, teresantol, standalone, santalene
Sassafras	*Sassafras albidum*	Lauraceae	Safrole, camphor, methyleugenol
Strawberries	*Fragaria ananassa*	Rosaceae	Ethyl esters, Palmitic acid,
Tuberose	*Palianthes tuberosa*	Asparagaceae	Methyl benzoate, butyric acid, augenol, nerol, farnesol, geraneol
Vetiver	*Chrysipogon zizanoides*	Poaceae	Citral, geraniol, α and β v

Contd….

Animal			
Ambergris	*Physeter catoden*	Physeteridae	Ambrene, epicoprostemolcoprostemone
Musk	*Moschus moschiferus*	Cervidae	Musckone, Cholesterine, Albuminoids, Resin
Castoreum	*Caster faber*	Castoridae	Volatile oil, Resin, Castorin, benzyl alcohol, methyl phenol, l-borneol.
Civet	*Viverrazibetha*	Viverridae	Civetone, Indole civetole ethylamine, propylamine.

3.3 Herbal Formulations

3.3.1 Conventional Dosage Forms

Dosage forms are pharmaceutical product in which mixture of drug substance (active substance) withexcipients (inactive components), is presented in the market for one or more resons like accurate dose, protection of drug from gastric P^H and enzymes, masking taste and odor to make palatable, optimal drug action, insertion of drugs into body cavities (rectal, vaginal) and or with use of desired vehicle for insoluble drugs. Following are examples of convntonal dosage forms:

Oral

- Pill, i.e. tablet or capsule
- Syrups
- Specialty tablet like buccal, sub-lingual, or orally-disintegrating
- Liquid solution or suspension or syrup
- Powder or liquid or solid crystals
- Pastes

Ophthalmic

- Liquid solution
- Eye solutions 1.Eye drops 2.Eye lotions b) ophthalmic suspensions C) ophthalmic ointments d)ophthalmic emulsions

Inhalation

- Aerosol
- Inhaler
- Nebulizer
- Smoking
- Vaporizer

Parenteral

- Intradermal (ID)
- Subcutaneous (SC)
- Intramuscular (IM)
- Intraosseous (IO)
- Intraperitoneal (IP)
- Intravenous (IV)

Topical

- Cream, gel, liniment or balm, lotion, or ointment,
- Ear drops
- Eye drops
- Skin patch
- Vaginal rings
- Dermal patch
- Powder/Talc

Suppository

- Vaginal (douche, pessary)
- Rectal
- Urethral suppositories
- Nasal suppositories

3.3.1.1 Syrup

Definition	Sweet, viscous, concentrated aqueous solutions of sucrose or other sugars (dextrose, sorbitol, glycerin and propylene glycol). Sucrose is partly hydrolysed into reducing sugars, levulose and dextrose. This helps in retarding oxidation
Types	◉ Simple Syrup ◉ Medicated syrup ◉ Flavouring or flavoured syrups ◉ Artificial Syrup ◉ Dry Syrup
Advantages	◉ Mask disagreeable testing (nauseous, saline or bitter) drugs., high viscosity, mouth feel, Good demulcents and soothing agents
Ingredients	◉ Sugar, Anti-microbial agents/preservatives, flavorant, colorant ◉ Syrup I.P. is a 66.7% w/w solution of sucrose whereas syrup USP is 85% w/v (corresponding to 64.74% w/w) solution of sucrose. When the concentration of the sucrose in the syrup is low then, the preservatives like glycerin, methyl paraben, benzoic acid, sodium benzoate.
Methods of preparation	◉ ***Hot process*** (for substances neither volatile nor heat labile)***:*** Weighed sucrose + purified water = heat. Strain and if required make up volume with boiled purified water Example: Syrup IP, Acacia syrup NF, Cocoa syrup NF, and Tolu syrup IP ◉ ***Percolation*** (Cold process, syrup USP preparation method***) :*** Sucrose in percolator and allow to pass purified water slowly through sucrose. The neck of the percolator is packed with loosely compressed cotton. Rate of percolation regulates the rate of dissolution of sucrose. ◉ ***Addition of a Medicating or Flavouring liquid to syrup:*** when fluid extracts, tinctures or other liquids are to be added to syrup. Alcohol also acts as preservative. ◉ ***Agitation without heat*** (for heat-labile constituents)***:*** Sucrose and other ingredients if + purified water = add in bottle = thorough agitation (manual or using mechanical agitators) of bottle. ◉ ***Preservation and storage*** O Store at a temperature not exceeding 25°C. O Store in well dried, completely filled and carefully stoppered bottles in a cool dark place. ◉ ***Evaluation:*** Physical appearance (color, odor, taste), pH, weight per ml and viscosity, Stability study

3.3.1.2 Mixture

Definition	A mixture is a liquid preparation meant for oral administration in which medicament or medicaments are dissolved, suspended or dispersed in a suitable vehicle. Although "mixture" term is also used for "suspension"
Advantages	▪ Easy to administer. ▪ Suitable for insoluble drug ▪ Suitable for immiscible drug ▪ More bioavailability compared to solid dosage form
Disadvantages	▪ More Incompatibilities ▪ Less stable ▪ Expensive ▪ Tedious storage and transport

Contd....

Types	
Simple mixture containing soluble substances	Drug + Vehicle
Mixture containing diffusible solids –	Do not dissolve in water, but on shaking they can be mixed.
Mixture containing indiffusible solids	Reduce the settling of particles the viscosity of the mixture is increased by adding some thickening agents like gum acacia, tragacanth or compound targacanth powder or their mucilage.
Mixture containing Precipitate forming liquids	Protective colloid is dispersed in the vehicle before the tincture is added
Mixture containing colloidal particle	Drug is added with alkali like NaOH and or mix by hydration to form colloidal mixture
Examples	
Simple mixture containing soluble substances	Orange syrup
Mixture containing diffusible solids –	Rhubarb powder
Mixture containing indiffusible solids	Aromatic chalk powder
Mixture containing Precipitate forming liquids	Myrrh Tincture Tolu Tincture
Mixture containing Slightly soluble liquid	Milk of magnesia
Storage	▪ Plain glass bottles with uniform internal diameter. ▪ Suitable removable cork to prevent spilling of Mixture.
Evaluation	▪ Physical appearance (color, odor, taste), pH, weight per ml and viscosity, Stability study

3.3.1.3 Tablet

Definition	Tablets are the solid unit dosage forms containing a medicament or mixtures of medicament and excipients (Diluents, Binders, Lubricants, Disintegrators, Wetting agents) compressed or molded into solid spherical, cylindrical shape having either flat or convex surface.
Types	**Monoherbal or poly herbal tablets** Compressed Tablets • Sugar coated Tablets • Film coated Tablets • Enteric coated Tablets • Effervescent Tablets • Chewable Tablets • Dispersible Tablets • Sustained release Tablets • Multilayer Tablets • Sublingual Tablets • Troches • Buccal Tablets • Implant Tablets • Hypodermic Tablets • Solution Tablets • Vaginal Tablets
Methods of Preparation	⦿ Wet granulation method: oldest and most widely used method involving steps weighing, mixing, granulation, screening the damp mass, drying, drying screening, lubrication, finally compression. ⦿ Dry granulation method (slugging, double compression or recompression method) for ingredients sensitive to moisture or elevated temperatures during drying. Essential steps : weighing, mixing, slugging, dry screening, lubrication and compression. ⦿ Direct compression: for a small group of crystalline chemicals. Simple, absence of granulating step, avoidance of moisture and drying steps, minimum material handling, rapidity of the total process and optimum possible bioavailability of the drugs from the resulting tablets.

Contd....

Evaluation parameters	
Physical nature	Shape, Size (diameter and thickness), Weight (size and weight determines the density), Score (or groove), Imprinting, Color
Content of active ingredient	As per assay procedure or suitable analytical method calculate active ingredient concentration
Uniformity	Average weight deviation has to calculate. 80 mg or less = 10 % More than 80 mg or less than 250 mg =7.5 % 250 mg or more = 5 %
Friability	Tablets are subjected to abrasion and shock by utilizing a plastic chamber to know wear and tear during handling and shipping which should not be more than 0.5-1%
Hardness	Force required for breaking tablet is measured using Monsanto tester, The strong –cob tester, The Pfizer tester , The erweka tester, The schleuniger tester
Disintegration	Tablet disintegration is the first step for a drug to become bioavailable. The tablet must first disintegrate and discharge the drug to the body fluids.
Dissolution test	If the rate of dissolution is lower than the rate of absorption, then the dissolution rate determines the bioavailability.

3.3.2 Novel Drug Delivery Systems (NDDSs)

Poor water solubility hence frequent dosing, more side effects, poor site-specific action, and poor bioavailability and thus drug release are major drawbacks of conventional formulations. To overcome these issues and to improve patient compliance, recently, novel drug delivery systems (NDDSs) and dosage forms have gained much attention mainly in chronic disease (Cancer, arthritis, immunodeficiency diseases etc.) due to their target specificity, high efficacy and stability.

- **Drawbacks of conventional dosage forms**
    - Poor patient compliance and missing the dose of drug.
    - Fluctuation in drug concentration lead to under medication or over medication and thus side effects
- **Advantages of novel drug delivery system**
    - Enhancement of solubility.
    - Increased bioavailability.
    - Protection from toxicity.
    - Enhancement of pharmacological activity.
    - Enhancement of stability.
    - Sustained delivery.
    - Protection from chemical and physical degradation

Following are few different NDDSs:

Different types of NDDSs	
Modified release dosage forms	Modified-release dosage is a mechanism that (in contrast to immediate-release dosage) delivers a drug with a delay after its administration (delayed-release dosage) or for a prolonged period of time (extended-release dosage) or to a specific target in the body (targeted-release dosage). Extended-release dosage consists of either sustained-release (SR) or controlled-release (CR) dosage. SR maintains drug release over a sustained period but not at a constant rate. CR maintains drug release over a sustained period at a nearly constant rate. Examples: controlled delivery (CD), controlled release (CR), delayed release (DR), extended release (ER, XL, XR, XT), immediate release (IR), long-acting (LA), long-acting release (LAR), modified release (MR), prolonged release (PR), sustained action (SA), sustained release (SR), timed release (TR)
Vesicular Carriers	Liposomes, Phytosomes, Niosomes, BilosomesTransfersomes, Ethosomes, Emulsones, Pharmacocomes, Invasomes, Layerosomes,
Micellar Carriers	Polymeric micelles, Dendrimers. Mixed micelles, Phospholipid based micelles
Particulate Carriers	Solid lipid nanoparticles, Nanostructured lipid carriers, Polymeric nanoparticles
Emulsified Carriers	Microemulsions, Nanoemulsions, Lipid emulsions
Other	Oral Films, Transdermal patch

Vesicular Carriers	
Liposomes	Liposomes, sphere-shaped nano-sized to microsized vesicles consisting of one or more phospholipid bilayers, were first described in the mid-60s. Very small globule size (0.025 µm to 2.5 µm) and hydrophobic as well as hydrophilic character makes liposomes choice of drug delivery. Liposomes are artificially prepared vesicles made of lipid bilayer which vastly improves drug absorption and bioavailability. Materials commonly used for the preparation of transferosomes are phospholipids (soya phosphatidyl choline, egg phosphatidyl choline), surfactant (tween 80, sodium cholate) for providing flexibility, alcohol (ethanol, methanol) as a solvent, dye for confocal scanning lasermicroscopy (CSLM) and buffering agent (saline phosphate buffer pH 7.4), as a hydrating medium. **Types**: On the basis of their size and number of bilayers, liposomes are classified as follows: Multilamellar vesicles (MLV) Unilamellar vesicles Large unilamellar vesicles (LUV) Small unilamellar vesicles (SUV) **Preparation Methods** Following are different methods in preparation of liposomes: • Passive loading techniques • Mechanical dispersion method • Sonication. • French pressure cell: extrusion. • Freeze-thawed liposomes.

Contd….

<table>
<tr>
<td></td>
<td>

- Lipid film hydration by hand shaking, non-hand. shaking or freeze drying.
- Micro-emulsification.
- Membrane extrusion.
- Dried reconstituted vesicles
- Solvent dispersion method
- Ether injection (solvent vaporization)
- Ethanol injection
- Reverse phase evaporation method
- Detergent removal method (removal of non-encapsulated material)
- Dialysis
- Detergent (cholate, alkyl glycoside, Triton X-100) removal of mixed micelles (absorption)
- Gel-permeation chromatography

Procedure: There are four basic stages in preparation of liposomes i.e. drying down lipids from organic solvent, dispersing the lipid in aqueous media, purifying the resultant liposome and analyzing the final product. Active loading technique: At present, there is no single universal encapsulation method that offers stable encapsulation of most drugs; each drug requires a different approach to manage all of its properties.

Evaluation parameters:

Liposomal drug delivery system involves following evaluation parameters:

Rheological properties like Viscosity

Electro kinetic properties like zeta potential, surface charge, polydispersity

Particle size, lamellarity

Drug entrapment efficiency and drug release.

</td>
</tr>
<tr>
<td>Phytosome</td>
<td>

Phytosome is a patented technology developed by a leading manufacturer of drugs and nutraceuticals, to incorporate standardized plant extracts or water soluble phytoconstituents into phospholipids to produce lipid compatible molecular complexes, called as phytosomes. In liposomes no chemical bond is formed; the phosphatidylcholine molecules surround the water soluble substance. There may be hundreds or even thousands of phosphatidylcholine molecules surrounding the water soluble compound. In contrast, with the phytosome process the phosphatidylcholine and the plant components actually form a 1:1 or a 2:1 molecular complex depending on the substance(s) complexed, involving chemical bonds.

Differnce Between Liposomes vs Phytosomes

<table>
<tr><th>S.no</th><th>Phytosome</th><th>Liposome</th></tr>
<tr><td>1</td><td>In this the active chemical constituent molecule are attaches through chemical bonds to their polar head of phospholipids</td><td>In this active principle is dissolved in the medium of cavity or in layer of membrane</td></tr>
<tr><td>2</td><td>Chemical bond are formed</td><td>No chemical bonds are formed.</td></tr>
<tr><td>3</td><td>In phytosome phosphatidylcholine and plant compound form 1:1 or 2:1 complex depending on substances.</td><td>In this hundred and thousand of phosphatidylcholine molecule surrounded by water soluble molecule.</td></tr>
<tr><td>4</td><td>Phytosomes are much better absorbed.</td><td>Comparatively with phytosome less absorbed</td></tr>
<tr><td>5</td><td>Content of phospholipid is less</td><td>Content of phospholipid is more</td></tr>
</table>

</td>
</tr>
</table>

Contd….

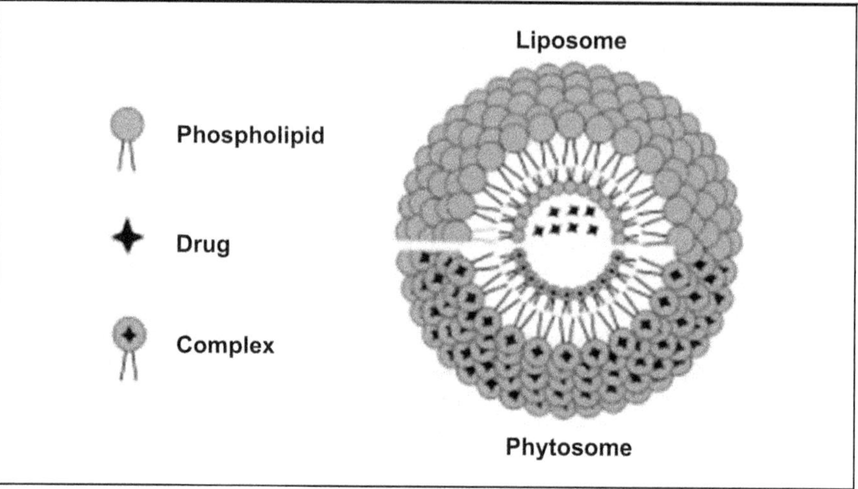

Preparation Methods of phytosomes

- Antisolvent preparation method
- Rotatory evaporation process
- Solvent ether-injection process.

Procedure: Generally phytosomes are prepared by reacting one mole of a phospholipid (natural or synthetic) such as phosphatidylcholine, phosphatidylethanolamine or phosphatidylserine with one mole of phytocomponent either alone or in the natural mixture in aprotic solvent such as dioxane or acetone from which complex can be isolated by precipitation or lyophilization or by spray drying. Common ratio range between these two moieties is 0.5-2.0 moles. The most preferable ratio 1:1 mole

Commonly used chemicals in phytosome preparation

Chemicals	Examples	Use
Phospholipid	Soyaphospotidylcholine, Eggphospotidylcholine, dipalmitoyl phosphatidylcholine, distrerylphospotidylcholine	Cellular vesical generating component
Solvent	Dioxane, acetone, methyl chloride.	Aprotic solvent
Non-solvent	Aliphatic hydrocarbon, n-Hexane	Complex precipitation
Alcohol	Ethanol, methanol	As a solvent
Color and dyes	Rhodamine 6G, DHPE-rhodamine, fluorescein, 6carboxy fluorescence.	Laser microscopy study
Buffering agent	Saline phosphate buffer 7%, ethanol tris buffer.	Hydrating medium

Evalaution Methods

- ***Determination of entrapment efficiency***: Entrapment efficiency of phytosome can be determined by ultracentrifugation technique, and drug entrapment percentage will be calculated by dividing actual amount and theoretical amount.
- ***Determination of vesical size and zeta potential***: It can be determined by dynamic light scattering which uses a computerized inspection system and photon correlation spectroscopy.

Contd....

	➢ ***Surface tension activity measurement*** : It can be measured by ring method using "Du Nouy ring tensiometer" the surface tension of drug will be measured. ➢ ***Spectroscopic evaluation***: It is help to confirm the formation of complexes as well as to study interaction between complexes. ➢ ***Determination of drug content***: Determine the drug content of phytosmes by UV spectrometer at drug lamda max. ➢ ***In vitro and in vivo evaluation***: this can be done according to therapeutic activity measurement parameters of biologically active phytoconstituents present in phytosome. ➢ ***Visualization***: visualization of phytosomes can be accomplished using scanning electron microscopy, or transition electron microscopy.
Niosomes	Niosomes are formations of vesicles by hydrating mixture of cholesterol and nonionic surfactants. In niosomes, the vesicles forming amphiphile is a non-ionic surfactant which is usually stabilized by addition of cholesterol and small amount of anionic surfactant such as diacetyl phosphate. Niosomes are preferred over liposomes because the former exhibit high chemical stability and economy. One of the reasons for preparing niosomes is the assumed higher chemical stability of the surfactants than that of phopholipids, which are used in the preparation of liposomes. Due to the presence of ester bond, phospholipids are easily hydrolysed.
Ethosomes	These are soft, malleable vesicles tailored for enhanced delivery of active agents. They are composed mainly of phospholipids, (phosphatidylcholine, Phosphatidyl serine, phosphatitidic acid), high concentration of ethanol and water. The high concentration of ethanol makes the ethosomes unique, as ethanol is known for its disturbance of skin lipid bilayer organization therefore, when integrated into a vesicle membrane it gives that vesicle the ability to penetrate the stratum corneum. Also because of their high ethanol concentration, the lipid membrane is packed less tightly than conventional vesicles but has equivalent stability, allowing a more malleable structure and improves drug distribution ability in stratum corneum lipids
Transfersomes	Transfersomes are specially optimized, ultradeformable (ultraflexible) lipid supramolecular aggregates, which are able to penetrate the mammalian skin intact. Each transfersome consists of at least one inner aqueous compartment, which is surrounded by a lipid bilayer with specially tailored properties, due to the incorporation of "edge activators" into the vesicular membrane. Surfactants such as sodium cholate, sodium deoxycholate, span 80 and Tween 80, have been used as edge activators.
Bilosomes	They are specialised delivery vehicles which protect vaccines from being broken down in the stomach, thereby enabling the oral delivery of vaccines as an alternative to administering treatment by injection. developed non-ionic surfactant vesicle (NISV) having liposome like structures and stabilized them with bile salts for the oral delivery of vaccines. These were called bilosome, bilosomes differ from the liposomes and niosomes in term of their composition, chemical stability and storage conditions. In order to avoid the problems during GI transit, bilosomes were developed which not only prevented antigens from degradation, but also enhanced mucosal penetration. Bilosome based vaccine produced both systemic as well as mucosal immune response which was equivalent to immune response produced by subcutaneous route
Emulsomes	Emulsome is a novel lipoidal vesicular system with an internal solid fat core surrounded by a phospholipid bilayer. Emulsomal formulations composed of solid lipid core material and stabilized by cholesterol and soya lecithin. The drug is loaded followed by sonication to produce emulsomes of small size. The polymer used for core material should be solid at room temperature (25°C).The high soya lecithin concentration stabilized the emulsomes in form of O/W emulsion.These fat cored lipid particles are dispersed in an aqueous phase. These systems are often prepared by melt expression or emulsion solvent diffusive extraction.

Contd….

Pharmacosome	They may be defined as a neutral molecule possessing both positive and negative charge, water-loving and fat-loving properties, and an optimum ratio of polyphenol with phospholipids in a complex form. The drugs are present in a dispersion form in these lipoidal drug delivery system conjugated by electron pair sharing's and electrostatic forces or by forming a hydrogen bond with lipids. Pharmacosome is derived from the word "Pharmakon" which means drug and "soma" meaning carrier. It means a vesicular system in which the drug is associated with the carrier. These lipid conjugated vesicles may exist as colloidal, nanometric size micelles, vesicles or may be in the form of hexagonal assembly enjoying a functional hydrogen atom banking upon the architecture of the complex. The drug molecule with a free carboxylic or functional hydrogen atom like amino, hydroxyl groups, is converted to an ester with the help of the hydroxyl moiety of the lipid, resulting in the formation of a prodrug.
Invasomes	invasomesare novel vesicular systems that exhibit improved transdermal penetration compared to conventional liposomes. These vesicles contain phospholipids, ethanol, and terpene in their structures; these components confer suitable transdermal penetration properties to the soft vesicles. The main advantages of these nanovesicles lie in their ability to increase the permeability of the drug into the skin and decrease absorption into the systemic circulation, thus, limiting the activity of various drugs within the skin layer.
Layersomes	The layersomes are conventional liposomes coated with one or multiple layers of biocompatible polyelectrolytes in order to stabilise their structure. The formulation strategy is based on an alternative coating procedure of positive poly(lysine) and negative poly(glutamic acid) (pGA) polypeptides on initially charged small unilamellar liposomes (SUVs). The size distribution and the zeta potential of the final entity depend on the number of polyelectrolyte layers and the charge of the last coating layer. The layer-by-layer self-assembly of polycations and polyanions has been largely applied to coat solid surfaces and consequently modulate their physicochemical properties. The major drawback of liposomes is their instability during storage or in biological media, which is related to surface properties. Different strategies were investigated to increase nanoparticle stability. One of them consists in the modification of their external surface by optimisation of the lipid composition of the membrane, by incorporation of bioadhesive molecule (chitosan) in their membrane, by the polymerization of a two-dimensional network in the hydrophobic core of the membrane, by coating with nonporous silica or by the addition of surface-active polymers.

Micellar Carriers	
Mixed micelles	The solubilization of lipid bilayer by surfactant is accompanied by morphological change of bilayer and emergence of mixed micelles. From the phase equilibrium perspective, the lipid, surfactant, water system is in two phase area during the solubilization a phase containing mixed micelles is in equilibrium with bilayer structure of laminar phase. In some cases, three phases are present the single micelles phase is replaced by a concentrated and dilute solution phase in the case of non-ionic surfactant. The lipid bilayer reach saturation when mixed micelles often flexible rod like or thread like start from it aqueous solution at the constant chemical proportion of surfactant.
Polymeric micelles	They are formed from self-aggregation of amphiphilic block / graft co-polymers with the hydrophobic part of the polymer on the inside (core) and hydrophilic on the outside

Contd....

(shell). In drug delivery, PM are classified under the "Nano carriers". A polymeric micelle usually consists of several hundred block copolymers and has a diameter of about 20-50 nm

They have Self-assembled supramolecular core-shell structure. Core is a dense region consisting of the hydrophobic part of the amphiphilic polymer. Core serves as a reservoir for drugs with low aqueous solubility. Shell consisting hydrophilic portion of the co-polymer. the morphology of micelles is the hydrophilic– hydrophobic balance of the block copolymer defined by the hydrophilic volume fraction, f (f>45% form PM)

Solid lipid nano-particle

Colloidal particles ranging in size between 10 & 1000 nm are known as nanoparticles. Solid lipid nanoparticle (SLNs) are new generation of submicron sized lipid emulsion where the liquid lipid(oil) has been substituted by a solid lipid.

Advantages of SLNs over polymeric NPs Polymeric Nanoparticles Solid Lipid Nanoparticles Residual Contamination Avoid residual contamination Possible toxicity problems No toxicity problems Expensive production & a lack of large scale production method Cost effective methods are available Lack of suitable sterilization method Feasible sterilization method available Not stable as compared to SLNs SLNs formulation stable for even three years have been development. General ingredients include solid lipids, emulsifier & water. Lipid contains triglycerides, partial glycerides, fatty acids, steroids, waxes Combination of emulsifier might prevent particle agglomeration, Emulsifier include soybean lecithin, egg lecithin, poloxamer etc.

Different methods of Nanoparticles preparation

- High shear homogenization:
  - Hot homogenization
  - Cold homogenization
- Ultrasonication/high speed homogenization:
  - Probe ultrasonication
  - Bath ultrasonication
- Solvent emulsification/evaporation
- Micro emulsion based SLN preparations
- SLN preparation by using supercritical fluid
- Spray drying method
- Double emulsion method

Ingredients Used in the Preparation of Nanoparticles

Name of the ingredients	Concentrations
Lipid	3.33% w/v
Phospholipids	0.6-1.5%
Glycerol	2-4%
Poloxamer 188	1.2-5% w/w
Soy phosphatidyl choline	95%
Compritol	10%
Cetyl palmitate	10% w/w
Isopropyl myristate	3.60%
PEG 2000	0.25%
PEG 4500	0.5%

Contd….

Name of the ingredients	Concentrations
Tween 85	0.5%
Ethyl oleate	30%
Sodium alginate	70%
Ethanol/butanol	2%
Tristearin glyceride	95%
PEG 400	5%
Tego care 450 (surfactant)	1.2% w/w
Pluronic F 68(non-ionic surfactant)	40%
Tween 80(non-ionic surfactant)	50%

Phospholipid-based micelles:	The self-assembly of amphiphilic surfactants in solution is an interesting phenomenon that has wide significance in fields ranging from fundamental biology to chemical engineering and biotechnology. Particularly interesting biological surfactant self-assemblies are formed by phospholipids. Besides their essential role in the cell membrane of most organisms, phospholipids are present and form various aggregates and colloidal assemblies in many bioproducts, including all plant oils and their derivatives, and have various industrial applications as surface-active components. A commonly employed phospholipid surfactant is lecithin, which is an amphiphilic substance mostly consisting of glycerol-based phospholipids extracted from food sources such as eggs and soybeans. This makes it biocompatible and nontoxic. Most widely studied and applied self-assembling lecithin systems include ternary mixtures of lecithin, water, and an organic solvent of low polarity (oil), which typically take the form of an emulsion with the hydrophobic tail of the lecithin molecule residing in the nonpolar oil phase and the hydrophilic headgroup being in contact with the water.
Dendrimers	Dendrimers are well-defined, multivalent molecules having branched structure of nanometer size. Dendrimers possess a distinct molecular architecture that consists of three different domains: (i) a central core (ii) branches (iii) terminal functional groups, present at the outer surface of the macromolecule, that dictates the nucleic acid complexation or drug entrapment efficacy. Dendrimers of defined size and structure can be engineered by a step-wise chemical synthesis approach, and that too with low polydispersity index. Generally, dendrimers are synthesized by two conceptually different approaches, the divergent and the convergent.

Particulate Carriers	
Nanostructured lipid carrier	NLC (Nanostructured lipid carrier) which are second generation of SLN. NLC composed of binary mixture of solid lipid and a spatially different liquid lipid as hybrid carrier. Average size between 10-500 nm. NLC consist of a mixture of specially blended solid lipid (long chain) with liquid lipid (short chain), preferably in a ratio of 70:30 to 99.9:01. Objectives of NLCTo overcome disadvantages of SLN such as Tendency for particle growth. Unpredictable gelation tendency. Poor drug loading capacity. Drug expulsion after polymeric transition during storage. High water content in dispersions have been observed i.e.70-99.9%. The Excipients used in NLC¬ Solid lipids A mixture of several chemical compounds which have high melting point (higher than 40°C). These solid lipids are well tolerated of GRAS status. Accepted for human use. Also in vivo

Contd....

	biodegradable. Liquid lipids (OIL) These solid lipids are well tolerated of GRAS status. Emulsifying agents It is an surfactant, which is adsorbed at interfaces and lowers the interfacial tension. UV blockers Help to protect the skin from the ultraviolet radiation of the sun. Lowering the risk of skin cancer. Sunscreen products contain either an organic chemical compound that absorbs UV light
Polymeric Nanoparticles:	Polymeric nanoparticles (PNP) They are solid colloidal particles ranging in size from 10 to 1000 nm (1μm). Drug may be dissolved, entrapped, encapsulated or attached to a nanoparticle matrix. Because these systems have very high surface areas, drugs may also be adsorbed on their surface. Polymer-based nanoparticles effectively carry drugs, proteins and DNA to target cells and organs. Their nanometer-size promotes effective permeation through cell membranes and stability in the blood stream. **Nanocapsules**: They are the systems in which the drug is confined to a cavity surrounded by a unique polymer membrane. **Nanospheres**: They are the matrix systems in which the drug is physically and uniformly dispersed.

Emulsified Carriers	
SMEDDS	Formulations that are developed using liquid lipid exist as either simple emulsions or self-emulsifying drug delivery systems (SEDDS). Depending upon the size, they are called as self-microemulsifying drug delivery system (SMEDDS) or self-nanoemulsifying drug delivery system (SNEDDS). These are isotropic, anhydrous, and single-phase system constituted of cosurfactant(s), surfactant(s), and oil(s) in addition to solubilize lipophilic bioactive. It effortlessly forms o/w emulsion upon dispersion in water phase following mild agitation. Self-emulsifying micro- and nanosystem increases the bioavailability of poorly soluble drugs. Nonionic surfactants with high hydrophilic–lipophilic balance (HLB) values are used in the formulation of SEDDS (Example-Tween, Labrasol, Labrafac CM 10, Cremophore). Cosurfactant/cosolvents like Spans, capyrol 90, Capmul, lauroglycol, diethylene glycol monoethyl ether (transcutol), propylene glycol, polyethylene glycol, polyoxyethylene, propylene carbonate, tetrahydrofurfuryl alcohol, polyethylene glycol ether (Glycofurol), etc., may help to dissolve large amounts of hydrophilic surfactants or the hydrophobic drug in the lipid base. These solvents sometimes play the role of the cosurfactants in the microemulsion systems.
Micro-emulsion	IUPAC defines micro-emulsion as dispersion made of water, oil, and surfactant(s) that is an isotropic and thermodynamically stable system with dispersed domain diameter varying approximately from 1 to 100 nm, usually 10 to 50 nm. The major components of micro emulsion system are:1) Oil phase 2) Surfactant (Primary surfactant) 3) Co-surfactant (Secondary surfactant) 4) Co-Solvent.
Nano-emulsion	**Nano-emulsion** Nano-emulsions are very similar to microemulsions that are dispersions of nano-scale particles but obtained by mechanical force unlike to microemulsions which forms spontaneously. Microemulsions and nano-emulsions are promising delivery for poorly water soluble drugs.

Subjective Questions

1. Define herbal cosmetics.
2. Give brief account on use of fixed oil or waxes inherbal cosmetics
3. Give brief account on use of colorants in herbal cosmetics
4. What are different herbal originated bleaching agents/perfumes?
5. What is mode of action of bleaching agents?
6. What is function of Antioxidants in Cosmetics?
7. What is Shikonin, Alizarin, Bixin?
8. How antioxidants are useful in oral hygiene products?
9. Write a note on herbal drugs used in hair care or oral hygiene.
10. Write a note on herbal colorants/sweeteners/binders/diluents/flavorants
11. How to prepare and evaluate herbal syrup?
12. How to prepare and evaluate herbal mixtures?
13. How to prepare and evaluate herbal tablets?
14. How to prepare and evaluate herbal phytosomes?
15. What is difference between liposomes and phytosomes?
16. Why there is need of NDDSs?
17. What is difference between defination of Syrup in IP and USP

Multiple Choice Questions (MCQs)/Objective Questions

1. Naturally occurring form of vitamin A is known as ....
   a. Tritinoin
   b. Tretin
   c. Retinoic acid
   d. both a and c
2. Retinoic acid improves hyper pigmentation and skin eruption with red pimples by ....
   a. Bleaching action
   b. Increasing rate of cell division
   c. Exerting anti inflammatory action
   d. None of the above
3. Which compound isolated from shellac is now preffered highly in place of alpha hydroxy acids in topical cosmetics?
   a. Glycolic acid
   b. Lactic acid
   c. Ascorbic acid
   d. Aleuritic acid

4. Boswellic acids are used in anti-inflammatory creams and lotions because
   a. It inhibits enzyme 5 – lipoxygenase
   b. It inhibits Histamine
   c. Inhibits fluid retention
   d. None of the above
5. Which one of the following herb acts as free radical scavenger and protects skin from UV radiation?
   a. Arjuna c. Amla
   b. Neem d. Ashoka
6. In herbal toothpaste, which ingredient acts as analgesic, antimicrobial and flavoring agent?
   a. Fennel c. pepper
   b. Cinnamon d. Clove
7. Which component of the herbal shampoo produces foam and acts as cleansing agent?
   a. Sodium lauryl sulphate c. Fenugreek
   b. Shikekai d. Neem
8. Which one of the herb is popular as mouth freshener?
   a. Clove c. Tulsi
   b. Papermint d. All of the above
9. Which one of the herb is a 'multipurpose' herb in skin and hair care?
   a. Neem c. Aloe vera
   b. Tulsi d. Cucumber
10. Which ingredient in herbal hair oil causes hair re-growth and improves hair loss?
    a. Hibiscus c. Neem
    b. Arnica d. Ritha
11. Which one of the following is not fixed oil used as carrier in herbal cosmetics?
    a. Coconut oil c. Jojoba oil
    b. Argon oil d. Tea tree oil
12. Which one of the essential oil exerts cooling effect in oral care formulations?
    a. Clove oil c. chamomile oil
    b. Peppermint oil d. camphor
13. Which method is preffered for extraction of fixed oils to be used in herbal cosmetics?
    a. steam distillation c. Hot press method
    b. cold press method d. All of the above

14. Coconut oil used in herbal cosmetics is obtained from.........
    a. Dry leaves of Cocus nucifera
    b. Kernels of fruit of cocus nucifera
    c. Bark of Cocus nucifera
    d. Roots of Cocus nucifera
15. *Daucus carota* is the biological source of ....
    a. Vitamin A
    b. Vitamin E
    c. Vitamin C
    d. Vitamin D
16. ....is non drying oil and widely used for production of firm and excellent white soap
    a. Olive oil
    b. Castor oil
    c. Arachis oil
    d. Chaulmoogra oil
17. ....wax is an ingredient of Paraffin ointment IP?
    a. Carnauba wax
    b. Yellow bees wax
    c. Lard
    d. Japan wax
18. Which gum is used as binding agent in formulation of herbal toothpaste?
    a. Gum acacia
    b. Tragacanth
    c. Guar gum
    d. All of the above
19. Rose oil, used as soothing agent as well as perfume in cosmetics is obtained from
    a. *Rosa damascena Mill*
    b. *Rosa gallica L*
    c. *Rosa moschata*
    d. All of the above
20. Colouring agent bixin used in herbal lipsticks and lipbalms is obtained from
    a. Beat root
    b. Lipstick pods
    c. Curcuma
    d. cochineal
21. *Stevia rebaudiana*, Family Astaraceae is biological source of
    a. Natural sweetener
    b. Natural colorant
    c. Flavoring agent
    d. Natural binder
22. Stevia is ....times sweeter than sucrose
    a. 10
    b. 100
    c. 200
    d. 300
23. Which one of the following is NOT nonsaccharide sweetening agent?
    a. Glycerrhizin
    b. Rebaudiana
    c. Sapodilla
    d. Tremalose
24. Which one of the following is Colour Index number of natural Beta carotene used in cosmetic formulations?
    a. CI40800
    b. CI75130
    c. CI73015
    d. E110

25. Which one of the dye is used as a pH indicator and as a colorant for oral and pharmaceutical topical preparations?
   a. Tartrazine
   b. Brilliant blue
   c. Indigo carmine
   d. Quinolline yellow

26. Which one of the coloring agent is highly unstable to light and air? And also requires special packaging for materials containing this colorant?
   a. Indigo carmine
   b. Turmeric
   c. Carmine
   d. Beta carotene

27. Which one of the following is first anthraquinones dye produced synthetically in 1869?
   a. Emodin
   b. Alizarin
   c. Purpurin
   d. Mungistin

28. Which one of the polysaccharide having Pharmaceutical industry utility is obtained from microbial fermentation process?
   a. Chitosan
   b. Tragacanth gum
   c. Pectin
   d. Pullulan

29. Psyllium mucilage is widely used in pharmaceutical industry as
   a. Binding agent
   b. Tablet disintegrator
   c. Sustained release
   d. All of the above

30. Most widely used flavoring agent used in pharmaceutical as well as food industry is
   a. Eugenol
   b. Menthol
   c. Citric acid
   d. None of the above

31. Which property should excipient Posses?
   a. Should have own pharmacological effect
   b. Should be compatible with active ingredient
   c. Both a and b
   d. None of the abovc

32. Most of the natural polysaccharides used as pharmaceutical excipients belong to family.....
   a. Apocynceae
   b. Leguminosae
   c. Labiatae
   d. Combretacae

33. Gellan gum is used in pharmaceutical industry as
   a. Binding agent
   b. Disintegrating agent
   c. Both a and b
   d. None of the above

34. Cellulose has application in pharmaceutical industry as ....
   a. Viscosity enhancer
   b. Laxative
   c. Binder
   d. Both a and c

35. Mimosa pudica is used as a......................in pharmaceutical formulations
    a. Binder
    b. Disintegrating agent
    c. Both a and b
    d. None of the above
36. What is Rosin?
    a. High molecular weight oleoresin
    b. Low molecular weight oleoresin
    c. Polysaccharide
    d. None of the above
37. Which of the pharmaceutical excipient belongs to category animal polysaccharide?
    a. Pullulan
    b. Xanthn gum
    c. Chitin
    d. None of the above
38. Which one of the excipient is used for preparation of capsule shell of folic acid?
    a. Alginate
    b. Pectin
    c. Both a and b
    d. None
39. Which of the following is anionic gum used as excipient?
    a. Karaya gum
    c. Arabic gum
    c. Guar gum
    d. Both a and b
40. Carrageen is obtained from
    a. Red algae
    b. Blue algae
    c. Fruits
    d. Seeds
41. Herbal syrups are prepared by ....
    a. Combining concentrated herbal infusions with sugar, honey or alcohol
    b. Combining concentrated herbal decoctions with sugar, honey or alcohol
    c. Both a and b
    d. None
42. What is the role of alcohol in Herbal syrups?
    a. Flavoring agent
    b. Stabilizer
    c. Preservative
    d. All of the above
43. Herbal cough syrups contains mainly......................as an expectorant
    a. Vasaka
    b. Ginger
    c. Garlic
    d. All of the above
44. Which one of the formulation is example of herbal mixture?
    a. Churna
    b. Bhasma
    c. Gutika
    d. None of the above
45. Herbal mixture should NOT contain ingredients having
    a. Agonistic activity
    b. Antagonistic activity
    c. Excipients
    d. therapeutic activity

46. Herbal mixtures should be free of ....
   a. Heavy metals
   b. Micro organisms
   c. Foreign particles
   d. All of the above
47. Herbal tablets active pharmaceutical ingredient is ....
   a. Raw herb or extract
   b. Standardized herb or extract
   c. Synthetic drug
   d. None of the above
48. In case of herbal formulations, standardization parameters for flow properties like Cars index and Angle of repose is applicable for .....
   a. Syrups
   b. Herbal mixture
   c. Tablets
   d. Bhasma
49. Angle of repose value in between 46 to 55 indicates flow property of herbal granules is .....
   a. Good
   b. Passable
   c. fairly passable
   d. Poor
50. For excellent flow property of herbal granules, Houser's ratio should be .....
   a. 1.35 -1.45
   b. 1.19 – 1. 25
   c. 1 -1.11
   d. 1.26 – 1.34
51. Cars index value 21 – 25% indicates flow property of granules .....
   a. Excellent
   b. Poor
   c. Good
   d. Passable
52. Liposomes are spherical structures with diameter.....................
   a. 0.01μm – 50 μm
   b. 0.01μm – 500 μm
   b. 0.01μm – 5000 μm
   c. 0.01μm – 1000 μm
53. Liposome phospholipids undergoes ....
   a. Oxidation
   b. Reduction
   c. Hydrolysis
   d. Both a and c
54. Liposomes can encapsulate
   a. Hydrophilic drugs
   b. Hydrophobic drugs
   c. Both a and b
   d. None of the above
55. Which of the following is NOT advantage of liposome?
   a. Bioavailability enhancement
   b. Short half life
   c. Solubility enhancement
   d. Programmed targeting

56. ....is widely used phospholipid in synthesis of herbal liposomes?
    a. Egg yolk
    b. Lecithin
    c. Milk
    d. None of the above

57. Which of the following is acute parameter in determination of circulation half life of liposomes?
    a. Vesicle size
    b. Phospholipid
    c. Active pharmaceutical ingredient
    d. Hydrophilic core

58. Intermediate sized unilaminar vesicles are prepared by ....
    a. Sonication
    b. Detergent analysis
    c. High pressure extrusion technique
    d. Both b and c

59. Liposomes enhance therapeutic activity of herbal extracts by ....
    a. Enhancement of target specificity of herbal extract
    b. Prevention of enzymatic degradation
    c. Enhancement of solubility of herbal extract
    d. All of the above

60. Liposomes are used specifically in treatment of ......
    a. Diabetes
    b. Cardiac disorders
    c. Cancer
    d. viral diseases

Answer Key

1.d	2. b	3. d	4. a	5. c	6. d	7. b	8.b	9. c	10. b
11. d	12. b	13. b	14. b	15. a	16. c	17. b	18. b	19. a	20. b
21. a	22. d	23. d	24. b	25. c	26. d	27. b	28. d	29. d	30. b
31. b	32. b	33. c	34. d	35. c	36. b	37. c	38. c	39. d	40. a
41.b	42. c	43. a	44. a	45. b	46. d	47. b	48. c	49. d	50. c
51. d	52. a	53. d	54. c	55. b	56. b	57. a	58. d	59. d	60. c

Unit 4

4.1 Evaluation of Drugs

4.1.1 ICH Guidelines for the Assessment of Herbal Drugs

Introduction

The International Council for Harmonisation of Technical Requirements for Pharmaceuticals for Human Use (ICH) is unique in bringing together the regulatory authorities and pharmaceutical industry to discuss scientific and technical aspects of drug registration. Since its inception in 1990, ICH has gradually evolved, to respond to the increasingly global face of drug development. ICH's mission is to achieve greater harmonisation worldwide to ensure that safe, effective, and high quality medicines are developed and registered in the most resource-efficient manner.

In November 2005, the ICH Steering Committee adopted a new codification system for ICH Guidelines. The purpose of this new codification is to ensure that the numbering / coding of ICH Guidelines is more logical, consistent and clear. Because the new system applies to existing as well as new ICH Guidelines a history box has been added to the beginning of all Guidelines to explain how the Guideline was developed and what is the latest version.

With the new codification revisions to an ICH Guideline are shown as (R1), (R2), (R3) depending on the number of revisions. Annexes or Addenda to Guidelines have now been incorporated into the core Guidelines and are indicated as revisions to the core Guideline (Example-., R1).

The ICH topics are divided into four categories and ICH topic codes are assigned according to these categories.

Q- Quality Guidelines

Harmonisation achievements in the Quality area include pivotal milestones such as the conduct of stability studies, defining relevant thresholds for impurities testing and a more flexible approach to pharmaceutical quality based on Good Manufacturing Practice (GMP) risk management.

Q1A - Q1F Stability

Q2 Analytical Validation

Q3A - Q3D Impurities

Q4 - Q4B Pharmacopoeias

Q5A - Q5E Quality of Biotechnological Products

Q6A- Q6B Specifications

Q7 Good Manufacturing Practice

Q8 Pharmaceutical Development

Q9 Quality Risk Management

Q10 Pharmaceutical Quality System

Q11 Development and Manufacture of Drug Substances

Q12 Lifecycle Management

S-Safety Guidelines

ICH has produced a comprehensive set of safety Guidelines to uncover potential risks like carcinogenicity, genotoxicity and reprotoxicity. A recent breakthrough has been a non-clinical testing strategy for assessing the QT interval prolongation liability: the single most important cause of drug withdrawals in recent years.

S1A - S1C Carcinogenicity Studies

S2 Genotoxicity Studies

S3A - S3B Toxicokinetics and Pharmacokinetics

S4 Toxicity Testing

S5 Reproductive Toxicology

S6 Biotechnological Products

S7A - S7B Pharmacology Studies

S8 Immunotoxicology Studies

S9 Nonclinical Evaluation for Anticancer Pharmaceuticals

S10 Photosafety Evaluation

S11 Nonclinical Safety Testing

E- Efficacy Guidelines

The work carried out by ICH under the Efficacy heading is concerned with the design, conduct, safety and reporting of clinical trials. It also covers novel types of medicines derived from biotechnological processes and the use of pharmacogenetics/genomics techniques to produce better targeted medicines.

E1 Clinical Safety for Drugs used in Long-Term Treatment

E2A - E2F Pharmacovigilance

E3 Clinical Study Reports

E4 Dose-Response Studies

E5 Ethnic Factors

E6 Good Clinical Practice

E7 Clinical Trials in Geriatric Population

E8 General Considerations for Clinical Trials

E9 Statistical Principles for Clinical Trials

E10 Choice of Control Group in Clinical Trials

E11 Clinical Trials in Pediatric Population

E12 Clinical Evaluation by Therapeutic Category

E14 Clinical Evaluation of QT

E15 Definitions in Pharmacogenetics / Pharmacogenomics

E16 Qualification of Genomic Biomarkers

E17 Multi-Regional Clinical Trials

E18 Genomic Sampling

M-Multidisciplinary Guidelines

Those are the cross-cutting topics which do not fit uniquely into one of the Quality, Safety and Efficacy categories. It includes the ICH medical terminology (MedDRA), the Common Technical Document (CTD) and the development of Electronic Standards for the Transfer of Regulatory Information (ESTRI).

M1 MedDRA Terminology

M2 Electronic Standards

M3 Nonclinical Safety Studies

M4 Common Technical Document

M5 Data Elements and Standards for Drug Dictionaries

M6 Gene Therapy

M7 Genotoxic Impurities

M8 Electronic Common Technical Document (eCTD)

M9 Biopharmaceutics Classification System-based Biowaivers

M10 Bioanalytical Method Validation

4.1.2 WHO Guidelines for the Assessment of Herbal Drugs

4.1.2.1 Introduction

Herbal medicines means: Finished, labelled medicinal products that contain as active ingredients, aerial or underground parts of plants, or other plant material, or combinations thereof, whether in the crude state or as plant preparations.

Plant material includes juices, gums, fatty oils, essential oils, and any other substances of this nature. Herbal medicines may contain excipients in addition to the active ingredients.

Medicines containing plant material combined with chemically defined active substances, including chemically defined, isolated constituents of plants, are not considered to be herbal medicines.

Exceptionally, in some countries herbal medicines may also contain, by tradition, natural organic or inorganic active ingredients which are not of plant origin.

The past decade has seen a significant increase in the use of herbal medicines. The objective of these guidelines is to define basic criteria for the evaluation of quality, safety and efficacy of herbal medicines and thereby to assist national regulatory authorities, scientific organizations and manufacturers to undertake an assessment of the documentation/submissions/dossiers in respect of such products.

As a general rule in this assessment, traditional experience means that long-term use as well as the medical, historical and ethnological background of those products shall be taken into account.

The definition of long-term use may vary according to the country but should be at least several decades.

Therefore, the assessment should take into account a description in the medical/ pharmaceutical literature or similar sources, or a documentation of knowledge on the application of an herbal medicine without a clearly defined time limitation.

Marketing authorizations for similar products should be taken into account.

Prolonged and apparently uneventful use of a substance usually offers testimony of its safety.

In a few instances, however, investigation of the potential toxicity of naturally occurring substances widely used as ingredients in these preparations has revealed previously unsuspected-potential for systematic toxicity, carcinogenicity and teratogenicity.

Regulatory authorities need to be quickly and reliably informed of these findings. They should also have the authority to respond promptly to such alerts, either by withdrawing or varying the licences of registered products containing suspect substances, or by rescheduling the substances to limit their use to medical prescription.

4.1.2.2 Assessment of Quality

Pharmaceutical assessment: This should cover all important aspects of the quality assessment of herbal medicines. It should be sufficient to make reference to a pharmacopoeia monograph if one exists. If no such monograph is available, a monograph must be supplied and should be set out as in an official pharmacopoeia. All procedures should be in accordance with good manufacturing practices.

- ***Crude plant material:*** The botanical definition, including genus, species and authority, should be given to ensure correct identification of a plant. A definition and description of the part of the plant from which the medicine is made (Example-leaf, flower, root) should be provided, together with an indication of whether fresh, dried or traditionally processed material is used.

  The active and characteristic constituents should be specified and, if possible, content limits should be defined.

  Foreign matter, impurities and microbial content should be defined or limited.

Voucher specimens, representing each lot of plant material processed, should be authenticated by a qualified botanist and should be stored for at least a 10-year period. A lot number should be assigned and this should appear on the product label.

- ***Plant preparations:*** Plant preparations include comminuted or powdered plant materials, extracts, tinctures, fatty or essential oils, expressed juices and preparations whose production involves fractionation, purification or concentration. The manufacturing procedure should be described in detail. If other substances are added during manufacture in order to adjust the plant preparation to a certain level of active or characteristic constituents or for any other purpose, the added substances should be mentioned in the manufacturing procedures.

  A method for identification and, where possible, assay of the plant preparation should be added. If identification of an active principle is not possible, it should be sufficient to identify a characteristic substance or mixture of substances (Example- "chromatographic fingerprint") to ensure consistent quality of the preparation.

- ***Finished product:*** The manufacturing procedure and formula, including the amount of excipients, should be described in detail. A finished product specification should be defined. A method of identification and, where possible, quantification of the plant material in the finished product should be defined. If the identification of an active principle is not possible, it should be sufficient to identify a characteristic substance or mixture of substances (Example- "chromatographic fingerprint") to ensure consistent quality of the product. The finished product should comply with general requirements for particular dosage forms.

  For imported finished products, confirmation of the regulatory status in the country of origin should be required. The WHO Certification Scheme on the Quality of Pharmaceutical Products Moving in International Commerce should be applied.

  Stability: The physical and chemical stability of the product in the container in which it is to be marketed should be tested under defined storage conditions and the shelflife should be established.

4.1.2.3 Assessment of Safety

This should cover all relevant aspects of the safety assessment of a medicinal product. A guiding principle should be that, if the product has been traditionally used without demonstrated harm, no specific restrictive regulatory action should be undertaken unless new evidence demands a revised risk–benefit assessment.

A review of the relevant literature should be provided with original articles or references to the original articles. If official monograph/review results exist, reference can be made to them.

However, although long term use without any evidence of risk may indicate that a medicine is harmless, it is not always certain how far one can rely solely on long-term usage to provide assurance of innocuity in the light of concern expressed in recent years over the long-term hazards of some herbal medicines.

Reported side-effects should be documented according to normal pharmacovigilance practices.

Toxicological studies: Toxicological studies, if available, should be part of the assessment. Literature should be indicated as above.

Documentation of safety based on experience: As a basic rule, documentation of a long period of use should be taken into consideration when assessing safety. This means that, when there are no detailed toxicological studies, documented experience of long-term use without evidence of safety problems should form the basis of the risk assessment.

However, even in cases of drugs used over a long period, chronic toxicological risks may have occurred but may not have been recognized.

The period of use, the health disorders treated, the number of users and the countries with experience should be specified.

If a toxicological risk is known, toxicity data must be submitted.

The assessment of risk, whether independent of dose or related to dose, should be documented. In the latter case, the dosage specification must be an important part of the risk assessment.

An explanation of the risks should be given, if possible. Potential for misuse, abuse or dependence must be documented. If long-term traditional use cannot be documented or there are doubts on safety, toxicity data should be submitted.

4.1.2.4 Assessment of Efficacy

This should cover all important aspects of efficacy assessment. A review of the relevant literature should be carried out and copies provided of the original articles or proper references made to them.

Research studies, if they exist, should be taken into account.

The pharmacological and clinical effects of the active ingredients and, if known, their constituents with therapeutic activity should be specified or described.

Evidence required supportingindications. The indication(s) for the use of the medicine should be specified. In the case of traditional medicines, the requirements for proof of efficacy should depend on the kind of indication.

For treatment of minor disorders and for non-specific indications, some relaxation in requirements for proof of efficacy may be justified, taking into account the extent of traditional use.

The same considerations may apply to prophylactic use. Individual experiences recorded in reports from physicians, traditional health practitioners or treated patients should be taken into account. Where traditional use has not been established, appropriate clinical evidence should be required.

Combination products: As many herbal remedies consist of a combination of several active ingredients, and as experience of the use of traditional remedies is often based on combination products, assessment should differentiate between old and new combination products.

Identical requirements for the assessment of old and new combinations would result in inappropriate assessment of certain traditional medicines.

In the case of traditionally used combination products, the documentation of traditional use (such as classical texts of Ayurveda, traditional Chinese medicine, Unani, Siddha) and experience may serve as evidence of efficacy.

An explanation of a new combination of well-known substances, including effective dose ranges and compatibility, should be required in addition to the documentation of traditional knowledge of each single ingredient. Each active ingredient must contribute to the efficacy of the medicine. Clinical studies may be required to justify the efficacy of a new ingredient and its positive effect on the total combination.

Intended use Product information for the consumer

Product labels and package inserts should be understandable to the consumer or patient. The package information should include all necessary information on the proper use of the product. The following elements of information will usually suffice:

- Name of the product ¨
- Quantitative list of active ingredient(s) ¨
- Dosage form ¨
- Indications ÿ dosage (if appropriate, specified for children and the elderly) general guidelines for methodologies on research and evaluation of traditional medicine
- Mode of administration
- Duration of use
- Major adverse effects, if any
- dosage information
- Contraindications, warnings, precautions and major drug interactions
- Use during pregnancy and lactation
- Expiry date
- Lot number
- Holder of the marketing authorization.

Identification of the active ingredient(s) by the Latin botanical name, in addition to the common name in the language of preference of the national regulatory authority, is recommended. Sometimes not all information that is ideally required may be available, so drug regulatory authorities should determine their minimal requirements.

Promotion Advertisements and other promotional material directed to health personnel and the general public should be fully consistent with the approved package information.

4.1.2.5 Utilization of these Guidelines

These guidelines for the assessment of herbal medicines are intended to facilitate the work of regulatory authorities, scientific bodies and industry in the development, assessment and registration of such products. The assessment should reflect the scientific knowledge gathered in that field. Such assessment could be the basis for future classification of herbal medicines in different parts of the world. Other types of traditional medicines in addition to herbal products may be assessed in a similar way. The effective regulation and control of herbal medicines moving in international commerce also requires close liaison between national institutions that are able to keep under regular review all aspects of production and use of herbal medicines, as well as to conduct or sponsor evaluative studies of their efficacy, toxicity, safety, acceptability, cost and relative value.

Preliminary evaluation	Sampling, Foreign matter determination, Determination of total fiber
Morphological evaluation	Qualitative evaluation of color, odor and taste, size, shape, extra features etc
Microscopical evaluation:	➢ Qualitative microscopy: histological evaluation of types and arrangements of tissues ➢ Quantitative microscopy: o Leaf constant: assessment of palisade ratio, vein-islet, vein termination, stomatal index, stomatal number o Lycopodium spore method ➢ Powder microscopy
Physical Qualitative evaluation	Solubility, refractive index, optical rotation, melting point, boiling point, density, viscosity, chromatographic and spectroscopic evaluation
Physical quantitative or Physicochemical evaluation	Ash value, extractive value, moisture content, volatile oil determination
Chemical evaluation	➢ Qualitative chemical evaluation: to detect different classes of phytochemicals ➢ Quantitative chemical evaluation: determination of phytochemicals, assay
WHO Specific Parameters	Swelling index, Foam index, Hemolytic index, Bitterness value , Total tannin value
Biological evaluation	
Toxicological evaluation	Microbial load determination, Aflatoxin detection, Pesticide residue determination, Radioactive contamination, Heavy metal detection
Pharmacological evaluation	In-vivo, ex-vivo evaluation (Animal, animal organ or tissue activities)
Analytical evaluation	Chromatographic (TLC, Paper, HPTLC, HPLC and GC data) and spectroscopic evaluation
Along with above parameters there is need to evaluate herbal formulation for specific pharmaceutical parameters, such as: tablet: weight variation, friability, disintegration, and dissolution.	

4.2 Stability Testing of Herbal Drugs

Definition	The test, which involves examining for and potency at suitable time intervals, is conducted for a period corresponding to the normal time that the product is likely to remain in stock or in use.
Current status	➢ In recent years, the pharmaceutical dosage forms are becoming mire and more complex and diverse. Many novel dosage forms and drug targeting systems have been introduced. Hence, designing of stability testing protocol for a particular product has become much difficult. In addition, finding a right approach for estimating shelf life has become challenging. ➢ Traditionally, multi temperature accelerated studies and Arrhenius approach were used for determination of shelf life. But, this is not applicable in all the situations. It is applicable only in cases where the drug degradation is reasonable and temperature dependant and in cases where the rate and order of reaction can determine.

Contd....

<table>
<tr><td></td><td>➢ Accelerating the decomposition process and extrapolating the result to normal storage conditions may make a prediction of the life of the product.</td></tr>
<tr><td>Purpose of stability testing</td><td>Stability testing of pharmaceutical products is done for the following purposes
I. To ensure the efficacy, safety and quality of active drug substance and dosage forms.
II. To establish shelf life or expiration period and to support label claims.</td></tr>
<tr><td>Stability components</td><td>The stability of a product is made up of two distinct components
1. The inherent stability of the contents of the immediate container. This refers to the stability of the contents when stored in an inert, impermeable container which it does not interact and which protects it completely from the ambient atmosphere.
2. The compatibility between the contents and the immediate container. This includes all interactions between the contents and container, such interactions may be any or all of the following:
a. Sorption of constituents of the contents by the container.
b. Leaching of constituents of the container into the contents.
c. Adverse effects on the container such as corrosion.
Contents-container compatibility also includes the effectiveness of the container in protecting the contents from atmospheric oxygen and/or water vapors and in retaining water and other volatile constituents of products.</td></tr>
<tr><td>Types of changes occur on storage:-</td><td><table><tr><td>Contents
➢ Physical: viscosity, texture,colour, odour, pH, loss of volatile constituents, uptake of water, oxygen or carbon dioxide.
➢ Chemical: Degradation of active constituents, Interaction between constituents, Loss of constituents by sorption by container.
➢ Microbiological: Loss of antimicrobial preservative efficacy, Microbial spoilage</td><td>Container
➢ Leakage
➢ Corrosion
➢ Stress cracking</td></tr></table></td></tr>
<tr><td>Specific objectives of stability testing</td><td>• While it is that the overall purpose of any stability test is to determine whether the contents are stable and the contents and the immediate container are compatible, the specific purpose of a particular test can often be more specifically defied. If the product under test is a new product, then it is necessary to carry out a full programme of stability and compatibility testing. In many instances, however, stability tests are conducted on modifications of products, the stability and container compatibility of which are already known. Thus, test may be required to investigate the effect on product stability of, for
1. A modification of the formula
2. A modification of the manufacturing process
3. A change in the specification of a raw material
4. A raw material from a new source of supply
5. A change to the immediate container
6. An immediate container from a new manufacturer
• When any such change has been made, it is necessary to conduct stability and compatibility tests on the modified product.</td></tr>
</table>

Contd....

Herbal Poduct stability	The maintenance of herbal product quality during storage is critical for guaranteeing therapeutic activity. Stability testing is used to evaluate how herbal products retain their properties under specified storage conditions stressed by heat, moisture, light, oxygen, various physical and chemical conditions (Example- vibration or freezing), and container-related factors. Herbal products are produced in various dosage forms (Example- tablets, powders, or liquids for oral administration or as creams for external application), and thus, stability testing of various dosage forms requires appropriate methods. The stabilities of finished herbal products can be determined by testing for properties susceptible to storage conditions and include physical (organoleptic characteristics, physical condition, particle size, etc.), chemical (assays of active components, pH, identification, etc.), microbial, and toxicological properties. These properties can all affect the qualities, safeties, or the efficacies of herbal products, and thus, the shelf lives of herbal products should be determined by stability testing .Furthermore, different stability protocols are used in different countries as herbal products are generally developed to meet national regulations. Global harmonization of stability testing has been recently emphasized in the context of herbal drug development, but the adoption of international standards can only be achieved by sharing national experiences and information
Mechanisms involved in change product	Loss of activity, Change in concentration of active component, Alteration in bioavaibility, Loss of content uniformity, Loss of elegance, Formation of toxic degradation product, Loss of packaging integrity.
Predictable changes in Herbal medicinal Product	Following predictable changes may occurs in herbal medicinal product during storage and in shelf life determination: Hydrolysis, Oxidation, Racemization, Geometric isomerization, Temperature, Moisture and Light

Storage conditions and sampling times for stability testing

Conditions	Sampling times	Parameters studied at each conditions
Long term testing $25^0C+2^0C/60\%RH+5\%RH$	0, 3, 6, 9, 12, 18, 24, 36, 48, 60 months	Organoleptic properties Assay pH Viscosity Particle size Weight loss
Accelerated testing $40^0C+2^0C/75\%RH+5\%RH$	3, 6 months	
Intermediate testing $30^0C+2^0C/60\%RH+5\%RH$	3, 6, 9, 12 months	
Freeze thaw stability	3 cycles over 24 hour each	

Types of stability and conditions required throughout the shelf life

Chemical	Each active ingredient retains its chemical integrity and labeled potency, within specified limits.
Physical	The original physical properties, including appearance, palatability, uniformity, dissolution and suspendability are retained.
Microbiological	Sterility or resistance to microbial growth is retained according to the specified requirement.
Therapeutic	The therapeutic effect remains unchanged.
Toxicological	No significant increase in toxicity occurs.

- These testing parameters and methods for finished herbal products are detailed in the guidelines and regulations issued by 5 global authorities and 15 countries, that is, the Association of Southeast Asian Nations (ASEAN), the Eurasian Economic Commission (EEC), the European Medicines Agency (EMA), the International Council for Harmonisation of Technical Requirements for Pharmaceuticals for Human Use (ICH), the World Health Organization (WHO), Australia, Brazil, Canada, China, Egypt, Hong Kong, India, Japan, Kenya, Republic of Korea, the Philippines, Qatar, Switzerland, USA, and Zambia.
- Physical, chemical, and biological stability tests were compared between different dosage forms, and the testing conditions (temperature and relative humidity) used for long-term, accelerated, or intermediate testing were included in the guidelines and regulations.
- Comparisons of global regulations and guidelines addressing stability testing are fundamental for the international harmonization of herbal product quality assessments.

Storage conditions used for long-term stability testing

Global community	Testing period (container type)	Storage conditions (temperature/relative humidity, RH)		
		In ambient storage	In refrigerator	In freezer
ASEAN	0, 3, 6, 9, 12, 18, 24 months, and annually thereafter	30°C ± 2°C/75% RH ± 5% RH (moisture-permeable container[1]) 30°C ± 2°C (moisture-impermeable container[2])	5°C ± 3°C	—
ICH	12 months (general container)	25°C ± 2°C/60% RH ± 5% RH or 30°C ± 2°C/65% RH ± 5% RH	5°C ± 3°C	−20°C ± 5°C
	12 months (semipermeable container)	25°C ± 2°C/40% RH ± 5% RH or 30°C ± 2°C/35% RH ± 5% RH	—	—
WHO	6 or 12 months (general case)	25°C ± 2°C/60% RH ± 5% RH or 30°C ± 2°C/65% RH ± 5% RH or 30°C ± 2°C/75% RH ± 5% RH	5°C ± 3°C	−20°C ± 5°C
	6 or 12 months (semipermeable case)	25°C ± 2°C/40% RH ± 5% RH or 30°C ± 2°C/35% RH ± 5% RH	—	—

Storage conditions used for accelerated stability testing

Global community	Testing period (container type)	Storage condition (temperature/relative humidity, RH)		
		In ambient storage	In refrigerator	In freezer
ASEAN	0, 3, and 6 months (including the initial and final time points)	40°C ± 2°C/75% RH ± 5% RH	25°C ± 2°C/60% RH ± 5% RH	—

Contd....

Global community	Testing period (container type)	Storage condition (temperature/relative humidity, RH)		
		In ambient storage	In refrigerator	In freezer
ICH	6 months (general container)	40°C ± 2°C/75% RH ± 5% RH	25°C ± 2°C/60% RH ± 5% RH	—
	6 months (semipermeable container)	40°C ± 2°C/not more than 25% RH	—	
WHO	6 months (general case)	40°C ± 2°C/75% RH ± 5% RH	25°C ± 2°C/60% RH ± 5% RH or 30°C ± 2°C/65% RH ± 5% RH or 30°C ± 2°C/75% RH ± 5% RH	—
	6 months (semipermeable case)	40°C ± 2°C/not more than 25% RH	—	—

Storage conditions used for intermediate stability testing

Global community	Testing period (container type)	Storage condition (temperature/relative humidity, RH)
ICH	6 months (general container)	30°C ± 2°C/65% RH ± 5% RH
	6 months (semipermeable container)	30°C ± 2°C/65% RH ± 5% RH
WHO	6 months (general case)	30°C ± 2°C/65% RH ± 5% RH
	6 months (semipermeable case)	30°C ± 2°C/35% RH ± 5% RH

4.3 Patenting and Regulatory Requirements of Natural Products

4.3.1 Intellectual Property Rights (IPR)

IPR are legal rights to intellectual creations of the mind like inventions, artistic works, symbols, names, images, and designs used in commerce.

History:

- The need for a system to protect IP internationally arose when foreign exhibitors refused to attend an International Exhibition of Inventions in Vienna in 1873 because they were afraid that their ideas would be stolen and exploited commercially in other countries.
- This led to the creation of the Paris Convention for the Protection of Industrial Property of 1883. The Paris Convention was the first major international treaty designed to help the people of one country obtain protection in other countries for their intellectual creations, in the form of industrial property rights.
- In 1886, copyright entered the international arena with the Berne Convention for the Protection of Literary and Artistic Works. The aim of this Convention was to help nationals

of its Member States obtain international protection of their right to control, and receive payment for, the use of literary and artistic works.

- Both the Paris Convention and the Berne Convention set up International Bureaus to carry out administrative tasks, such as organizing meetings of the Member States.
- In 1893, these two small bureaus united to form an international organization called the United International Bureaus for the Protection of Intellectual Property – best known by its French acronym, BIRPI.
- Based in Berne, Switzerland, with a staff of seven, BIRPI was the predecessor of what is today known as the World Intellectual Property Organization or WIPO.

WIPO is a specialized agency of the UN, with a mandate to administer IP matters recognized by the UN Member States. There are about 21 international treaties in the field of intellectual property, which are administered by WIPO.There was thus a need for harmonization and predictability for disputes to be settled more systematically. The World Trade Organization (WTO) Agreement on Trade-Related Aspects of Intellectual Property Rights (TRIPS Agreement) came into force in 1995, brought with it a new era in the multilateral protection and enforcement of IP rights.

Thus, IPR matters to everyone and it involves following main types of IPs:

- ***Patent***: It is protection to one's invention (novel, non-obviousness and utility) for technological, economical advances as well as promotion to creativity with award of solely benefits. A patent is a set of exclusive rights granted by a state to a person for a fixed period of time in exchange for the regulated, public disclosure of certain details of a device, method, process or composition of matter (substance) known as an invention which is new, inventive and useful. *Patents are of three types* :
    - ***Utility patents:*** which relate to a new or improved machine, article of manufacture, a composition of matter, or a process.
    - ***Design patents:*** which relate to manufacturing of new, useful, and ornamental or aesthetic article.
    - ***Plant patents:*** which relate to a new asexually reproducible variety of plant.
- ***Copyright:*** These are legal rights granted to a work of authorship or creator Example- poems, theses, plays and other literary works, motion pictures, choreography, musical compositions, sound recordings, paintings, drawings, sculptures, photographs, computer software, radio and television broadcasts, and industrial designs.

  Copyright does not cover ideas and information themselves, only the form or manner in which they are expressed.

  Several exclusive rights typically attach to the holder of a copyright:
    - to produce copies or reproductions of the work and to sell those copies (including, typically, electronic copies)
    - to import or export the work
    - to create derivative works (works that adapt the original work)
    - to perform or display the work publicly

- to sell or cede these rights to others
- to transmit or display by radio or video

➢ ***Industrial design***: These are eye appealing designs of useful articles (ornamental or aesthetic) despite of distinctive or functional necessity Example- teapot

➢ ***Trademark:*** It is distinctive and deceptive sign to distinguish goods and services Example- Star of Mercedes, logo of university, brand names

- ™ (for an unregistered trade mark to promote or brand goods)
- ℠ (for an unregistered service mark to promote or brand services)
- ® (for a registered trademark)

A trademark is typically a name, word, phrase, logo, symbol, design, image, or a combination of these elements. There is also a range of non-conventional trademarks comprising marks which do not fall into these standard categories, such as those based on colour, smell, or sound (like jingles). A trademark cannot be offensive.

➢ ***Trade secret***: A trade secret is information that: is not generally known to the public. It confers some sort of economic benefit on its holder (where this benefit must derive specifically from its not being generally known, not just from the value of the information itself); is the subject of reasonable efforts to maintain its secrecy. Trade secrets are not protected by law in the same manner as trademarks or patents. Instead, trade secrets are protected under state laws

➢ ***Geographical indication***: indication and appellation of origin of goods and service Example- made in India, Champagne.

Here we will see more details on patents.

4.3.1.1 Patent

A patent is an intellectual property relating to inventions and is the grant of exclusive right, for limited period, provided by the Government to the patentee, in exchange of full disclosure of his invention, for excluding others, from making, using, selling, importing the patented product or process producing that product for those purposes. An invention must meet the following three criteria to be eligible for grant of patent:

(i) ***Novelty:*** An invention will be considered novel, a) if it does not form the state of the art or has not been described orally and b) if it has not been published or not used before the date of filing the patent application

(ii) ***Inventiveness (Non-obviousness)***: The invention is not obvious to a person skilled in the art in the light of the prior publication/knowledge/docu-ment.

(iii) ***Usefulness***: An invention must possess industrial applicability for the grant of patent.

What can be patented?

Anything which is new, non-obvious and useful such as Process, product (Machine, Article of manufacture, Composition of matter) and Improvement of any of the process or product can be patented in every country.

What cannot be patented in India?

As per section-3of Indian Patent's Act, 1970 following are exceptions to patent:

- Section 3 (a): Frivolous inventions
- Section 3 (b): Inventions which are contrary to Law or Mortality or injurious to public health
- Section 3 (c): Mere discovery of a scientific principle or formulation of an abstract theory.
- Section 3 (d): The mere discovery of a new form of a known substance which does not result in the enhancement of the known efficacy of that substance or the mere discovery of any new property or new use for a known substance or of the mere use of a known process, machine or apparatus unless such known process results in a new product or employs at least one new reactant is not an invention.
- Section 3 (e): A substance obtained by a mere admixture resulting only in the aggregation of the properties of the components thereof or a process for producing such substance is not an invention.
- Section 3 (f): Mere arrangement or re-arrangement of known devices
- Section 3 (h): Method of agriculture or horticulture
- Section 3 (i): Any process for the medicinal, surgical, curative, prophylactic diagnostic therapeutic or other treatment of human being or any process for a similar treatment of animals to render them free of disease or to increase their economic value or that of their products is not patentable
- Section 3 (j): Plants and animals in whole or any part thereof other than micro-organisms but including seeds, varieties and species and essentially biological processes for production or propagation of plants and animals are not inventions.
- Section 3 (k): A mathematical or business method or a computer program per se or algorithms are not inventions and hence not patentable.
- Section 3 (l): A literary, dramatic, musical or artistic work or any other aesthetic creation whatsoever including cinematographic works and television productions is not patentable.
- Section 3 (m): A mere scheme or rule or method of performing mental act or method of playing game is not patentable.
- Section 3 (n): A presentation of information is not patentable.
- Section 3 (o) Topography of integrated circuits is not patentable.
- Section 3 (p) An invention which in effect, is traditional knowledge or which is an aggregation or duplication of known properties of traditionally known component or components is not patentable.

Who may apply for patent?

- A patent may be applied by the name(s) of the actual inventor(s).
- For ordinary patent: any person residential to country, claiming to be first inventor
- For patent of addition: applicant of original patent
- For convention application: Patent applicant
- PCT application: same as of ordinary patent applicant

Types of Patent

Ordinary Application

The first application for patent filed in the Patent Office without claiming priority from any application or without any reference to any other application under process in the Patent office is called an ordinary application.

Convention Application

When an applicant files a patent application, claiming a priority date based on the same or substantially similar application filed in one or more of the convention countries, it is called a convention application. To get a convention status, an applicant should file the application before any of the patent offices within 12 months from the date of first application in the convention country.

Patent of Addition

Patent of addition is an application made for a patent in respect of any improvement or modification of an invention described or disclosed in the complete specification already applied for or has a patent. In order to be patentable an improvement, should be something more than a mere workshop improvement and must independently satisfy the test of invention. The major benefit is the exemption of renewal fee so long as the main patent is renewed. A patent of addition lapses with the cessation of the main patent.

Divisional Application

A divisional application is one which has been "divided" from an existing application. The applicant, at any time before the grant of a patent can file a further application, if he so desires or if an objection is raised by the examiner on the ground that the claims disclosed in the complete specification relates to more than one invention. A divisional application can only contain subject matter in the application from which it is divided (its parent), but retains the filing and priority date of that parent. A divisional application is useful if a unity of invention objection is issued, in which case the second invention can be protected as a divisional application.

PCT- International Application

The Patent Cooperation Treaty or PCT is an international agreement for filing patent applications. PCT- international application should be filed within 12 months of priority date in Form PCT/RO/101. World intellectual property organization Geneva forwards your application to respective patent offices. ISR (International Search Report), IPER (International Preliminary Examination Report which is optional) are conducted before entering national phase.

PCT- National Application

The PCT-national phase must follow the international phase. The applicant must individually 'enter into the national phase'. i.e. file a national phase application in each county he wishes to enter. The applicant can enter the national phase in up to 138 countries within 30-31 months (depends on the laws of the designated countries) from the international filing date or priority date (whichever is earlier). If the applicant does not enter the national phase within the prescribed time limit, the international application loses its effect in the designated or elected states.

After 30 months from the filing date of the PCT-international application or from the earliest priority date of the application if a priority is claimed, the international phase ends and the international application enters in national and regional phase. However, there is nothing called as a 'world patent'. The PCT application does not provide for the grant of an international patent, it simply provides a streamlined process for the patent application process in many countries at the same time. Some of the benefits of the system are: It simplifies the process of filing patent applications i.e., an applicant can file a single international patent application in one language with one receiving patent office in order to simultaneously seek protection for an invention in up to 138 countries throughout the world. It provides internationally recognized priority date, which has an effect in each of the countries designated. Delays the expenses associated with applying for patent protection in various countries. PCT gives 30 to 31 months time to enter into various countries from the priority date or international filing date whichever is earlier unlike the convention method which gives only 12 months time to file for a patent application in the country of interest from the priority date. Hence, the PCT route allows the inventor more time to assess the commercial viability of his/her invention

It provides an international search report. The results of this search are very valuable to the applicant. They allow the applicant to make more informed choices early in the patent process, and to amend the application to deal with any conflicting material, before the major expenses of the national phase of the patent process begin. Provides an option of an International Preliminary Examination Report that is forwarded to the elected Offices and the applicant, the report containing an opinion as to whether the claimed invention meets certain international criteria for paten-tability. These reports give the applicant a fair idea about the patentability of the invention before incurring charges for filing and prosecution in each individual country.

4.3.2 Patenting aspects of Traditional Knowledge and Natural Products

- The traditional knowledge (TK) can be said as the knowledge of practice and the skills developed or sustained and passed from generation to generation within a community which forms a part of its cultural or spiritual identity often.
- Innovations based on TK may benefit from patent, trademark, and geographical indication protection, or be protected as a trade secret or confidential information.
- But successful documentation of a traditional knowledge requires enactment of new legislations to cope up issues in documentation of indigenous products and the traditional knowledge as such products being patented in other countries and this finally leads to **biopiracy** of traditional knowledge by other countries.

Various aspects of TK Patenting

- **Defensive protection**: From the example of turmeric and neem, it is decided that patent applicants should in some way have to disclose TK (and genetic resources) used in the claimed invention
- **Equitable benefit-sharing**: share the benefits arising from the commercialization of this TK-based drug.

- **Prior informed consent (PIC):** TK holders should be fully consulted before their knowledge is accessed or used by third parties
- **Unfair competition and trade practices laws:** These allow for action to be taken against false or misleading claims that a product is authentically indigenous, or has been produced or endorsed by, or otherwise associated with, a particular traditional community.
- **The law of confidentiality and trade secrets:** This has been used to protect non-disclosed TK, including secret and sacred TK.
- **Customary laws and practices:** Define custodial rights and obligations over TK, including obligations to guard it against misuse or improper disclosure; they may determine how TK is to be used, how benefits should be shared, and how disputes are to be settled, as well as many other aspects of the preservation, use and exercise of knowledge.
- **Convention on Biological diversity (CBD) Law of Costa Rica in 1993:** Sovereign rights over biological resources and communities rights over their knowledge also providing sharing of benefits arising from the utilization of the genetic resources.
- **FAO 1945:** Agriculture of the Food and Agriculture Organization adapted Farmer's right law in 1989
- **UPOV1961:** International Union for the Protection of New Varieties of Plants
- **Sui generis law, 2002:** The sui generis regime of Peru was established by Law No. 27, 811 of 2002, whose objectives are to protect TK, to promote fair and equitable distribution of benefits, to ensure that the use of the knowledge takes place with the prior informed consent of the indigenous peoples, and to prevent misappropriation. Protection is afforded to collective knowledge of indigenous peoples associated to biological resources. The law grants indigenous peoples the right to consent to the use of TK. The law also foresees the payment of equitable compensation for the use of certain types of TK into a national Fund for Indigenous Development or directly to the TK holders. For instance,
- **UNCCD:** UN Convention to Combat Desertification
- **Traditional Knowledge Digital Library project (TKDL) 2001:** An initiative of several Indian Government agencies for documentation of traditional medicinal knowledge
- **Traditional Knowledge Resource Classification (TKRC):** Classification system for the purpose of systematic arrangement, dissemination and retrieval.

Structure of TKRC

The TKRC is mainly divided into the following sections: A – Ayurveda B – Unani C – Siddha Y – Yoga

Section A ie Ayurveda is divided into the following classes:

- 01 – Pharmaceutical preparations (Kalpana)
- 02 – Personal Hygiene Preparations
- 03 – Dietary (Food / Food stuff or Beverages)
- 04 – Biocides, Fumigatives (Dhupana, Krimighna)

The Pharmaceutical preparations are divided into following sub-classes based on the material used.

- 01A – Based on Plants (Audbhida)
- 01B – Based on Animals (Jangama)
- 01C – Based on Minerals (Parthiva)
- 01D – Characterised by Diseases (Roga)
- 01E – Characterised by Actions (Karma)
- 01F – Mode of Administration
- 01G – Miscellaneous

Thus, the sub-class A01A represents Pharmaceutical preparations (Kalpana) based on plants (Audbhida) Group A01A-1/00 is for Whole Medicinal Plants (Audbhida) There are group codes and subgroup codes for the rest of the Sub Classes. Similarly, classification has been developed for Unani, Siddha and Yoga systems.

Example: A01A-1/1326 is the TKRC code for the plant Nigella sativa. Nigella sativa belongs to the family Ranunculaceae which is classified under the sub-group, A61K 36/71 in the IPC classification. Therefore, the TKRC code A01A-1/326 is linked to A61K 36/71 and Nigella sativa can in turn be searched using either of the above codes.

4.3.3 Bioprospecting and Biopiracy

- Bioprospecting can be defined as the systematic search for and development of new sources of chemical compounds, genes, micro-organisms, macro-organisms, and other valuable products from nature. So, in brief, bioprospecting means looking for ways to commercialize biodiversity.
- Lately, exploration and research on indigenous knowledge related to the utilization and management of biological resources has also been included into the concept of bioprospecting.
- Bioprospecting should be regulated, both at national and international level, based on the principles of the :Convention on Biological Diversity (CBD) conservation of biodiversity, sustainable use of its components and fair and equitable sharing of the benefits arising out of the utilization of genetic resources.
    - A comprehensive bioprospecting policy should contain at least the following, complementary elements:
    - Legislation and regulation for access to genetic resources based on prior informed consent, fair and equitable sharing of the benefits, capacity building, financing, assessment or situation analysis of biodiversity, participation in considering both stakeholders' interests and safeguardsing weaker parties and or Monitoring and evaluation
    - Bioprospecting may involve biopiracy which means the exploitative appropriation of indigenous forms of knowledge by commercial factors, and can include the patenting of already widely used natural resources, such as plant varieties, by commercial entities.

- 'Biopiracy' is being used to describe the exploitation and appropriation of biological and genetic resources and/or associated (traditional) knowledge without the approval or consent of their holders, and without adequate compensation.

4.3.4 Biopiracy Case

Neem

Over 60 patents have been granted in the US and Europe relating to neem so far. Neem extracts can be used against hundreds of pests and fungal diseases that attack food crops; the oil extracted from its seeds can be used to cure cold and flu; and mixed in soap, it provides relief from malaria, skin diseases and even meningitis.

In 1994, European Patent Office (EPO) granted a patent (EPO patent No.436257) to the US Corporation W.R. Grace Company and US Department of Agriculture for a method for controlling fungi on plants by the aid of hydrophobic extracted Neem oil. In 1995, a group of international NGOs and representatives of Indian farmers filed legal opposition against the patent. They submitted evidence that the fungicidal effect of extracts of Neem seeds had been known and used for centuries in Indian agriculture to protect crops, and therefore, was unpatentable.The European Patent Office revoked the same patent in Europe based on India's petition, but the U.S. patent remains valid. [Because in US, use of invention outside the US does not destroy novelty: Knowledge of neem is from India but there is the novelty of the invention is that it increases the shelf life of the neem pesticide].

Curcuma

- The US Patent (No. 5,401,504) has been given to the healing properties of turmeric, known for centuries to Indians. On March 28, 1995 two researchers from the University of Mississippi Medical Center acquired a patent (US Patent No. 5,401 ,504) on the process of using turmeric as a wound healing agent in the US.65
- In 1996, the Council of Scientific and Industrial Research of India (CSIR) requested that the patent be revoked, on the basis that turmeric powder is widely known and used in India for its wound healing properties, and that a great deal of research has been carried out by Indian scientists that confirms the existence of these properties.
- Eventually, the patent was indeed revoked on the basis of lack of novelty. CSIR succeed in challenging the patent, because it was able to provide relevant scientific literature, including an ancient Sanskrit text and a paper published in 1953 in the Journal of the Indian Medical Association.
- This event is frequently billed as the first case of successfully reversing a biopiracy patent.

4.3.5 Farmer's Right

The Protection of Plant Variety and Farmers Right Act, 2001 (PPVFR Act) is an Act of the Parliament of India that was enacted to provide to grant intellectual property rights as effective system for protection of plant varieties, the rights of farmers and plant breeders, and to encourage the development and cultivation of new varieties of plants. The period of protection for field crops is 15 years and for trees and vines is 18 years and for notified varieties it is 15 years from the date of notification under section 5 of Seeds Act, 1966. The International Union for the Protection of New Varieties of Plants or UPOV is an intergovernmental organization with headquarters in Geneva, Switzerland. The UPOV Convention was adopted in 1961 as a result of the Diplomatic Conferences held in Paris in 1957 and 1961. The UPOV Convention entered into force in 1968 with the ratification of Germany, the Netherlands and the United Kingdom. The UPOV Convention was amended in 1972, 1978 and 1991. UPOV, which continues to be the only internationally harmonized, effective sui generis system of plant variety protection, is continuing to expand.In UPOV, rights are granted only to the breeder, which in today's context means the seed companies. There is no concept of Farmers' Rights in the UPOV (International Union for the Protection of New Varieties of Plants) system, particularly under 1991 Act. The PPVFR Act provides a balance between breeder's right and farmer's right, the provisions for compulsory licensing, researcher's rights, and exclusion of certain varieties from registration.

Definition

Farmers' Rights consist of the customary rights of farmers to save, use, exchange and sell farm-saved seed and propagating material, their rights to be recognized, rewarded and supported for their contribution to the global pool of genetic resources as well as to the development of commercial varieties of plants, and to participate in decision making on issues related to crop genetic resources.

When did the concept of *Farmers' Rights* first appear?

The idea of Farmers' Rights came up in the early 1980s as a countermove to the increased demand for plant breeders' rights, as voiced in international negotiations. The purpose was to draw attention to the unremunerated innovations of farmers that were seen as the foundation of all modern plant breeding. The concept was first brought up in international negotiations in 1986.

Why Farmers' Rights matter?

- Plant genetic diversity is probably more important for farming than any other environmental factor, simply because it is the factor that enables adaptation to changing environmental conditions such as plant diseases and climate change.
- Thus, as a precondition for the maintenance of this diversity, Farmers' Rights are crucial for ensuring present and future food security in general, and in the fight against rural poverty in particular.
- Farmers' Rights are a precondition for the maintenance of crop genetic diversity, which is the basis of all food and agriculture production in the world.

Basically, realizing Farmers' Rights means enabling farmers to maintain and develop crop genetic resources as they have done since the dawn of agriculture, and recognizing and rewarding them for this indispensable contribution to the global pool of genetic resources

What are plant genetic resources for food and agriculture (PGRFA)?

- PGRFA is defined in the International Treaty on Plant Genetic Resources for Food and Agriculture as any genetic material of plant origin of actual or potential value for food and agriculture.

- This means that the genetic material of all the various crops grown around the world today, as well as any genetic material that may prove to be of value to food production and agriculture, are encompassed by the term.

4.3.6 Plant Breeder's Right

- Plant Breeder's Rights are a form of Intellectual Property (IP). They grant a limited commercial monopoly to breeders of new plant varieties. PBR allows a breeder the right to exclude others from a range of activities including producing and reproducing a protected variety. PBR is personal property and can be assigned, sold and transferred to other parties.
- Patents and plant breeders' rights are separate intellectual property rights with different conditions of protection, scope and exceptions.
- Breeders can use plant breeders' rights, patents, trademarks or other forms of intellectual property rights, or a combination to the extent that such systems are available in the territory concerned.
- Nowadays, with recent technological developments, for example the rising number of gene-related patents and rapid progress in the field of genetic engineering, patents and plant breeders' rights are more interlinked.
- The existence of the Protection of New Varieties of Plants (UPOV) Convention can be attributed largely to two organizations, the International Association for the Protection of Industrial Property (AIPPI), and the International Association of Plant Breeders (ASSINSEL).
- The Conference, which convened in May 1957 in Paris, established the basic principles of plant breeders' rights that were later incorporated into the International Union for the Protection of New Varieties of Plants (UPOV), which is based in Geneva and has a close association with WIPO.

What are rights?

- Plant Breeders' Rights (PBRs) are used to protect new varieties of plants that are distinguishable, uniform, and stable. A PBR is legally enforceable and gives the owner, exclusive rights to commercially use it, sell it, direct the production, sale, and distribution of it, and receive royalties from the sale of plants.
- In many countries PBR lasts for up to 25 years for trees and vines and 20 years for other species.

What is a plant variety?

- A plant variety represents a more precisely defined group of plants, selected from within a species, with a common set of characteristics. To be eligible for protection, the new variety must be shown to be distinct, uniform, and stable. In a comparative trial the variety must be clearly distinguishable from any other variety, the existence of which is a matter of common knowledge.

Why is plant variety protection necessary?

- Successful breeding requires great skill and knowledge. In addition, large-scale breeding calls for significant investment in land, specialized equipment (for example, greenhouses, growth chambers and laboratories), and skilled, scientific manpower.
- It takes a long time to develop a successful plant variety (10 to 15 years in the case of many plant species). Yet not all new plant varieties are successful and, even where the varieties show significant improvements, changes in market requirements may eliminate the possibility of a return on investment.
- This makes it necessary to balance the benefits with the return of the original high investment. Generally, however, plant breeding results in the availability of varieties with increased output and improved quality for the benefit of the society.
- Sustained and long-term breeding efforts are only worthwhile if there is a chance to be rewarded for the investment made. To recover the costs of this research and development, the breeder may seek protection to obtain exclusive rights for the new variety.
- At the same time, a new variety, once released, can often be easily reproduced by others. The original breeder is thus deprived of the fair opportunity to benefit from his or her investment. It is, therefore, critical to provide an effective system of plant variety protection, which encourages the development of new varieties of plants thereby benefiting the breeder and society at large.

4.4 Regulatory Issues

4.4.1 Regulations in India

Regulatory bodies are agencies which look after implementation of the legislation related to safety, efficacy and quality of drugs. They work under the Ministry of Health and Family Welfares. Each country has its own regulatory body. WHO (World Health Organization) and ICH (International Conference on Harmonization) are some important organizations who proposed guidelines for the Quality Standards of Herbal products. Department of AYUSH concentrates on the overall governance, education, regulation, development and growth of ISM in the India and abroad. The department has few subordinate offices, several autonomous bodies in the form of research councils, professional council, pharmacopoeia laboratories, national institutes, academy and hospitals.

In India, the national policy on T&CM is the National Policy on Indian Systems of Medicine and Homeopathy,issued in 2002. National legislation on T&CM includes the Indian Medicines Central Council Act 1970, theHomeopathy Central Council Act 1973 and the Drugs and Cosmetics Act of 1940 (amended in 2009).

The Government of India created a separate department known as the Department of Indian Systems of Medicine and Homeopathy in 1995, later renamed as the Department of ayurveda, Yoga, Unani, Siddha andHomeopathy (AYUSH), to serve as the national office for T&CM, which is administered under the MoH. Theindependent Ministry of AYUSH was formed in 2014.

There are a number of expert committees for T&CM in the country, the important ones being the pharmacopoeiacommittee, the Drug Control Cell, and the ayurveda Siddha and Unani Technical Advisory Board.

There are four separate councils for research under AYUSH: the Central Council for Research in ayurvedaand Siddha, the Central Council for Research in Unani Medicine, the Central Council for Research in Yogaand Naturopathy, and the Central Council for Research in Homeopathy.

A national plan for integrating T&CM into national health delivery began in 2014. Government and publicresearch funding is allocated towards T&CM.

Historical developments in herbal medicines in India	
1940	Drug and Cosmetic Act 1940 and Drug and Cosmetic Rule
1959	Govt of India recognized traditional Indian System of Medicine (ISM) and updated Drug and Cosmetic Act
1962	Several expert committees for different ISM
1969	Separate chapter related to Ayurveda, Siddha and Unani drugs was inserted by act 13 of 1964 in the Act
1970	Central Council of Indian Medicine (CCIM) is constituted
1970	Pharmacopoeial Laboratory of Indian Medicine was formed to ensure standardization and testing of ASU drugs
1983, 1987, 1994 and 2002	Drug and Cosmetic Act 1940 modified again with some substitutions
1995	Department of Indian Medicine and Homeopathy (ISM & H) was formed
2002	National Policy on Indian Systems of Medicine & Homoeopathy
2003	Department of Indian Medicine and Homeopathy (ISM & H) was renamed as Department of Ayurveda, Yoga and Naturopathy, Unani, Siddha and Homoeopathy (AYUSH)
2006 and 2008	Guideline for evaluation and analysis of drugs under ISM was given under Drug and Cosmetic Rule 1945
2008	Manufacturing units to maintain record of the raw material in the Performa schedule TA by 30th June of the succeeding financial year
2009	AYUSH department in collaboration with Quality Council of India (QCI) introduced certification scheme for AYUSH drug products
2009	NMPB Guidelines and standard for Good Field Collection Practices for Indian Medicinal Plants
2012	Sowa Rigpa system of medicine is incorporated in the CCIM
2003	Department of Indian Medicine and Homeopathy (ISM & H) was renamed as Department of Ayurveda, Yoga and Naturopathy, Unani, Siddha and Homoeopathy (AYUSH)
2013	Good clinical practice guidelines for clinical trials to have a well-programmed clinical study Siddha and Unani Medicine (GCP-ASU).
2014	Separate ministry on AYUSH was formed
2018	General guidelines forDrug development ofAyurvedic formulations
2018	AYUSH General Guidelines For Safety/Toxicity Evaluation Of Ayurvedic Formulations 2018

Contd....

Regulatory status of herbal medicines

Herbal medicines are regulated under ayurveda, Siddha and Unani drugs provision in the Drugs andCosmetics Act. They are categorized as prescription medicines and non-prescription medicines, and aresold with medical claims, health claims and nutrient content claims. Regulations for herbal medicines wereupdated in 2006 and 2017, and the list of registered herbal medicines was updated in 2016. The herbalmedicines included in the NEML were updated in 2013.

The Ayurveda pharmacopoeia of India, the Unani pharmacopoeia of India and the Siddha pharmacopoeiaof India are used and are legally binding. There are also monographs on single herbs and formularies. TheIndian herbal pharmacopoeia is also used but is not legally binding.

GMP exist for ayurveda, Unani and Siddha drugs, which include herbal medicines. There are exclusive regulationsfor GMP, separate from those for conventional pharmaceuticals, that apply to the manufacturing of herbalmedicines to ensure their quality. Adherence to manufacturing information in pharmacopoeias and monographsis required. Compliance mechanisms include periodic inspections by authorities at the manufacturing plants orlaboratories, and the requirement for manufacturers to submit samples of their medicines to a governmentapproved laboratory for testing and to assign a person to the role of ensuring compliance. Licences givento manufacturing units are renewed every 3 years, to ensure compliance with GMP. Traditional use withoutdemonstrated harmful effects is considered sufficient for safety assessment of herbal medicines.

Herbal medicines are also included under Schedule E of the Drugs and Cosmetics Rules. There is a separateessential drug list for ayurveda and Unani medicines; inclusion of a herbal medicine is based on its traditionaluse and long-term historical use, as well as disease-wise classification.

Herbal medicines categorized as prescription medicines are sold in pharmacies; herbal medicines categorizedas non-prescription medicines, self-medication or OTC medicines are sold in pharmacies and other outlets,and by licensed practitioners.

Practices, providers, education and health insurance

There are national and state level regulations that apply to providers of ayurvedic medicine, homeopathicmedicine and Unani medicine.

T&CM providers practise in both public and private sector clinics and hospitals. The national Governmentissues the T&CM licence required to practise. Licences and certificates are both issued after graduation andsubsequent completion of compulsory rotating internship. Bachelor's, master's, PhDs and clinical doctorate degrees in T&CM are available at the university level.

Regulations for homeopathy practitioners were updated in 2014 and the list of registered TM practitioners was updated in 2016. A consumer education programme for self-help care using T&CM has beenin place since 1997. T&CM services are reimbursed by both public and private health insurance as at end2016. Numbers of T&CM practitioners registered (as at 1 January 2016) under each practice are: ayurveda,419 217; Unani, 48 196; Siddha, 8528; naturopathy, 2220; and homeopathy, 293 307. The total numberis 771 468 (6.4 per 10 000 population).

The International Drug Monitoring Program of World Health Organization (WHO) has made certain guidelines for herbal drugs evaluation and quality control analysis. The WHO has done various efforts for the improvement of herbal drugs in the context of their safety and efficacy.

WHO Guideleines for herbal drugs	
2000	WHO - General Guidelines for Methodologies on Research and Evaluation of Traditional Medicine
2000	WHO Guidelines For Assessment, Evaluation Of Toxicity, Safety And Efficacy Of Herbal Medicines
2003	WHO Good Agricultural and Collection Practices [GAP, GCP, GACP]
2018	WHO guidelines on good herbal processing practice for herbal medicine
2019	WHO Good Storage and Distribution Practices

ASU-DTAB, ASU-DCC

- Central Drugs Standard Control Organization (CDSCO) under Directorate General of Health Services of Ministry of Health & Family Welfare Government of India forms Drugs Technical Advisory Board (DTAB)' and 'Drugs Consultative Committee (DCC)' to give recommendations if required on the matters of administration of the Drugs and Cosmetics Act and Rules there under.
- **Similarly there exists** Ayurveda, Siddha, Unani Drugs Technical Advisory Board (ASUDTAB) under separate Chapter IV-A in the Drugs & Cosmetics Act, 1940 which regulates the manufacture and sale, packaging and labeling of ASU drugs for domestic use and export and penalty for manufacture and sale of ASU drugs in contravention of these rules and for misbranded, adulterated and spurious ASU drugs.
- A separate Ayurveda, Siddha and Unani Technical Advisory Board (ASU-DTAB) has been constituted to advise the Central and State Governments on technical matters relating to regulation of ASU drugs by the Central Government comprising. :
    - Officials and nominees of central government,
    - Pharmacognosists
    - Phytochemists
    - Members of the Ayurveda Pharmacopoeia Committee, Siddha Pharmacopoeia Committee and Unani Pharmacopoeia Committee
    - representatives of teachers, practitioners and

ASU Drugs industry person nominated by the Central Government

- The Central Government has also constituted an Ayurveda, Siddha and Unani Drugs Consultative Committee (ASUDCC) under the Act to advise the Central and State Governments and the ASUDTAB on any matter for the purpose of securing uniformity though out India in the administration of Drugs & Cosmetics Act, 1940 as it relates to ASU drugs.
- A specific law, the Drugs & Magic Remedies Act, 1954, is also in place for prevention of objectionable advertisements & publicity relating to certain drugs and magic remedies for treatment of certain identified diseases and disorders.

4.4.2 Regulation of Manufacture of ASU Drugs

- Good Manufacturing Practices (GMP) for ASU drugs were notified on 23rd June, 2000 under Schedule - T of the Indian Drugs & Cosmetics Act, 1940 and Rules, 1945: which seeks mandatory compliance from the licensed manufacturers with regard to raw-materials, manufacturing area, manufacturing processes, record keeping, storage of raw-materials and finished products and quality testing.
- Must to ensure strict compliance of GMP by ASU drugs manufactures or cancel the license of non-GMP compliant units.
- Strict compliance by State Drug Controllers/Licensing Authorities for display of all the ingredients along with the quantities contained in the formulations on the label/container or a leaflet inserted inside the container since 2005.
- Exporters of purely herbal ASU drugs have been directed to mandatory testing for heavy metals and either conspicuously display on the container of purely herbal ASU drugs words "Heavy metals within permissible limits" or furnish the above certificate from authorized laboratories.
- Use of permissible excipients, preservatives for increasing the shelf-life of ASU drugs and draft rules for expiry date has been notified.
- The issue of safety of herbo-mineral/herbo-metallic Bhasmas/Compounds is also being addressed by the Central Government through a following project:
- A project has been sanctioned for chemical analysis and safety studies of eight most widely used Rasaushadhis/Bhasmas, namely, Kajjali, Rasmanikya, Nag Bhasma, Rasasindoor, Basantkusumkar Ras, ArogyavardhiniVati, Mahayograj Guggul and Mahalaxmi Vilas Ras by CSIR laboratories under the Golden Triangle Project within a time frame of 18 months.

4.4.3 Provisions in Drugs & Cosmetics Acts & Rules with Special Reference to ASU Drugs

Drugs & Cosmetics Act 1940 Chapter IV-A (section 33-B to 33-N): Provides provisions related to Ayurveda, Siddha and Unani Drugs

- The First Schedule -List of scheduled books: 98 books of different systems of medicines : Ayurveda-54, Siddha-30, Unani-14
- The Second Schedule: Standards which to be complied with by imported drugs and by drugs manufactured for Sale, Stocked or Exhibited for Sale or Distributed
- Schedule A: Different types of forms, particularly 24D, 24E, 25D, 25E, 26D, 26E, 26E-1, 47, 48, 49
- Schedule B-1 Fees for the test or analysis by Pharmacopoeial Laboratory for Indian Medicine or the Govt. Analyst
- Schedule E-1 List of poisonous substances under ASU Systems of Medicine
- Schedule FF Standards for Opthalmic Preparations
- Schedule T Good Manufacturing Practices for ASU Medicines
- Schedule Y Requirements and Guidelines for permission to import and / or manufacture of New drugs for sale or to undertake clinical trials

Drugs & Cosmetics Rules 1945

- Part XVI (Rule 151-160): Manufacture for sale of Ayurvedic (including Siddha) or Unani Drugs
- Part XVI-A (Rule 160 A - 160 J): Approval of institutions for carrying out tests on ASU Drugs and Raw material used in their manufacture
- Part XVII (Rule 161) : Labeling, Packing and Limit of Alcohol in ASU Drugs
- Part XVII (Rule 161-B): Shelf life or date of expiry for ASU Medicines
- Part XVIII (Rule 162-167): Government analysts and Inspectors for ASU Drugs
- Part XIX (Rule 168-170) Standards of ASU Drugs
- (**Proposed**) Schedule Z Requirements and Guidelines related to mandatory clinical trials of ASU drugs to manufacture ASU Drugs for sale

Subjective Questions

1. How to perform stability testing of herbal drugs
2. Define IPR? What are different types of IPR
3. What is patent? What are different patenting aspects of natural products?
4. How geographical indication is important IPR?
5. Can we have patent granted worldwide?
6. Who can register geographical indication?
7. How long does a patent last?
8. How long does a copyright last?
9. What is biopropsecting? Explain with examples
10. What is boipiracy?Explain with examples
11. What is Farmer's right? Which rights are covered and why?
12. What is Breeder's right? Which rights are covered and why?
13. How ASU DTAB and ASU DCC work to regulate herbal drugs?
14. How manufacturing of herbal drugs get regulated?
15. What is (proposed) schedule Z?

Multiple Choice Questions (MCQs)/Objective Questions

1. Source of mycotoxin is ..

   a. Aspergillus
   b. Penicillium
   c. Fusarium
   d. All of the above

2. Which one of the mycotoxins are classified as Group 1 human carcinogen by the International agency for research on Cancer?
   a. Ochratoxins
   b. Fumonisins
   c. Aflatoxins
   d. All of the above
3. Quality assessment for microbial contamination of herbal drugs to be used for parental purpose is must to eliminate risk of ......
   a. Endotoxins
   b. Aflatoxins
   c. Soil particles
   d. Exotoxins
4. According to WHO guidelines, 2-4-D is classified under the category ......
   a. Chlorinated hydrocarbon pesticides
   b. Chlorinated phenoxyalkanoic acid herbicides
   c. Carbamate insecticide
   d. Amino acid herbicide
5. Which one of the following is NOT pesticide of plant origin according to WHO?
   a. Derris rotenoids
   b. Tobacco extracts
   c. Pyrethrum extract
   d. Datura extract
6. According ICH guidelines for residual solvents in herbal products, Benzene comes under
   a. Class 3
   b. Class 2
   c. Class 1
   d. Class 4
7. According to ICH guidelines, Class 2 of residual solvents indicates .....
   a. Solvents to be avoided for extraction
   b. Solvents having low toxic potential
   c. Limited toxic potential solvents
   d. Non toxic solvents
8. As per WHO guidelines, The maximum amounts of toxic metals and non meals in medicinal plant materials can be given based on..........
   a. Provisional Tolerance Intake
   b. Provisional Inhibitory Intake
   c. Provisional non tolerable intake
   d. None of the above
9. As per WHO guidelines, the intake of residues from herbal materials should account ....of total intake from all sources
   a. Not less than 1%
   b. Not more than 1 %
   c. Not more than 5%
   d. Not less than 5%
10. According to WHO recommendation, limit for toxic lead in herbal medicines is ....
    a. 1 mg/kg
    b. 10 mg/kg
    c. 0.3 mg/kg
    d. 100 mg/kg

11. Which microbial contamination should be completely absent in Herbal products and herbal materials according to WHO guidelines?
    a. E. Coli
    b. Mould
    c. Shigella
    d. Salmonella
12. Which agar is recommended as a medium of moderate or high selectivity for isolation of shigella?
    a. Slmonella shigella agar
    b. Xylose lysine desoxycholate agar medium
    c. Agar-agar medium
    d. None of the above
13. It is recommended that, for herbal medicine product containing natural product or herbal drug preparation with known therapeutic activity, the variation in component during the proposed shelf life should not exceed........
    a. ±10
    b. ± 5
    c. ±15
    d. ± 20
14. Stress testing in stability study helps to identify
    a. Tolerance of the product
    b. Degradation of the product
    c. Shelf life of product
    d. None of the above
15. Which of the following is predictable change can occur in herbal medicinal product during storage?
    a. Racemization
    b. Polymerization
    c. Oxidation
    d. All of the above
16. The process in which one enantiomer of a compound converts to other enantiomer is called as .....
    a. Geometric isomerization
    b. Racemization
    c. Polymerization
    d. All of the above
17. Herbal drug substances should be tested at .... with no requirement for intermediate/accelerated testing
    a. 30°C/65 per cent relative humidity
    b. 25°C/60 per cent relative humidity
    c. 40°C/75 per cent relative humidity
    d. None of the above
18. Stability data can be generated by using modern analytical methods like ....
    a. HPLC
    b. HPTLC
    c. Both a and b
    d. None of the above

19. Which is an obligatory requirement in the registration process of all medicinal products including Herbal medicinal products?

    a. Analytical testing
    b. Stability studies
    c. chemical testing
    d. None of the above

20. Vinblastin rapidly biotransforms into ....in presence of UV light.

    a. Reserpine
    b. Ajmalicine
    c. Vincristine
    d. Vindoline

21. A government authority or license conferring a right or title for a set period especially the sole right to exclude others from making or selling an invention is known as.......

    a. Patent
    b. copyright
    c. Trademark
    d. None of the above

22. Intellectual property rights allows the owner of intellectual property to.....

    a. Get the benefits of his own creativity
    b. Prevents others from using, dealing or tampering his creativity by using lawsuits
    c. Both a and b
    d. None of the above

23. Which one of the following does not comes under intellectual property?

    a. Patent
    b. Copyright
    c. Trademark
    d. Brand

24. Any information of commercial value concerning production or sales operations which is not generally known is called as ....

    a. Trade mark
    b. Trade secret
    c. Copyright
    d. All of the above

25. Copyright is generally related to .....

    a. Innovation
    b. Artistic work
    c. Goods and services
    d. All of the above

26. 'Coca cola' is excellent example of ....

    a. Trademark
    b. Trade secret
    c. Trade name
    d. Copyright

27. Protection of Plant Varieties and Farmer's Right act was enacted in India in ....year

    a. 1999
    b. 2000
    c. 2001
    d. 2003

28. Which section in Farmers right act provides safeguard against innocent infringement?

    a. Section 18
    b. Section 42
    c. Section 20
    d. Section 40

29. Farmer's Right act is established to provide .....
    a. Protection of plant varieties
    b. Protect rights of farmers and plant breeders
    c. Encouragement to develop new varieties of plants
    d. All of the above
30. In which year, Farmer's Right gained formal recognition by FAO Conference?
    a. 1999
    b. 1989
    c. 1979
    d. 2009
31. The International treaty which recognizes the enormous contribution of local and indigenous community and farmers worldwide to develop and conserve crop diversity is known as....
    a. Farmer's Act
    b. Farmers right
    c. Both a and b
    d. None of the above
32. Farmers right is the International treaty strictly related to.........
    a. Plant genetic resources for food and agriculture
    b. Plant genetic resources for Medicinal plants
    c. Both a and b
    d. None of the above
33. A form of intellectual property right that allows plant breeders to protect new varieties of plants known as .....
    a. Farmers right
    b. Breeders right
    c. Nursery rights
    d. None of the above
34. Exploitation of natural sources for small molecules, macromolecules, biochemical and genetic information to develop in to valuable commercial products is known as ....
    a. Biopiracy
    b. Bioprospecting
    c. Biodiversity
    d. All of the above
35. Digitoxin production from Digitalis herb and its commercialization as cardiotonic drug is example of .....
    a. Biopiracy
    b. Bioprospecting
    c. Drug discovery
    d. None of the above
36. ....happen when researcher or research organization take biological resources without official sanction largely from less affluent country and marginalized people
    a. Bioprospecting
    b. Biopiracy
    c. Infringement
    d. All of the above

37. Historically biopiracy is linked to ....
    a. Colonialization
    b. Colonialism
    c. Both a and b
    d. None of the above
38. Which one of the following is known case of biopiracy?
    a. Neem
    b. Ashoka
    c. Datura
    d. All of the above
39. In........... tragedy of US patent on use turmeric powder and its administration was happened?
    a. 2000
    b. 1999
    c. 1995
    d. 1990
40. .... took legal opposition from India on patent for Neem filed by USA ?
    a. The Indian council for Scientific and Industrial Research (CSIR)
    b. Research Foundation for Science, Technology and Ecology, New Delhi
    c. Indian Institute of Science
    d. Indian Institute of Technology
41. Ayurvedic, Siddha and Unani Drugs Technical Advisory Board (ASU DTAB) comes under .... section of Drugs and Cosmetics Act 1940.
    a. Section 33D
    b. Section 33C
    c. Section 33E
    d. Section 33EE
42. The Ayurvedic Siddha and Drugs Consultative Committee (ASU DCC) comes under .... section of Drugs and Cosmetics Act 1940.
    a. Section 33D
    b. Section 33C
    c. Section 33E
    d. Section 33EE
43. Which is the highest statutory decision making body on technical matters related to drugs in the country?
    a. DCC
    b. DTAB
    c. IPC
    d. NPPA
44. DTAB is constituted as per ....
    a. Drugs and Cosmetics Act 1940
    b. Drugs and Cosmetics Act 1945
    c. Drugs and Cosmetics Act 1948
    d. Drugs and Cosmetics Act 1958
45. Function of DTAB is to advise Central and State Governments for....
    a. Uniform implementation of act
    b. Technical /Policy matters of ASU drugs
    c. Makes and amends regulatory provisions
    d. None of the above

46. Ayurvedic formulary of India contains ……
    a. 985 formulations
    b. 1229 formulations
    c. 399 formulations
    d. 1000 formulations
47. National Formulary of Unani Medicine consists of …….
    a. 1329 formulations
    b. 1329 formulations
    c. 1229 formulations
    d. 1429 formulations
48. Siddha Formulary of India contains ……
    a. 100 Formulations
    b. 399 Formulations
    c. 300 Formulations
    d. 200 Formulations
49. ……………………….based on compliance to the standards more than the domestic regulatory requirements
    a. AYUSH premium Mark
    b. AYUSH standard Mark
    c. Both a and b
    d. None of the above
50. ……………………..broadly based on compliance to WHO-GMP/USFDA criteria or GMP prescribed by importing country or fulfillment of quality requirements as per international norms
    a. AYUSH premium Mark
    b. AYUSH standard Mark
    c. Both a and b
    d. None of the above
51. In which year ASU drugs are included in Drugs and Cosmetics Act?
    a. 1985
    b. 1983
    c. 1995
    d. 1993
52. Which schedule in Drugs and Cosmetics Act 1940 deals with requirements to sale or undertake clinical trials of ASU drugs?
    a. Schedule T
    b. Schedule Z
    c. Schedule Y
    d. Schedule X
53. According to Schedule Z, Ayurvedic dosage form Churna should have shelf life of ……….
    a. 1 Year
    b. 2 Years
    c. 3 Years
    d. 4 years
54. Dosage forms 'Mandura and Lauha Kalpana' should have shelf life of ……
    a. 5 years
    b. 10 years
    c. 15 years
    d. 20 years
55. Scheme of pharmacovigilance for safety monitoring of AYUSH drugs surveillance of misleading advertisements implemented since
    a. November 2018
    b. November 2019
    c. November 2017
    d. November 2016

56. Which certificate is mandatory for export oriented ASU herbal drugs manufacturing?
    a. WHO GMP
    b. WHO GMP COPP
    c. GMP
    d. None of the above
57. How many monographs of single drugs are included in Siddha Pharmacopoeia?
    a. 150
    b. 298
    c. 139
    d. 645
58. Unani pharmacopoeia is composed of ....
    a. 298 monographs of single drugs
    b. 139 monographs of single drugs
    c. 645 monographs of single drugs
    d. None of the above
59. State licensing authority for ASU drugs must be a technical officer as per ....
    a. Rule 170 of D & C Rule
    b. Rule 168 of D & C Rule
    c. Rule 169 of D & C Rule
    d. Rule 165 of D & C Rule
60. How much GMP compliant AYUSH drug manufacturing units are present in Maharashtra?
    a. 834
    b. 391
    c. 734
    d. 634

Answer Key

1. d	2.c	3. a	4. b	5. d	6. c	7. c	8. a	9. b	10. b
11. c	12. b	13. b	14. b	15. d	16. b	17. b	18. c	19. b	20. c
21.a	22. c	23. d	24. b	25. b	26. b	27. c	28. b	29. d	30. b
31. b	32. c	33. b	34. b	35. b	36. b	37. b	38. a	39. c	40. b
41. b	42. a	43. b	44. a	45. b	46. a	47. a	48. b	49. b	50. a
51. b	52. b	53. b	54. b	55. c	56. b	57. c	58. a	59.a	60. a

Unit 5

5.1 General Introduction to Herbal Industry

Plant products and their derivatives constitute about 50% of modem drugs. There has been a quest to develop new drugs /formulation despite of being a costly and low success rate process. In recent years the research have focused on drug discovery from herbal medicines or botanical source by gaining leads from traditional literatures, folklore claims, database etc.

As Traditional Systems have long history of herbal usage in management of disease, the success rate of their development as therapeutic approach is comparatively higher than that of the synthetic counterpart. Examples of plant products and derivatives used by the pharmaceutical industry include paclitaxel, vincristine, vinblastine, artemesinin, camptothecin, podophyllotoxin, etc.

5.1.1 Herbal Industry: Present Scope

Numerous herbal products (drugs, food, nutraceuticals, cosmetics, agrochemicals, toiletry preparations etc) have entered the international market through exploration of ethnopharmacology and traditional medicine. The global herbal medicine market size was valued at USD 71.19 billion in 2016 and is expected to exhibit profitable growth over the forecast period. Many countries from all over the world especially from Asia, Africa, and Latin America etc. rely on traditional herbal medicines for their primary health care need. The majority of leading herbal industries, specialized in herbal drugs are over 100 years old. China and India are the top exporting countries and Hong Kong, Japan, USA and Germany are the leading importers.

India has 15 Agroclimatic zones and 17000-18000 species of flowering plants of which 6000-7000 are estimated to have medicinal usage in folk and documented systems of medicine, like Ayurveda, Siddha, Unani and Homoeopathy. About 960 species of medicinal plants are estimated to be in trade of which 178 species have annual consumption levels in excess of 100 metric tones. The domestic trade of the AYUSH industry is of the order of Rs. 80 to 90 billion (1US$ = Rs.50). The Indian medicinal plants and their products also account of exports in the range of Rs. 10 billion.

Effectiveness over long period of time, easy availability, low cost, prevention is better than cure trend, and comparatively being devoid of serious toxic effects (time tested). Nature has provided the complete store house of remedies to cure all ailments of mankind

Export Value plants		**Import value Plants**	
Botanical names	**Parts used**	**Botanical name**	**Parts used**
Acorus calamus	Rihizome	*Aloe vera*	Dried leaf
Argemone Mexicana	Fruit	*Adhatodavasica*	Whole plant
Curcuma amada	Rhizome	*Cinnamomum iners*	Bark and leaf
Curcuma longa	Rhizome	*Curcuma aromatic*	Rhizome
Curcuma aromatic	Wild turmeric	*Garcinia indica*	Fruit
Cassia lanceolata	Leaves	*Gloriosa superb*	Tuber and seed

Contd....

Export Value plants		Import value Plants	
Botanical names	**Parts used**	**Botanical name**	**Parts used**
Glycyrrhiza glabra	Root	*Juniperus communis*	Fruit
Withaniasomnifera	Vegetable rennet	*Myrica nagi*	Bark
Myrica nagi	Leaf	*Strycnosnux-vomica*	Bark and seed
Piper longum	Fruit	*Phyllanthus amarus*	Fruit
Rubia cordifolia	Madder root	*Ricinus communis*	Seed
Symplocosracemosa	Bark	*Rauvolfia serpentina*	Root
Swertia chirata	Whole plant	*Ocimum sanctum*	Leaf and essential oil
Terminalia chebula	Bark and seed	*Tylophorapurpuria*	Root
Wedelia calendula	Leaf and root	*Vinca rosea*	Leaf, seed and stem

5.1.2 Future Prospects

- Global Herbal Medicine Market is expected to register a CAGR of 5.88% during forecast period upto 2027.Asia Pacific herbal medicine market is predicted to record strong CAGR over 2020-2026, attributable to heavy investments in countries like China and India for research & development of effective drugs originated from herbs and plants.
- Multiple applications of herbal medicines are expected to enhance the market growth.
- Medicinal plants have evolved over the centuries as essential parts of African civilization and are widely recognized today as representing its rich cultural and scientific heritage. The increasing demand for medicinal plant products has renewed interest in the pharmaceutical industry in the production of herbal health care formulations, herbal-based cosmetic products, and herbal nutritional supplements.
- Worldwide there will be growing demand for herbal and other traditional forms of medicines and other products due to awareness about prevention is better than cure.
- International promotion of herbal drugs is getting explored through exhibitions and targeted branding.
- There is increase in advancement in herbal drug patenting which will surely promote herbal market.
- More elaborate guidelines on quality control of herbal drugs by WHO, ICH and various authorities of many countries are boosting herbal industry growth. There is improved supply of standardized and certified raw materials, extracts and markers.
- Awareness regarding SOPs, GLP, GAP, GACP, GSP guidelines and government facilities among growers and manufacturers is responsible for future rise international export-import market.
- Unified protocols, timelines, and guidelines and harmonization among the pharmacopoeias and regulations across countries will also improve import-export market scenario
- Scientific evidences for safety and efficacy of many herbal products will be available

- Increase in substantial research investments and funding will expected to offer significant market expansion opportunities in future.
- Arkopharma, Bayer AG, BEOVITA, Hishimo Pharmaceuticals, Schaper &Brümmer, ZeinPharma Germany GmbH, Venus Pharma GmbH, Himalaya Global Holdings Ltd, and Dr. Willmar Schwabe India Pvt. Ltd.are the major players in Herbal Medicine Market.

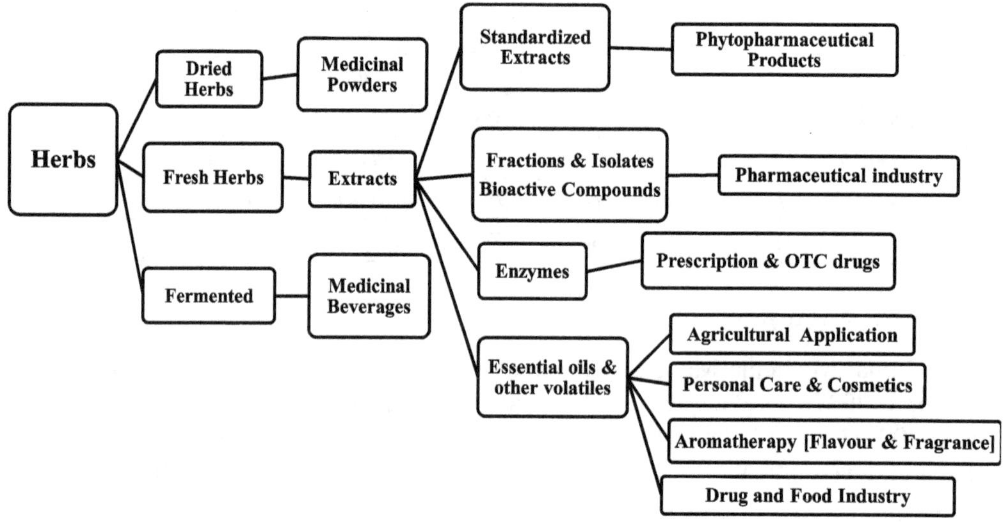

Fig. 5.1 Herbal industry Segments

5.2 Plant Based Industries in India

Dabur India Ltd. (1884)	Name is derived from owner name DaktarBurman. For the past 130 years, It has been dedicated to providing nature-based solutions for a healthy and holistic lifestyle. It is World's largest ayurveda company. Dabur Chyawanprash (herbal honey) has a market share of 70% and chewable Hajmola Digestive Tablets has an 88% share. Other major products are Dabur Amla Hair Oil, Dabur Lal Tail, (Ayurvedic massage Oil), Dabur Gripe Water and Dabur JanamGhuntiVatika (Shampoo), Babool, Meswak, and Honitus. Dabur has joined hands with online marketplace Snapdeal to set up an e-store, called LiveVEDA, for its range of Ayurvedic products. Dabur's home care portfolio includes Mosquito Repellents (Odomos), Air Fresheners (Odonil) and Toilet Cleaners (Sanifresh). During fiscal 2015-16, your Company recorded consolidated sales of 8436.0 crore growing by 8.1%.
Sri Baidyanath Ayurvedic Bhawan Ltd. (1917)	Pandit Ram Dayal Joshi established Shree BaidyanathAyurved Bhawan Private Limited in 1917 to combine the resources of AYURVEDA with modern research and manufacturing technology. More popularly known as Baidyanath, it is one of India's most respected companies, manufacturing the largest range of Ayurvedic products in the world. There is a range of over 700 Ayurvedic products at10 manufacturing centers. Most of products are patented. Herbal teas, massage oils, Chyawanprash, Shikakai (soap pod) Shampoo, Lal DantManjan (Tooth Powder), Amala hair oil, Gulabari are few of the well known products of Baidyanath.

Contd....

Zandu Pharmaceutical (1919)	Zandu Pharmaceutical Works Ltd. was named after venerable Mahatma ZanduBhattji to whom it owes its origin. ZanduBhattji's real name was Karunashankar; he was the son of legendary Vaidya VithalBhattji, a personal physician to Ranmal, the then King of Jamnagar. Zandu is a strong player in the balm, Ayurvedic OTC and classical range. Company is specialised in Rheumatology, Gynaecology and CNS (Central nervous system). In 2008, Emami, acquired Zandu Pharmaceuticals Works Ltd, from the Parikh family, keeping in mind the huge synergy between the Emami and Zandu brands in various categories. With acquisition, Emami acquired brands like Zandu Balm, Pancharista, NityamChurna apart from the other Zandu ayurvedic range of products. Zandu balm, Fair and Handsome, Boroplus and Navratna among the top brands in the country.
Himalaya Drug Company (1934)	The Himalaya Drug Company is a company established by M Manal in 1930 and based in Bangalore, India. It produces health care products under the name Himalaya Herbal Healthcare whose products include ayurvedic ingredients. It is spread across locations in India, the United States, the Middle East, Asia and Europe, while its products are sold in 92 countries across the world. Serpinaantihypertensive drug is the first natural antihypertensive produced by company in 1934. Liv-52 (flagship product), a liver protector launched in 1955. The Neem Face Wash is also one of their most popular and well known products. 200 million Himalaya products enter the homes of consumers around the world with a range of over 300 healthcare and personal care products including brands like Liv.52, Liv 52-HB, Cystone, and Bonnisan.
Charak Pharmaceuticals (1947)	Charak is established in 1947 by Shroff Brothers: Shri D.N. Shroff and Dr. S.N. Shroff. Company products are well accepted in more than 35 countries worldwide. Evanova (Safe alternative in the management of menopausal symptoms), Danil Oil (natural cytostatic and antifungal antidandruff hair oil) and many products for different ailments based of evidence and standardisation are popular.
Natural Remedies Pvt Ltd (1951)	Natural Remedies founded by R.K. Agarwal is one of the leading herbal pharmaceutical company in India, headquartered at Bangalore, in the state of Karnataka. The company is a manufacturer and supplier of standardized herbal extracts, pure phytochemicals and herbal veterinary healthcare products which are validated, effective, safe and consistent. It has a significant presence in major markets and footprints worldwide. Natural Remedies has successfully carved its place in Veterinary industry as India's No. 1, herbal veterinary healthcare company.
Vicco Laboratories (1952)	Founded in 1952 by late Shri K.V.Pendharkar, the VICCO Group has emerged today as makers of the best internationally known products of the Ayurveda, the ancient Indian system of natural medicines. Having production units at Dombivli, Nagpur and Goa in India. Company has established strong foothold in almost every developed country in Asia, Europe, America, Africa and Australia. Name is derived from Vishnu Industrial Chemical Company, Mumbai. Vajradanti Paste, Vajradanti Powder, Turmeric Multipurpose Cream, Turmeric Skin cream (Oil Base), Turmeric WSO (without sandalwood oil) Cream are famous products of company. Vajradanti SF (Sugar free) is latest product.
Emami Group (1974)	In 1995, Kemco Chemicals, the partnership firm led by Mr. R S Agarwal and Mr. R S Goenka was converted into a Public Limited Company under the name and style of Emami Ltd. In 1998, Emami Ltd was merged with Himani Ltd and its name was changed to Emami Ltd as per fresh certificate of incorporation dated September1, 1998. In 2000, with a view to concentrate on its core FMCG business, Emami's investment undertaking was demerged and Pan EmamiCosme Ltd. issued its fully

Contd....

	paid up shares to shareholders of Emami in the ratio of 1:1. In 2003 a new factory unit was set up at Amingaon, Guwahati. Emami Talcum, Emami Vanishing Cream and Emami Cold Cream and glycerine soap are popular products. Boroplus is not only the largest selling Antiseptic Cream in India but also in Russia, Ukraine, and Nepal. The next flagship brand of the company Navratna Cool Oil. In 2005 Emami created a marketing history in India by launching Fair and Handsome, the first fairness cream for men.
Universal /Unijules Medicaments (1984)	It has established itself as one of the preferred healthcare solution providers in the field of New Drug Delivery Systems (NDDS) while keeping its grass roots expertise like Mother Tinctures, classical herbals alive offering time tested benefits to the common man. Famous products: Karnim (Anti-diabetic supplement), Herbokam (Anti-stress formula), Chetak (Stimulant), Tonabilin (Iron supplement), Minitone, U-Gyanetone, and Unicough Syrup
Ayur Herbals (1984)	Ayur has more than 155 variants in Hair, Skin and Face Care Products. But it all started with a single product- Hair Removing Wax. Due to low price and high quality cosmetic products, Ayur is very famous brand in India as well as Asia. Ayur rose water, hot wax, cold wax, face packs, tea tree face wash etc are famous products.
Hamdard Laboratories (1906)	Hamdard Laboratories , is a Unani and Ayurvedic pharmaceutical company in India having branches in Bangladesh & Pakistan. It was established in 1906 by Hakeem Hafiz Abdul Majeed in Delhi, and became a waqf (non-profitable trust) in 1948. Some of its most famous products include Sharbat RoohAfza, Safi, RoghanBadam Shirin, Sualin, Joshina and Cinkara. It is associated with Hamdard Foundation, a charitable educational trust.
Patanjali Ayurved (2006)	Baba Ramdev established the Patanjali Ayurved Limited at Haridwar in 2006 along with Acharya Balkrishna with the objective of establishing science of Ayurveda in accordance and coordination with the latest technology and ancient wisdom. Annual turnover of the year 2016-17 of this company to be estimated ₹10,216 crore (US$1.6 billion). The company manufactures more than 900 products including 45 types of cosmetic products and 30 types of food products. According to Patanjali, all the products manufactured by Patanjali are made from Ayurveda and natural components Patanjali have also launched beauty and baby products. Patanjali Ayurvedic manufacturing division has over 300 medicines for treating a range of ailments and body conditions, from common cold to chronic paralysis.

5.3 Plant Based Institutes in India

CSIR	▸ The Council of Scientific and Industrial Research (CSIR) is a contemporary R & D organization. CSIR has a dynamic network of 38 national laboratories, 39 outreach centres, 3 innovation complexes and 5 units. ▸ CSIR covers a wide spectrum of science and technology – from radio and space physics, oceanography, geophysics, chemicals, drugs, genomics, biotechnology and nanotechnology to mining, aeronautics, instrumentation, environmental engineering and information technology. ▸ On an average CSIR files about 200 Indian patents and 250 foreign patents per year. About 13.86% of CSIR patents are licensed - a number which is above the global average. CSIR holds the 17th rank in Asia and leads the country at the first position

Contd....

NBRI	▶ The CSIR-National Botanical Research Institute (NBRI) - is amongst one of the constituent research institutes of CSIR, New Delhi. Originally set up as the National Botanic Gardens (NBG) by the State Government of Uttar Pradesh (U.P.), it was taken over by the CSIR in 1953. Consequently, the NBG was renamed as the NBRI, i.e., The National Botanical Research Institute in 1978. ▶ Following are different areas of R and D and infrastructure: 1. Botanic Garden and Distant Research Centers 2. Plant Diversity, Systematics and Herbarium 3. Plant Ecology and Environmental Science 4. Genetics and Molecular Biology 5. Plat Microbe Interaction and Pharmacognosy 6. Science and Technology Support Services
CIMAP	▶ Central Institute of Medicinal and Aromatic Plants, popularly known as CIMAP, is a frontier plant research laboratory of CSIR. Established originally as Central Indian Medicinal Plants Organisation (CIMPO) in 1959. ▶ CIMAP is steering multidisciplinary high quality research in biological and chemical sciences and extending technologies and services to the farmers and entrepreneurs of medicinal and aromatic plants (MAPs) with its research headquarter at Lucknow and Research Centres at Bangalore, Hyderabad, Pantnagar and Purara. ▶ Research Centres at different agro-climatic zones of the country to facilitate multi-location field trials and research. ▶ CIMAP has extended its wings overseas with scientific collaboration agreements with Malaysia. ▶ Mint varieties released and agro-packages developed and popularised by CIMAP has made **India** the global leader in **mints** and related industrial products. ▶ CIMAP has released several varieties of the MAPs, their complete agro-technology and post harvest packages which have revolutionised MAPs cultivation and business scenario of the country.
CDRI	▶ Central Drug Research Institute (CDRI) is a constituent laboratory of Council of Scientific and Industrial Research (CSIR), inaugurated on 17th Feb 1951 with a vision to strengthen and advance the field of drug research and development in the country. ▶ Today, it has become a unique model for modernized drug research in India – having everything under one roof, from synthesis, screening, development studies, process up-scaling to clinical studies. ▶ Unique achievements of the institute includes discovery and development of 12 new drugs, of which, Arteether (Brand Name: E-mal), BESEB (Brand Name: Memory Sure), Centchroman (Brand Name: Saheli) are currently in market; transferred more than 130 indigenous technologies to the pharmaceutical companies, a significant contribution in the metamorphosis of the Indian Pharma Industry. Institute obtained more than 350 Indian patents and 90 international patents.
NCL, Pune	National Chemical Laboratory (CSIR-NCL), Pune, established in 1950, is a constituent laboratory of CSIR. CSIR-NCL is a science and knowledge based research, development and consulting organization. It is internationally known for its excellence in scientific research in chemistry and chemical engineering as well as for its outstanding track record of industrial research involving partnerships with more than 55 industries (Like Alembic, Cadilla, CIPLA, Dabur, Emcure, FDC, Glenmark, Lupin, Orchid Chemicals, Ranbaxy, RPG Life Sciences, USV Limited etc) from concept to commercialization.

Contd....

NMPB	The National Medicinal Plants Board (NMPB) set-up in November 2000 by the Government of India has the primary mandate of coordinating all matters relating to medicinal plants and support policies and programmes for growth of trade, export, conservation and cultivation.
Indian Agricultural Research Institute (IARI)	This institute deals with genetics and plant breeding; plant pathology; microbiology; post harvest technology
Agarkar Research Institute, Pune, Maharashtra	This institute deals with biodiversity and palaeobiology, bioenergy, bioprospecting, development biology, genetics and plant breeding, nanobioscience
NBPGR	**National Bureau of Plant Genetic Resources (NBPGR)** institute deals with Plant Genetic Resources (PGR) Management and Use, policy issues on exchange of genetic resources: quarantine, intellectual property rights (IPR); assessing economic value; conflicts over ownership management and use; national and international treaties / legislation; CBD, IT-PGRFA, GPA, PVP and FR Act, biodiversity act etc, genomics and bioinformatics: genomic resources generation, use and conservation, genetically modified (GM) crops; GM detection techniques.
Jamia Hamdard university, Delhi	▸ The history of Jamia Hamdard begins with the establishment of a small Unani clinic in the year 1906 by Hakeem Hafiz Abdul Majeed, one of the well-known practitioners of Unani System of Medicine of his time. ▸ Hakeem Hafiz Abdul Majeed had a vision of making the practice of Unani Medicine into a scientific discipline so that Unani medicines could be dispensed in a more efficacious manner to patients. He gave the name "Hamdard" to his venture which means "sympathy for all and sharing of pain". ▸ Hamdard College of Pharmacy was set up with the objective of providing education and training in all branches of pharmacy. ▸ Jamia Hamdard offers postgraduate and doctoral programmes in several disciplines for which advanced facilities are available. ▸ Hamdard Laboratories , is a Unani and Ayurvedic pharmaceutical company associated with Hamdard Foundation, a charitable educational trust. ▸ Some of most famous products include Sharbat RoohAfza, Safi, RoghanBadam Shirin, Sualin, Joshina and Cinkara.

5.4 Schedule T – Good Manufacturing Practice of Indian Systems of Medicine

5.4.1 Components of GMP (Schedule – T)

Componenets

Objectives **Part-I** 1. Requirement 1.1. General Requirements ▸ Location and surroundings- ▸ Buildings ▸ Water Supply ▸ Disposal of Waste ▸ Containers' Cleaning- ▸ Storage ▸ Raw Materials stores ▸ Packaging Materials stores ▸ Finished Goods Stores ▸ Working Space ▸ Health, Clothing, Sanitation and Hygiene of Workers ▸ Medical Services ▸ Machinery and Equipments ▸ Batch Manufacturing Records ▸ Distribution Records 1.2 Requirement for Sterile Product (A) Manufacturing Areas (B) Precautions against contamination and mix:	**PART-II** A. List of recommended machinery, equipment and minimum manufacturing premises for Ayurved and Sidhha B. List of recommended machinery, equipment and minimum manufacturing premises for Unani C. List of equipment recommended for in-house quality control section D. Supplementary guidelines for manufacturing of Herbo-mineralmetallic compounds of ASU 2. Manufacturing Process Areas 3. Quality Control 4. Product recalls 5. Medical Examination of the employees 6. Self- Inspection 7. Dosage form of Rasaushadhis 8. Area Specification/requirement for an applicant companies only to have GMP of Herbo-mineralmetallic compounds of ASU

Objectives of GMP

- Raw materials used in the manufacture of drugs arc authentic, of prescribed quality and are free from contamination.
- The manufacturing process is as has been prescribed to maintain the standards.
- Adequate quality control measures are adopted.
- The manufactured drug which is released for sale is of acceptable quality.

However, under IMCC Act 1970 registered Vaidyas, Siddhas and Hakeems who prepare medicines on their own to dispense to their patients and not selling such drugs in the market are exempted from the purview of G.M.P.

PART-I

- Factory Premises:

- The manufacturing plant should have adequate space for:
  - Receiving and storing raw material
  - Manufacturing process areas
  - Quality control section
  - Finished goods store
  - Office
  - Rejected goods/drugs store

1. Requirements

1.1 General Requirements	
Location and surroundings-	Avoid contamination from open sewerage, drain, public lavatory or any factory which produces disagreeable or obnoxious odour or fumes or excessive soot, dust or smoke
Buildings	Hygienic conditions and should be free from cobwebs and insects/rodents, adequate provision of light and ventilation, floor and the walls should not be damp or moist
Water Supply	Pure and of potable quality, Adequate provision of water for washing
Disposal of Waste	Prejudicial to the workers or public health water shall be disposed off after suitable treatment as per guidelines of pollution control authorities
Containers' Cleaning	Separate arrangement for washing, cleaning and drying of such containers.
Storage	Proper ventilation and shall be free from dampness, separate space for material, such as raw material, packaging material and finished products
Raw Materials stores	Different containers for different raw materials, metals, minerals, animal source, fresh herbs, dry herbs, volatile oils, extracts, resins, excipients etc 'First in first out procedure, properly identified and labled container used for raw material storage with clear remark such as Batch No. or Lot. No., date of receipt or UNDER TEST' or 'APPROVED' or 'REJECTED
Packaging Materials stores	Bottles, jars, capsules should be cleaned and dried before packing
Finished Goods Stores	Should be labeled "Quarantine", or "Approved Finished Goods Stock," maintain Distribution records
Working Space	Adequate space (manufacture and quality control), eliminate any risk of mix-up, cross-contamination
Health, Clothing, Sanitation and Hygiene of Workers	Workers should be free from contagious diseases, clean uniform, facilities for changing their clothes and to keep their personal belongings, Separate lavatories to be used by men and women
Medical Services	Adequate facilities for first aid, Medical examination of workers once a year, maintain record
Machinery and Equipments	Based on product and size, manually operated or operated semi-automatically suitable equipment s for crushing, grinding, powdering, boiling, mashing, burning, roasting, filtering, drying, filling, labeling and packing, standard operational procedures (SOPs), adequate space between machines
Batch Manufacturing Records	Raw materials and their quantities obtained from the store, quality tests conducted during the various stages of manufacture, manpower responsible, finished products store including dates

Contd....

Distribution Records	Records of sale and distribution of each batch up to 5 years of the exhausting of stock to facilitate prompt and complete recall of the batch, if necessary
Record of Market Complaints	Record of data received on such market complaints, investigations carried out by, any corrective action initiated to prevent recurrence of such market complaint, submit such records once in a period of six months to Licensing Authority ; *adverse reaction* and investigation if any record in separate register,
Quality Control	Provide 150 sq feet area facility for quality control section in his own premises or through Government-approved testing laboratory, verify raw materials, monitor in process, quality checks and control the quality of finished product, shelf life and storage records
1.2 Requirement for Sterile Product	
(A) Manufacturing Areas	Sterile products: dust free and ventilated with an air supply, aseptic manufacture: HEPA Filters, mix-up between non-sterile products
(B) Precautions against contamination and mix:	Separate operations in a separate block, suitable exhaust, laminar flow sterile air system for sterile products,

PART-II

- A. List of recommended machinery, equipment and minimum manufacturing premises required for the manufacture of various categories of ayurvedic, siddha system of Medicines
- B. List of machinery, equipment and minimum manufacturing premises required for the manufacture of various categories of unani system of medicines
- C. List of equipment recommended for in-house quality control section (Alternatively, unit can get testing done from the Government approved laboratory)
- D. Supplementary guidelines for manufacturing of rasaushadhies or rasamaraunthukul and kushtajat (herb-mineral-metallic compound) of ayurveda, siddha and unani medicines.

2. Manufacturing Process Areas

Specified areas for Manufacturing of Bhasma and Kupipakawa and Rasaaushadhi preparations

Bhatti or Heating Devise Section for Bhasma and Rasaaushadhi	100 sq. feet for heating, burning, putta and any heat related work with proper ventilation, exhaust and chimney
Grinding, Drying and Processing Section for BhasmaandRasaaushadhi	10sq.feet
Rasaushadhis Related Store:	100 sq. ft.

Records of appropriate temperature attained during the entire process of using pyrometer and, pyrograph

3. Quality Control

- A. In Process Quality Control
  - (a) Shodhan Register with following details
  - (b) Bhavana and Putta Register with following details:
  - (c) Grinding Records Register: (Finished Products/Intermediate Procedure)
  - (d) Packing details:
- B. Product Quality Control: as per official Pharmacopoeia or Schedule books for texts

4. **Product recalls**
   - Literature inserted inside the products package should indicate the name, address of the manufacturing unit or email or telephone number for reporting of any adverse drug reaction by physicians or patients.
   - On receipt of such Adverse Drug Reaction report, it will be the responsibility of the manufacturer to ensure the recall the product from the market.
   - Standard operating procedures (SOP) should be included for storage of recalled Rasaushadhies in a secure segregated area, complying with the requirements specified for storage, till their final disposal.
5. **Medical Examination of the employees**
   - Medically examined periodically at least once a year.
   - Annual examination reports of the employees shall be made available to statuary inspectors during Good Manufacturing Practices inspections
6. **Self- Inspection**
   - The release of Rasaushadhis should be under the control of a person who has been trained in the specific features of the processing and quality assurance of Rasaushadhis Personnel
7. **Dosage form of Rasaushadhis**
   - It should be in acceptable dosage forms such as, churna, vati, guti, tablet, capsule etc. after adding suitable permissible fillers or binding agents as permissible under the Ayurvedic Pharmacopoeia of India or Indian Pharmacopoeia as updated from time to time.
   - Label must indicate the Ayurveda/Siddha/ Unani medicine in one Tablet or Pill or Capsule in addition to the filters. However for hospital bulk pack, it will not be applicable and label will not be applicable and label will clearly indicate the "Hospital Pack".
8. Area Specification/requirement for an applicant companies only to have GMP of Rasaushadhies or Rasamaraunthukul and Kushtajat (Herbo-mineralmetallic compounds) of Ayurveda, Siddha and Unani Medicines:

Forms

- SCHEDULE-TA (See Rule 157-A) Form for record of utilization of raw material by Ayurveda or Siddha or Unani Licensed manufacturing units
- FORM 1A Memorandum to the pharmacopoeial laboratory for indian medicine (plim)uring the financial year.
- FORM 2A Certificate of test or analysis from the pharmacopoeial laboratory for indian medicine or government analyst
- FORM 15 (To be seen in context of section 33EEC) Order under section 22(1)(c) of the drugs and cosmetics act, 1940 requiring a person not to dispose of stock in his possession
- FORM 16 Receipt for stock of drugs or cosmetics for record, register, document or material object seized under section 22(1) (c) or 22(1)(cc) of the drugs and cosmetics act,1940
- FORM 17 Intimation to person from whom sample is taken

- FORM 17-A Receipt for samples of drugs or cosmetics taken where fair price tendered thereof under sub-section (1) of section 23 of the drugs and cosmetics act, 1940 is refused
- FORM 18-A Memorandum to government analyst
- FORM 24-D Application for the grant / renewal of a license to manufacture for sale of ayurvedic / siddha or unani drugs
- FORM 24-E Application for grant or renewal of a loan license to manufacture for sale /ayurvedic (including siddha) or unani drugs
- FORM 25-D License to manufacture for sale of ayurvedic(including siddha) or unani drugs
- FORM 25-E Loan license to manufacture for sale of ayurvedic (including siddha) or unani drugs
- FORM 26-D Certificate of renewal of license to manufacture for sale of ayurveda/ siddha or unani drugs
- FORM 26-E Certificate of renewal of loan license to manufacture for sale of ayurveda/ siddha or unani drugs
- FORM 26E-I Certificate of Good Manufacturing Practices (GMP) to Manufacturer of Ayurveda, Siddha or Unani Drugs
- FORM 35 Form in which the inspection book shall be maintained
- FORM 47 Application for grant or renewal of approval for carrying out tests on ayurvedic, siddha and unani, drugs or raw materials used in the manufacture thereof on behalf of licensees for manufacture for sale of ayurvedic , siddha and unani drugs.
- FORM 48 Approval for carrying out tests or analysis on Ayurvedic, Siddha and Unani drugs or raw materials used in the manufacture thereof on behalf of licensee s for manufacture for sale of Ayurvedic , Siddha and Unani drugs.
- FORM 49 Certificate of renewal for carrying out tests or analysis on Ayurvedic, Siddha and Unani drugs or raw materials used in the manufacture thereof on behalf of licensees for manufacture for sale of Ayurvedic, Siddha and Unani drugs.

Subjective Questions

1. What is scope and future of herbal industry?
2. What are the major hurdles faced by herbal industry?
3. Write a brief account on plant based industries involved in work on medicinal and aromatic plants in India
4. Name patented herbal products of CDRI?
5. Discuss contribution of CSIR in marketed herbal product development.
6. Name the herbal formulations developed by AYUSH.
7. Which institute has made India the global leader in mints and related industrial products?

8. Write a brief account on plant based institutions involved in work on medicinal and aromatic plants in India
9. Write a brief account on Schedule T.

Multiple Choice Questions (MCQs)/Objective Questions

1. India is one of the leading countries in supply of ......
   a. Lavender oil
   b. Clove oil
   c. Lemon grass oil
   d. Castor oil
2. Regional Research Laboratory - Council of Scientific and Industrial Research, Jammu works on ......
   a. Dioscorea composita
   b. Claviceps purpurea
   c. Catharanthus rosus
   d. Both a and b
3. Extensive work on anticancer drug is going on in ....
   a. Regional Research Laboratory - Council of Scientific and Industrial Research, Jammu
   b. Central Institute of Medicinal and Medicinal plants, CSIR, Lucknow
   c. National Botanical Research Institute, CSIR, Lucknow
   d. All of the above
4. Research work on Chamomile oil is going on in which Institute?
   a. Regional Research Laboratory - Council of Scientific and Industrial Research, Jammu
   b. Central Institute of Medicinal and Medicinal plants, CSIR, Lucknow
   c. National Botanical Research Institute, CSIR, Lucknow
   d. All of the above
5. Which of the following is India's most trusted herbals Industry?
   a. Dabar
   b. Himalaya
   c. Lotus Herbals
   d. Vicco
6. India's largest Ayurvedic medicine supplier, Dabur India Ltd was established in
   a. 1984
   b. 1884
   c. 1994
   d. 1894
7. Which one of the India based company is popular in US for drug Liv -52?
   a. Dabur
   b. Himalaya
   c. Vicco
   d. Baidyanath
8. Which Indian Ayurvedic Company is best known internationally for its Toothpaste product?
   a. Dabur
   b. Vicco
   c. Baidyanath
   d. Patamnjali

9. The Ayurvedic market of India valued more than ....in 2018.
   a. INR 300 million
   b. INR 300 billion
   c. INR 100 million
   d. INR 200 billion

10. Regulations and requirements for manufacture of Ayurvedic, Sidha and Unani products are provided in
    a. Schedule Z
    b. Schedule T
    c. Schedule Y
    d. Schedule M

11. Recommended minimum manufacturing space according to Schedule Z, required for Churna preparation is
    a. 100 Sq. ft
    b. 200 Sq. ft
    c. 500 Sq. ft
    d. 1200 Sq. ft

12. Recommended minimum manufacturing space required for Unani medicines is
    a. 1200 sq ft
    b. 1600 sq. ft
    c. 800 sq.ft
    d. 1000 sq. ft

13. Quality control department of ASU should have minimum of one person with Sidha/Unani/Ayurveda qualification recognized under ....
    a. Schedule I of Indian Medicine Central Council Act 1970
    b. Schedule II of Indian Medicine Central Council Act 1970
    c. Schedule III of Indian Medicine Central Council Act 1970
    d. Schedule I V of Indian Medicine Central Council Act 1970

14. Legal provisions related to GMP are described under …
    a. Drug and Cosmetics Rules 1945, rule 151 to 160
    b. Schedule T
    c. Both a and b
    d. None of the above

15. Which form should be issued for getting license of manufacturing and sale of Ayurveda and Unani Drugs?
    a. Form 25-D
    b. Form 25 –C
    c. Form 21 - C
    d. Form 21 – D

16. For how many years, Certificate of Good Manufacturing Practices shall be issued to manufacture of ASU drugs in compliance with requirements given in Schedule T?
    a. 3 Years
    b. 4 years
    c. 5 Years
    d. 10 Years

17. Which is the key deterrent to the growth of the market?
    a. Adverse whether condition
    b. Excessive use of insecticides and pesticides
    c. Both a and b
    d. None of the above
18. Which guidelines are based on the principles of the WHO guidelines for the assessment of herbal medicines?
    a. EEC
    b. USFDA
    c. ICH
    d. None
19. In DTAB, ex officio member is ....
    a. Director General of health services, India
    b. Drug Controller of India
    c. Director of Central Drug Laboratory
    d. None of the above
20. In Asava/Arishtas, the upper limit of alcohol as self generated alcohol should not be ....
    a. Less than 12%
    b. More than 12%
    c. Less than 10%
    d. More than 10%

Answer Key

1. c	2. d	3. b	4. c	5. b	6. b	7. b	8. b	9. b	10. b
11. a	12. b	13. b	14. c	15. a	16. c	17. c	18. a	19. b	20. b

Further Reading

1. A.N.M. Alamgir. Therapeutic Use of Medicinal Plants and Their Extracts: Volume 1. [Pharmacognosy- Volume 1]. Springer International Publishing. 2017
2. Alice Kurian, M. Asha Sankar Medicinal Plants. New India Publishing Agency. 2007
3. Amitava DasguptaHandbook of Drug Monitoring Methods-Therapeutics and Drugs of Abuse. Humana Press. 2007
4. Amritpal Singh Saroya. Contemporary Phytomedicines. CRC Press. 2017
5. Amritpal Singh. Regulatory and Pharmacological Basis of Ayurvedic Formulations. CRC Press. 2017
6. Anil K. Sharma, Raj K. Keservani, Surya Prakash Gautam. Herbal Product Development-Formulation and Applications. Apple Academic Press Incorporated. 2020
7. Aronson JK. Defining 'nutraceuticals': neither nutritious nor pharmaceutical. Br J Clin Pharmacol. 2017 Jan;83(1):8-19.
8. Ashok Katdare, Mahesh Chaubal.Excipient Development for Pharmaceutical, Biotechnology, and Drug Delivery Systems. CRC Press. 2006
9. Ashraf Mozayani, Lionel RaymonHandbook of Drug Interactions-A Clinical and Forensic Guide. Humana Press. 2004
10. Ashutosh Kar. Pharmacognosy And Pharmacobiotechnology. New Age International (P) Limited. 2003
11. Ayurvedic pharmacopoeia of India Part-I vol.I, 2001.
12. Azhar Ali Farooqi, B. S. Sreeramu. Cultivation Of Medicinal And Aromatic Crops. Universities Press (India) Pvt. Limited. 2004
13. Bansal G, Suthar N, Kaur J, Jain A. Stability Testing of Herbal Drugs: Challenges, Regulatory in Compliance and Perspectives. Phytother Res. 2016;30(7):1046-58.
14. Barbara Steinhoff. Regulatory Situation of Herbal Medicines-A Worldwide Review. World Health Organization, Traditional Medicine Programme. 1998
15. Bertram Katzung. Bertram Katzung. Basic & Clinical Pharmacology. McGraw-Hill Education.
16. Beverly McCabe-Sellers, Eric H. Frankel, Jonathan J. Wolfe. Handbook of Food-Drug Interactions. CRC Press. 2003
17. Biren Shah, Avinash Seth. Textbook of Pharmacognosy and Phytochemistry. Elsevier Health Sciences. 2014
18. C. S. Shah, J. S. Qadry. A Textbook of Pharmacognosy. Messrs B.S. Shah 1971

19. C.K. Kokate, Purohit, Gokhlae. Text book of Pharmacognosy, 37th Edition, Nirali Prakashan, Pune. 2007

20. Charis M. Galanakis. Nutraceuticals and Natural Product Pharmaceuticals. Elsevier Science.2019

21. Cultivation and Utilization of Medicinal Plants. Regional Research Laboratory, Council of Scientific & Industrial Research. 1982

22. Darrell Addison Posey, Graham Dutfield. Beyond Intellectual Property-Toward Traditional Resource Rights for Indigenous Peoples and Local Communities. International Development Research Centre (Canada). 1996.

23. Debasis Bagchi, Sreejayan Nair. Developing New Functional Food and Nutraceutical Products. Elsevier Science. 2016

24. Deepa Goel, Shomini Parashar. IPR, Biosafety and Bioethics. Pearson Education India. 2013

25. Deore SL, Khadabadi SS, Baviskar BA. Pharmacognosy and Phytochemistry-A Comprehensive Approach. PharmMed Press, Hyderabad. 2nd Edition, 2018.

26. Deore SL. Pharmacognosy and Phytochemistry: A Companion Handbook. PharmMed Press, Hyderabad. . 2nd Edition, 2017.

27. Dossett ML, Cohen EM, Cohen J. Integrative Medicine for Gastrointestinal Disease. Prim Care. 2017 Jun;44(2):265-280.

28. Durgesh Nandini Chauhan, Madhu Gupta, Nagendra Singh Chauhan, Vikas Sharma. Novel Drug Delivery Systems for Phytoconstituents. CRC Press.2019

29. Dwyer JT, Coates PM, Smith MJ. Dietary Supplements: Regulatory Challenges and Research Resources. Nutrients. 2018 Jan 4;10(1):41.

30. Elizabeth M. Williamson, Karen Baxter, Samuel Driver. Stockley's Herbal Medicines Interactions-A Guide to the Interactions of Herbal Medicines, Dietary Supplements and Nutraceuticals with Conventional Medicines. Pharmaceutical Press.2009

31. FDA 2012. Code of Federal Regulations Title 21, Part 111. Current Good Manufacturing Practice in Manufacturing, Packaging, Labeling, or Holding Operations for Dietary Supplements. Food and Drug Administration.

32. Federici E, Multari G, Gallo FR, Palazzino G. Le droghe vegetali: dall'uso tradizionale alla normativa [Herbal drugs: from traditional use to regulation]. Ann Ist Super Sanita. 2005;41(1):49-54. Italian.

33. Graham Dutfield, Uma Suthersanen. Global Intellectual Property Law. Edward Elgar Publishing, Incorporated. 2008

34. GS Kumar. KN Jayaveera. A Textbook of Pharmacognosy and Phytochemistry. S Chand & Company Limited. India. 2014.

35. Gunnar Samuelsson. Drugs of Natural Origin-A Textbook of Pharmacognosy. Apotekarsocieteten. 1999

36. Gupta PD, Daswani PG, Birdi TJ. Approaches in fostering quality parameters for medicinal botanicals in the Indian context. Indian J Pharmacol. 2014;46(4):363-71.
37. H. Ansari. Essentials of Pharmacognosy. Second edition, Birla publications, New Delhi, 2007
38. H. Panda Medicinal Plants Cultivation & Their Uses. Asia Pacific Business Press. 2002
39. H. Panda The Complete Technology Book on Herbal Beauty Products with Formulations and Processes. NIIR Project Consultancy Services. 2005
40. H. Panda. Perfumes And Flavours Technology Handbook. NIIR Project Consultancy Services. 2010
41. H.Pande. Herbal Cosmetics. Asia Pacific Business press, Inc, New Delhi.
42. Hand Book of Ayurvedic Medicines with Formulations (a Complete Hand Book of Ayurvedic and Herbal Medicines). Engineers India Research Institute [EIRI]2006
43. Heinrich M. Quality and safety of herbal medical products: regulation and the need for quality assurance along the value chains. Br J Clin Pharmacol. 80(1):62-6. 2015
44. Helmut Buschmann, Jörg Holenz, Raimund Mannhold, Yogeshwar Bachhav. Innovative Dosage Forms-Design and Development at Early Stage. Wiley. 2019
45. Indian patent office website-http://www.ipindia.nic.in/index.htm
46. Indian Pharmacopeia 2018, Ghaziabad: Indian Pharmacopeia Commission; 2018.
47. International Organisation for Standardization. Guide 30/Amd. 1 – Revision of Definitions for Reference Material and Certified Reference Material. ISO copyright office, Geneva, Switzerland. 2008.
48. International Organisation for Standardization. Guide 31 - Reference Materials - Contents of Certificates and Labels. ISO copyright office, Geneva, Switzerland. 2000a
49. International Organisation for Standardization. Guide 32 - Calibration in Analytical Chemistry and Use of Certified Reference Materials. ISO copyright office, Geneva, Switzerland. 1997
50. International Organisation for Standardization. Guide 33 - Uses of Certified Reference Materials. ISO copyright office, Geneva, Switzerland. 2000b.
51. International Organisation for Standardization. Guide 34 - General Requirements for the Competence of Reference Material Producers. ISO copyright office, Geneva, Switzerland. 2009.
52. International Organisation for Standardization. Guide 35 – Reference Materials - General and Statistical Principles for Certification. ISO copyright office, Geneva, Switzerland. 2006
53. J.C. Tarafdar, K.P. Tripathi, M. Kumar. Organic Agriculture. Scientific Publishers. 2012
54. James Bobbers, Marilyn KS, VE Tylor. Pharmacognosy & Pharmacobiotechnology. Williams & Wilkins. 1996.

55. Jean Bruneton. Pharmacognosy, Phytochemistry, Medicinal Plants. Technique & Documentation. 1999

56. José Rodríguez Pérez. The FDA and Worldwide Current Good Manufacturing Practices and Quality System Requirements Guidebook for Finished Pharmaceuticals. ASQ Quality Press. 2014

57. K. Chopra. Medicinal Plants-Conservation, Cultivation and Utilization. Daya Publishing House . 2007

58. K. Mangathayaru. Pharmacognosy: An Indian perspective. Pearson Education India. 2013

59. Kaliya A. Text Book of Industrial Pharmacognosy. CBS Publishers & Distributors, Delhi. 2009

60. Kendall Jefferson. Pharmacognosy and Phytotherapy. Foster Academics.2019

61. Kerryn Phelps, Craig Hassed. Herb-drug Interactions-General Practice: The Integrative Approach Series. 2012

62. Khadabadi SS, Deore SL, Baviskar BA. Experimental Phytopharmacognosy. Nirali prakashan, Pune. 1st Edition, 2019.

63. Kim JH, Lee K, Jerng UM, Choi G. Global Comparison of Stability Testing Parameters and Testing Methods for Finished Herbal Products. Evid Based Complement Alternat Med. 2019;20;2019:7348929.

64. Luqi Huang. Molecular Pharmacognosy. Springer Netherlands. 2012

65. M.P. Singh, Himadri Panda. Medicinal Herbs with Their Formulations. Daya Publishing House. 2005

66. Michael Heinrich, Elizabeth M. Williamson, Joanne Barnes, Simon Gibbons, Jose Prieto-Garcia Fundamentals of Pharmacognosy and Phytotherapy E-Book. Elsevier Health Sciences. 2017

67. Michael Heinrich, Joanne Barnes, Simon Gibbons. Fundamentals of Pharmacognosy and Phytotherapy. Churchill Livingstone/Elsevier. 2012

68. Mitchell Bebel Stargrove, Jonathan Treasure, Dwight L. McKee. Herb, Nutrient, and Drug Interactions-Clinical Implications and Therapeutic Strategies. Mosby/Elsevier. 2008

69. Mohammad Ali. Text book of Pharmacognosy. CBS Publishers & Distribution, New Delhi.2019

70. Moulin AM. The herbal pharmaceutical industry in India - Drug reformulation and the market (edited by Jean-Paul Gaudillière and Laurent Pordié)]. Med Sci (Paris). 2016;32(10):895-897.

71. N P S Sengar, Ashwini Singh, Ritesh Agrawal. A Textbook of Pharmacognosy. PharmaMed Press. 2018

72. Neelesh Malviya, Sapna Malviya. Herbal Drug Technology. CBS India. 2018

73. Neeraj Pandey, Khushdeep Dharni. Intellectual Property Rights. PHI Learning. 2014

74. Nirmal Joshee, Prahlad Parajuli, Sadanand A. DhekneyMedicinal Plants-From Farm to Pharmacy. Springer International Publishing. 2019

75. P. K. Chattopadhyay. Herbal Cosmetics & Ayurvedic Medicines (EOU) (3rd Revised Edition). NIIR Project Consultancy Services. 2013

76. Parintek Innovations. Unfolding Intellectual PRoperty Rights-A Practical Patent Guide for Researchers, Academicians and start-ups. Notion Press. 2019

77. Peter Ulvskov. Patenting in Biotechnology-A Laboratory Manual. Polyteknisk Boghandel og Forlag. 2019.

78. Prabuddha Ganguli. Gearing Up for Patents-The Indian Scenario. Universities Press. 1998

79. Pulok K. Mukherjee. Evidence-Based Validation of Herbal Medicine. Elsevier Science. 2015

80. Pulok K. Mukherjee. Quality Control and Evaluation of Herbal Drugs-Evaluating Natural Products and Traditional Medicine.. Elsevier Science. 2019

81. Pulok K. Mukherjee. Quality Control of Herbal Drugs-An Approach to Evaluation of Botanicals. Business Horizons. 2002

82. Qu L, Zou W, Wang Y, Wang M. European regulation model for herbal medicine: The assessment of the EU monograph and the safety and efficacy evaluation in marketing authorization or registration in Member States. Phytomedicine. 2018 Mar 15;42:219-225.

83. R. O. B. Wijesekera, R. O. Wijesekera. The Medicinal Plant Industry. CRC-Press. 1991

84. R.D. Choudhary. Herbal drug industry. First Edn, Eastern Publisher, New Delhi. 1996

85. Rajesh K. Kesharwani. Anil K. Sharma. Nutraceuticals and Dietary Supplements-Applications in Health Improvement and Disease Management. Apple Academic Press. 2020

86. Ram Dev Chaudhuri. Herbal Drugs Industry-Practical Approach to Industrial Pharmacognosy. Eastern Publishers.1996

87. Ramesh Gupta. Nutraceuticals-Efficacy, Safety and Toxicity. Elsevier Science. 2016

88. Rangari VD. Pharmacognosy& Phytochemistry. Career Publication, Nashik. 2008

89. Ravindra Sharma. Agro-Techniques of Medicinal Plants. Daya Publishing House . 2004.

90. Reif K, Sievers H, Steffen J-P. The role of chemical reference standards as analytical tools in the quality assessment of botanical materials – A European perspective. Herbal Gram. 2004;63: 38-43.

91. S. S. Agarwal, M. Paridhavi. Herbal Drug Technology. Universities Press. 2012

92. S. S. Handa. Pharmacognosy. Vallabh Prakashan, New Delhi. 1989

93. S. S. Purohit, S. P. Vyas.A Scientific Approach : Including Processing and Financial Guidelines. Agrobios (India). 2004

94. Sahoo N, Manchikanti P.Herbal drug regulation and commercialization: an Indian industry perspective.J Altern Complement Med. 2013 Dec;19(12):957-63.

95. Santini A, Cammarata SM, Capone G, Ianaro A, Tenore GC, Pani L, Novellino E. Nutraceuticals: opening the debate for a regulatory framework. Br J Clin Pharmacol. 2018 Apr;84(4):659-672.

96. Serdar Oztekin, Milan Martinov. Medicinal and Aromatic Crops-Harvesting, Drying, and Processing. CRC Press. 2014

97. Serna-Thomé G, Castro-Eguiluz D, Fuchs-Tarlovsky V, Sánchez-López M, Delgado-Olivares L, Coronel-Martínez J, Molina-Trinidad EM, de la Torre M, Cetina-Pérez L. Use of Functional Foods and Oral Supplements as Adjuvants in Cancer Treatment. Rev Invest Clin. 2018;70(3):136-146.

98. Simone Badal Mccreath. Rupika Delgoda. Pharmacognosy-Fundamentals, Applications and Strategies. Elsevier Science. 2017

99. Sissi Wachtel-Galor. Herbal Medicine-Biomolecular and Clinical Aspects, Second Edition. CRC Press. 2011.

100. T. C. Denston. A Textbook of Pharmacognosy. Read Books. 2012

101. The British Pharmacopeia. London: Medicines and Healthcare Products Regulatory Agency; 1993.

102. The Complete Technology Book On Flavours, Fragrances And Perfumes. NIIR Project Consultancy Services. 2007

103. Uma J. Lele, William Lesser, Gesa Horstkotte-Wesseler. Intellectual Property Rights in Agriculture-The World Bank's Role in Assisting Borrower and Member Countries. World Bank. 2000

104. United States Pharmacopoeia and National Formulary, USP 25 NF 19/National Formulary 20, Rockville, MD, U. S. Pharmacopoeial Convention, Inc. 2002.

105. W.C.Evans, Trease and Evans Pharmacognosy, 16th edition, W.B. Sounders & Co., London, 2009.

106. Website- Farmer's right- http://www.fao.org/plant-treaty/areas-of-work/farmers-rights/en/

107. Website-pps.who.int/iris/handle/10665/42783

108. WHO Guidelines on Good Agricultural and Collection Practices (GACP) for Medicinal Plants By World Health Organization, WHO · 2003

109. WHO. Guidelines for Good Clinical Practice (GCP) for Trials on Pharmaceutical Products. World Health Organization, WHO Technical Series, No. 850, 1995, Annex 3.

110. WHO. Guidelines for the Assessment of Herbal Medicines. World Health Organization, 1991

111. WHO. Joint FAO/WHO Expert Committe on Food Additives: Evaluation of Certain Food Additives - WHO Technical Report Series, No. 952 - 69th Report. World Health Organization. 2009.

112. WHO. WHO Expert Committee on Specifications for Pharmaceutical Preparations - WHO Technical Report Series, No. 885 – 35th Report. 1999

113. WIPO Website-https://www.wipo.int/portal/en/index.html

114. World Health Organization Research Office for the Western Pacific. Research Guidelines for Evaluating the Safety and Efficacy of Herbal Medicines. 1993.

115. World Health Organization. Quality Control Methods for Medicinal Plant Materials. 1998

116. WTO Website-https://www.wto.org/

117. Yashwant Pathak. Handbook of Nutraceuticals Volume I.Ingredients, Formulations, and Applications. CRC Press.2010

118. Zhou S, Chan E, Pan SQ, Huang M, Lee EJ. Pharmacokinetic interactions of drugs with St John's wort. J Psychopharmacol. 2004 Jun;18(2):262-76.

Part - II

Practical Manual

Know Subject: Pharmacognosy

The term 'pharmacognosy' (combination of two Greek words i.e. *pharmakon* means drug and *gnosis* means knowledge) means acquiring knowledge of drugs was coined in 1815 by C. A. Seydler, German medical student in his thesis title "*Analyetica Pharmacognostica*". Pharmacognosy is defined as scientific and systematic study of structural, physical, chemical and biological characters of crude drugs along with history, method of cultivation, collection and preparation for the market. The American Society of Pharmacognosy defines pharmacognosy as "the study of the physical, chemical, biochemical and biological properties of drugs, drug substances or potential drugs or drug substances of natural origin as well as the search for new drugs from natural sources. It is also called as study of crude drugs.

Thus pharmacognostical studies of plant drugs involves study of synonyms, vernacular names, Biological sources, distribution, morphology, histology, chemistry, qualitative test, various physicochemical tests, pharmacological actions along with commercial varieties, substitutes, adulterants and any other quality control parameters of the drugs.

However, this subject is as old as pharmacy and mankind evolution; recently it is evolved as a multidisciplinary subject focusing many modern disciplines like ethanobotany, ethanopharmcology, phytotherapy, phytochemistry, chemo-taxanomy, biotechnology, clinical trials, herbal drug interaction and even novel drug delivery systems like phytosomes rather only botanical and taxanomical descriptions. Recent advances in extraction methods, analytical hyphenated techniques, screening methods continues to hasten major changes in this subject. Modernization of conventional and/or traditional dosage forms is opening doors to industrial Pharmacognosy.

Due to most recent technologies and innovative chemical concepts, many new drugs or drug candidates still originated from natural products or derivatives thereof. Even in this era of nanotechnology, natural drugs are important part of primary health care which is giving pharmacognosy professionals new possibilities to exploit the huge diversity designed and generated by nature.

There is a shortage of established scientists engaged in pharmacognosy research, which tends to involve subject matter beyond the conventional scientist's knowledge base. Hence, actual secret of opportunities in pharmacognosy research is that only the tip of the iceberg seems to have been discovered yet.

Following materials are required for Pharmacognosy laboratory work.

- Napkin
- Needle
- Filter paper
- Camel hair brushes
- Stains
- Watch glass
- A sharp razor blades
- Forceps
- Micro-slide
- Cover slip

Instructions for Students

Students shall read the points given below for understanding theoretical concepts and practical applications.

1. Students should wear white Apron, Cap, Mask, Gloves and Slipper before entering in to laboratory.
2. Students should keep their belongings in locker which are not required during practical like bag, Extra files etc.
3. Students should always carry Laboratory Manual, rough notebook, and practical requirements without fail.
4. Listen carefully to the lecture given by teacher about importance of subject, curriculum philosophy, graphical structure, skills to be developed, information about equipment, instruments, procedure, method of continuous assessment, tentative plan of working laboratory and total amount of work to be done in a year.
5. Students should perform the practical only at the place which allocated to him/her. (No change can be done without permission of subject teacher)
6. Students shall undergo study visit of laboratory for types of equipment, instruments, material to be used, before performing experiment
7. Read write up of each experiment to be performed, a day in advance.
8. Organize the work in the group and make a record of all observations.
9. Understand the purpose of experiment and its practical applications.
10. Write the answer of the questions allotted by teacher during practical hours if possible or afterwards, but immediately.
11. Students should not hesitate to ask any difficulty faced during conduct of practical.
12. The students shall study all the questions given in the laboratory manual and practice to write the answers to these questions
13. Students shall develop maintenance skill as expected by the industries.
14. Students should develop the habits of pocket discussion, group discussion related to the experiments so that exchanges of knowledge, skills could take place.
15. Students shall attempt to develop related hands on skills and gain confidence.
16. Students shall visit nearby workshops, workstation, industries, technical exhibitions, trade fair etc. even not included in the lab manual. In short, students should have exposure to the area of work right in the student's hood.
17. Students shall insist for the completion of recommended laboratory work, industrial visits, answers to the given questions, etc
18. Students shall develop habits of evolving more ideas, innovations skills etc. than included in the scope of manual

19. Students shall develop technical magazines, proceedings of seminars, refers websites related to the scope of the subjects and update their knowledge and skills.
20. Students should develop the habit of not to depend totally on the teachers but to develop self learning techniques
21. Students should develop the habit to react with the teacher without hesitation with respect to the academic involved.
22. Students should develop the habit to submit the practical exercise continuously and progressively on the scheduled dated and should get the assessment done
23. Student should be well prepared while submitting the write up of the experiments. This will develop the continuity of the studies and he will be over laded at the end of the term.
24. Students should clean platform before leaving the laboratory.

Index

Sr. No	Aim	Date	Page	Marks	Sign
1.	To perform preliminary phytochemical screening of given sample crude drug: Senna				
2.	To perform preliminary phytochemical screening of given sample crude drug: Licorice				
3.	To determine alcohol content of Asava and Arista				
4.	To evaluate excipients of natural origin: Agar, Tragacanth, Beeswax, Castor oil				
5.	To prepare and evaluate skin lightening cream containing standardized licorice extract				
6.	To prepare and evaluate skin lightening lotion containing standardized licorice extract				
7.	To prepare and evaluate herbal shampoo containing standardized extract of Reetha (Sapindus mukorosii) fruit				
8.	To prepare and evaluate standardized Licorice extract containing cough syrup				
9.	To prepare and evaluate Senna syrup containing standardized senna fluid extract				
10.	To prepare and evaluate Senna mixture containing standardized senna fluid extract				
11.	To determine total phenolic content in given crude drug sample				
12.	To determine total alkaloid content in given crude drug sample				
13.	To perform monograph analysis of Castor Oil				
14.	To perform monograph analysis of Clove Oil				
15.	To evaluate herbal drug (Licorice) as per Monograph analysis from recent Pharmacopoeias [Indian Pharmacopoeia 2018, The Ayurvedic Pharmacopoeia of India-2001, British Pharmacopoeia-1993, USP 26, NF 21]				

Aim: 1. To perform preliminary phytochemical screening of given sample crude drug: Senna

Requirements: All pharmacognosy chemical tests reagents, test tubes, Gas burners, water bath

Theory:

Preliminary phytochemical evaluation is the step after extraction in order to identify different classes of constituents that can be present in extracts i.e. carbohydrates, proteins, lipids, flavonoids, tannins, glycosides, alkaloids or essential oils.

Always choose a solvent of extraction whose solubility and/or polarity is same as that of the constituents i.e. to obtain polar components use polar solvents only. After detecting the particular class, one can perform specific chemical tests for whole crude drug or individual constituents to confirm any known drug or component.

<table>
<tr><th>Class of Drugs</th><th>Procedure</th><th>Inference</th><th>Observation (Positive/Negative)</th></tr>
<tr><td colspan="3">Carbohydrates</td><td></td></tr>
<tr><td>Molisch's test
[Dissolve 3.75 g of 1-naphthol in 25 ml of Ethanol 99%.]</td><td>Mix 1 ml reagent in 2 ml of test solution. Add 1 ml of concentrated sulfuric acid.</td><td>Red to violet ring depending on the amount of sugar appears at the junction of the two liquids.</td><td></td></tr>
<tr><td>Iodine test for starch</td><td>Mix 0.5 ml of iodine solution with 1 ml of the test solution.</td><td>Starch gives deep blue color.</td><td></td></tr>
<tr><td>Fehling's test
[Fehling's "A" is 7 g copper(II) sulfate pentahydrate dissolved in distilled water containing 2 drops of dilute sulfuric acid. Fehling's "B" is 35g of potassium tartrate and 12g of NaOH in 100 ml of distilled water. These two solutions should be stoppered and stored until needed.]</td><td>Mix 1 ml of Fehling's solution 'A' with 1 ml of Fehling's solution 'B' and 1 ml of test solution. Then, boil it.</td><td>Yellow to red precipitate indicates presence of reducing sugars</td><td></td></tr>
<tr><td>Benedict's test
[Benedict's reagent is prepared by mixing 17.3 grams of copper sulfate pentahydrate, 100 grams of sodium carbonate, and 173 grams of sodium citrate in distilled water (required quantity).]</td><td>Mix 2 ml of Benedict's reagent with 2 ml test solution. Boil it in a water bath.</td><td>Formation of red, yellow or green colored precipitate depending on the sugar concentration indicates presence of reducing sugars</td><td><table>
<tr><th>Colour of the Precipitate</th><th>Aproximate percentage of Reducing Sugar</th></tr>
<tr><td>Green</td><td>0.5%</td></tr>
<tr><td>Yellow</td><td>1%</td></tr>
<tr><td>Orange</td><td>1.5%</td></tr>
<tr><td>Red</td><td>2%</td></tr>
</table></td></tr>
</table>

Contd...

Class of Drugs	Procedure	Inference	Observation (Positive/Negative)
Barfoed's test [Barfoed's reagent is 0.33 molar solution of copper (II) acetate in 1% acetic acid solution.]	Mix 2 ml of Barfoed's reagent with 1 ml of the test solution. Boil it and wait.	Brick-red precipitate of monosaccharides.	
Seliwanoff's test for ketohexoses [Seliwanoff's Reagent is 110 mg of Resorcinol in 220 ml of 3N HCl.]	Mix 2 ml of Seliwanoff's reagent with 1 ml of test solution. Boil.	Deep red color due to ketohexoses.	
Bial's test for pentoses [Bial's reagent is 0.4 g orcinol, 200 ml of concentrated hydrochloric acid and 0.5 ml of a 10% solution of ferric chloride.]	Mix 5 ml of Bial's reagent with 1 ml of test solution. Warm slowly.	Green color precipitate due to pentoses.	
Proteins			
Biuret test [Biuret reagent is prepared by mixing 1.5 gram of pentavalent copper sulphate (CuSO4), 6 gram of Sodium potassium tartarate (chelating agent) in 500 ml of distilled water and 375 ml of 2 molar Sodium hydroxide Mix and make final volume to 1000 ml by adding distilled water.	Mix 2 ml test solution with 2 ml Biuret reagent.	Violet to pink color	
Millon's test [Millon's reagent is Mercuric Nitrate-160 g, Mercurous Nitrate-160 g, Conc. Nitric acid-400 ml and Distilled water-600 ml	Mix 2 ml test solution with 2 ml Millon's reagent. Boil it.	Red color	
Lead acetate test	Mix 2 ml test solution with 2 ml of 40% NaOH and 0.5 ml lead acetate solution. Boil it.	Black to brown color	

Contd...

Class of Drugs	Procedure	Inference	Observation (Positive/Negative)
Amino Acids			
Ninhydrin test [Ninhydrin reagent is 0.2 grams of ninhydrin in 10ml of either ethanol or acetone]	Mix 2 ml test solution with 1 ml of 5% ninhydrin solution. Boil for 5 minutes in water bath.	Blue or purple color.	
Tyrosine test	Mix 2 ml test solution with 1 ml Millon's reagent and boil the solution.	Dark red color.	
Alkaloids			
Dragendorff's reagent (Potassium Bismuth iodide)	Mix 2 ml of reagent with 2 ml filtrate of plant drug extract.	Reddish brown precipitate.	
Modified Dragendorff's reagent (Kraut's reagent) (Potassium Bismuth iodide + Nitric acid)	Mix 2 ml of reagent with 2 ml filtrate of plant drug extract.	Precipitate	
Hager's reagent (Picric acid)	Mix 2 ml of reagent with 2 ml filtrate of plant drug extract.	Yellow color precipitate	
Mayer's reagent (Potassium mercuric iodide)	Mix 2 ml of reagent with 2 ml filtrate of plant drug extract.	Cream colored precipitate	
Wagner's reagent (Potassium iodide)	Mix 2 ml of reagent with 2 ml filtrate of plant drug extract.	Reddish brown precipitate.	
Glycosides			
General test	**Solution A:** Extract sample powder with alcohol or water, and then, add Fehling Solution. **Solution B:** Add sulfuric acid and then add Fehling Solution to water or alcoholic extract	If solution B has dark color than solution A (if sugar content is high in solution B than solution A), it indicates the presence of glycosides. **Note**: Acid hydrolyzes glycone and aglycone moiety and thus, sugar content is increased in solution B.	
Cardiac Glycosides			
Kedde's test [Kedde Reagent A: Dissolve 3,5-dinitrobenzoic acid (2 g) in 90% ethanol). Kedde Reagent B: Dissolve sodium hydroxide (5 g) in distilled water 000 ml)]	Mix 1 ml of test solution with 2 ml reagent.	Blue to purple color	

Contd...

Class of Drugs	Procedure	Inference	Observation (Positive/Negative)
Baljet reagent (Bufadienolides)	Mix 2–3 mg of sample in 2 ml sodium picrate solution.	Yellow and orange to deep red color	
Keller-kiliani test for digitoxose sugar	To the alcoholic extract of sample, add 5 ml of water and 0.5 ml of strong solution of lead acetate. Filter and treat the clear filtrate with equal volume of chloroform, and evaporate to yield dry residue. Add glacial acetic acid, 0.5 ml of ferric chloride solution, and 2 ml of concentrated sulfuric acid.	The initial red-brown layer changes to blue green.	
Legal's test (Cardenolides)	Mix 1 ml of test solution with 2 ml pyridine and sodium nitroprusside.	Pink or red color	
Raymond test (alkaline m-dinitrobenzene)	Mix alcoholic extract of sample in 0.1 ml of Raymond's reagent and add 2-3 drops of 20% NaOH solution.	Violet color changes to blue	
Flavonoids			
Shinoda test	Add magnesium powder and a few drops of concentrated HCl or H_2SO_4 to 2 ml of sample solution.	Flavones, flavonols and xanthones: Orange, pink, red, and purple. Flavanones and flavononols: weak pink to magenta colors, or no color at all.	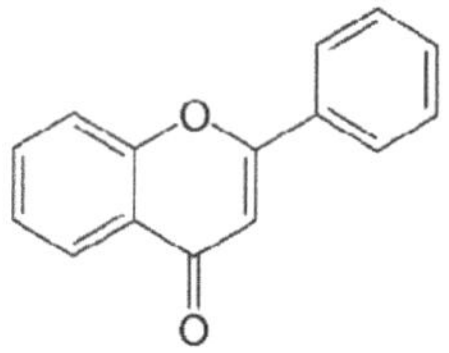 •
Modified Shinoda test	The procedure is same as above except the use of zinc powder instead of magnesium.	Flavanonols: Deep-red to magenta color	
Sulphuric acid	Add 3 ml of H_2SO_4 in sample.	Flavones and flavonols: Deep yellow color. Chalcones and aurones: Red or red-bluish. Flavanones: Orange to red colors.	
Lead acetate	Mix test solution with lead acetate.	Yellow precipitate	
Alkali test	Treat test solution with increasing amount of NaOH.	Yellow coloration which decolorizes after addition of acid	

Contd...

Class of Drugs	Procedure	Inference	Observation (Positive/Negative)
Tannins			
Ferric chloride test	Mix 2 ml of test solution with 5% of ferric chloride solution.	Blue, blue-black or blue-green color reaction	
Gelatin-salt test	Prepare three test tubes of extract solution. To the first, add 1% solution of NaCl; to the second, add 1% NaCl and 5% gelatin solution; and to the third, add $FeCl_3$ solution.	Formation of a precipitate in the second treatment suggests the presence of tannins and a positive response after addition of $FeCl_3$ to the third portion supports this inference.	
Lead acetate test	Mix test solution with lead acetate solution.	White precipitate	
Bromine water test	Mix test solution with bromine water.	Discoloration of original solution	
Dilute iodine test	Mix test solution with dilute iodine solution.	Red color to solution	
Triterpenoids			
Liebermann–Burchard test	Mix 2 ml test extract with 1 ml chloroform, 1 ml acetic anhydride, and add one drop concentrated H_2SO_4.	Blue-green to red-orange color. A bluish-green or blue color indicates presence of steroids, and a pink-violet color indicates terpenoids.	
Noller's test	Mix 2 ml test extract with small quantity of tin and thionyl chloride.	Pink coloration indicates the presence of triterpenoids.	
Sannie test	Mix 2 ml extract with stannous chloride, acetic acid and carbon tetrachloride (6:50:50). Heat at $100^{O}C$	Brown color	
Steroids			
Liebermann test	Mix 2 ml test extract with 2 ml acetic anhydride. Boil and add 0.5 ml of H_2SO_4.	Blue color.	
Zimmermann test (% dinitrobenzene)	Mix 2 ml test extract with 1 ml of 2N KOH in alcohol and 1 ml 1% dinitrobenzene in alcohol. After 10 min add this mixture to 8 ml alcohol.	Violet color	
Salkowski reaction	Dissolve 1–2 mg of the sample in 1 ml of $CHCl_3$ and add 1 ml concentrated H_2SO_4.	**Chloroform** layer shows red color and acid layer shows green fluorescence	

Contd...

Class of Drugs	Procedure	Inference	Observation (Positive/Negative)
Saponins			
Foam test	Shake aqueous solution of a saponin containing sample producing foam, which is stable for 15 seconds or more.	Foam lasts for more than 15 seconds	
Hemolysis test	Mix red blood sample with sufficient quantity of extract solution. Shake and observe.	Clear red solution	
Anthraquinone Glycosides			
Borntrager's test o-glycosides	Take a little quantity of aqueous solution of sample; add H_2SO_4, then add CCl_4 or ether in it. Separate the organic layer and shake with dilute ammonia.	Rose pink color of ammonia layer.	
Modified anthraquinone test for C-glycosides	Take little quantity of aqueous solution of sample; add ferric chloride solution, HCl, and then add CCl_4 or ether. Separate the organic layer and shake with dilute ammonia.	Rose pink color of ammonia layer	
Cyanogenetic Glycosides			
Sodium picrate test (Guignard picrate test)	Take the aqueous test solution of sample in test tube and add dilute H_2SO_4; suspend sodium picrate treated filter paper.	Hydrogen Cyanide (HCN) turns the paper to brick red color due to formation of sodium iso-perpurate.	
Mercurous nitrate test	Mix 2 ml test extract solution with 3% aqueous mercurous nitrate solution.	Formation of metallic mercury	
Guaiacum test	Dip strip of paper in guaiacum resin, then, moisten with dilute $CuSO_4$ and exposed to cut surface of crude drug.	Paper turns to blue due to HCN.	
Coumarin Glycosides			
Odour test	Take the odour of powder or extract.	Aromatic smell.	
Alkali test	Mix the test solution with alkali.	Blue green fluorescence	

Contd...

Class of Drugs	Procedure	Inference	Observation (Positive/Negative)
Fluorescence filer paper test	Take the moist powder of drug in test tube, cover test tube with alkali moist filter paper. Heat the test tube and observe paper under UV light.	Yellow green fluorescence	
Gum	Take the powder of gum sample and add HCl to hydrolyze the polysaccharides. Now, perform Fehling's or Benedict's test.	Positive test.	
Mucilage			
Ruthenium red test	Treat the powder with ruthenium red.	Red color	
Swelling test	Dissolve the powder in water.	Powder swells	
Fatty Oil			
Filter paper test	Press the powder between filter paper.	Permanent oily spot.	
Solubility test	Mix oil in alcohol.	Insoluble	
Essential Oil			
Sudan red III test	Treat the test solution with Sudan red III.	Red color	
Tincture alkana test (Alkanna tinctoria roots)	Treat the test solution with tincture alkana.	Red color	
Solubility test	Dissolve the oil in alcohol.	Completely soluble	

Result: Preliminary phytochemical screening of following sample crude drug was performed and following phytochemical class constituents are found present:

Questions

1. What are the chemical tests for identification of protcin?
2. What are the chemical tests for identification of carbohydrate?
3. Killer killani test is used for identification of..........?
4. Which test is useful for cardenolide detection?
5. Give the composition of Wagner's reagent?
6. Give the composition of Hager's reagent?
7. Give the composition of Mayer's reagent?
8. Give the composition of Dragendroff's reagent?
9. What is difference between Liebermann and Liebermann- Burchard test?
10. How to differentiate volatile and non-volatile oil by chemical tests?
11. What is difference between Shinoda and modified Shinoda test?

Aim: 2. To perform preliminary phytochemical screening of given sample crude drug: Rauwolfia

Requirements: All pharmacognosy chemical tests reagents, test tubes, Gas burners, water bath

Theory:

Preliminary phytochemical evaluation is the step after extraction in order to identify different classes of constituents that can be present in extracts i.e. carbohydrates, proteins, lipids, flavonoids, tannins, glycosides, alkaloids or essential oils. Always choose a solvent of extraction whose solubility and/or polarity is same as that of the constituents i.e. to obtain polar components use polar solvents only. After detecting the particular class, one can perform specific chemical tests for whole crude drug or individual constituents to confirm any known drug or component.

Class of Drugs	Procedure	Inference	Observation (Positive/Negative)
Carbohydrates			
Molisch's test	Mix 1 ml reagent in 2 ml of test solution. Add 1 ml of concentrated sulfuric acid.	Red to violet ring depending on the amount of sugar appears at the junction of the two liquids.	
Iodine test for starch	Mix 0.5 ml of iodine solution with 1 ml of the test solution.	Starch gives deep blue color.	
Fehling's test	Mix 1 ml of Fehling's solution 'A' with 1 ml of Fehling's solution 'B' and 1 ml of test solution. Then, boil it.	Yellow to red precipitate indicates presence of reducing sugars	
Benedict's test	Mix 2 ml of Benedict's reagent with 2 ml test solution. Boil it in a water bath.	Formation of red, yellow or green colored precipitate depending on the sugar concentration indicates presence of reducing sugars	
Barfoed's test	Mix 2 ml of Barfoed's reagent with 1 ml of the test solution. Boil it and wait.	Brick-red precipitate of monosaccharides.	
Seliwanoff's test for ketohexoses	Mix 2 ml of Seliwanoff's reagent with 1 ml of test solution. Boil.	Deep red color due to ketohexoses.	
Bial's test for pentoses	Mix 5 ml of Bial's reagent with 1 ml of test solution. Warm slowly.	Green color precipitate due to pentoses.	
Proteins			
Biuret test	Mix 2 ml test solution with 2 ml Biuret reagent.	Violet to pink color	
Millon's test	Mix 2 ml test solution with 2 ml Millon's reagent. Boil it.	Red color	
Lead acetate test	Mix 2 ml test solution with 2 ml of 40% NaOH and 0.5 ml lead acetate solution. Boil it.	Black to brown color	

Contd...

Class of Drugs	Procedure	Inference	Observation (Positive/Negative)
Amino Acids			
Ninhydrin test	Mix 2 ml test solution with 1 ml of 5% ninhydrin solution. Boil for 5 minutes in water bath.	Blue or purple color.	
Tyrosine test	Mix 2 ml test solution with 1 ml Millon's reagent and boil the solution.	Dark red color.	
Alkaloids			
Dragendorff's reagent (Potassium Bismuth iodide)	Mix 2 ml of reagent with 2 ml filtrate of plant drug extract.	Reddish brown precipitate.	
Modified Dragendorff's reagent (Kraut's reagent) (Potassium Bismuth iodide + Nitric acid)	Mix 2 ml of reagent with 2 ml filtrate of plant drug extract.	Precipitate	
Hager's reagent (Picric acid)	Mix 2 ml of reagent with 2 ml filtrate of plant drug extract.	Yellow color precipitate	
Mayer's reagent (Potassium mercuric iodide)	Mix 2 ml of reagent with 2 ml filtrate of plant drug extract.	Cream colored precipitate	
Wagner's reagent (Potassium iodide)	Mix 2 ml of reagent with 2 ml filtrate of plant drug extract.	Reddish brown precipitate.	
Glycosides			
General test	Solution A: Extract sample powder with alcohol or water, and then, add Fehling Solution. Solution B: Add sulfuric acid and then add Fehling Solution to water or alcoholic extract	If solution B has dark color than solution A (if sugar content is high in solution B than solution A), it indicates the presence of glycosides. Note: Acid hydrolyzes glycone and aglycone moiety and thus, sugar content is increased in solution B.	
Cardiac Glycosides			
Kedde's test Kedde Reagent A: Dissolve 3,5-dinitrobenzoic acid (2 g) in 90% ethanol 000 ml). Kedde Reagent B: Dissolve sodium hydroxide (5 g) in distilled water 000 ml).	Mix 1 ml of test solution with 2 ml reagent.	Blue to purple color	
Baljet reagent	Mix 2–3 mg of sample in 2 ml sodium picrate solution.	Yellow and orange to deep red color	

Contd...

Class of Drugs	Procedure	Inference	Observation (Positive/Negative)
Keller-kiliani test for digitoxose sugar	To the alcoholic extract of sample, add 5 ml of water and 0.5 ml of strong solution of lead acetate. Filter and treat the clear filtrate with equal volume of chloroform, and evaporate to yield dry residue. Add glacial acetic acid, 0.5 ml of ferric chloride solution, and 2 ml of concentrated sulfuric acid.	The initial red-brown layer changes to blue green.	
Legal's test (Cardenolides)	Mix 1 ml of test solution with 2 ml pyridine and sodium nitroprusside.	Pink or red color	
Raymond test (alkaline m-dinitrobenzene)	Mix alcoholic extract of sample in 0.1 ml of Raymond's reagent and add 2-3 drops of 20% NaOH solution.	Violet color changes to blue	
Flavonoids			
Shinoda test	Add magnesium powder and a few drops of concentrated HCl or H_2SO_4 to 2 ml of sample solution.	Flavones, flavonols and xanthones: Orange, pink, red, and purple. Flavanones and flavononols: weak pink to magenta colors, or no color at all.	
Modified shinoda test	The procedure is same as above except the use of zinc powder instead of magnesium.	Flavanonols: Deep-red to magenta color	
Sulphuric acid	Add 3 ml of H_2SO_4 in sample.	Flavones and flavonols: Deep yellow color. Chalcones and aurones: Red or red-bluish. Flavanones: Orange to red colors.	
Lead acetate	Mix test solution with lead acetate.	Yellow precipitate	
Alkali test	Treat test solution with increasing amount of NaOH.	Yellow coloration which decolorizes after addition of acid	
Tannins			
Ferric chloride test	Mix 2 ml of test solution with 5% of ferric chloride solution.	Blue, blue-black or blue-green color reaction	
Gelatin-salt test	Prepare three test tubes of extract solution. To the first, add 1% solution of NaCl; to the second, add 1% NaCl and 5% gelatin solution; and to the third, add $FeCl_3$ solution.	Formation of a precipitate in the second treatment suggests the presence of tannins and a positive response after addition of $FeCl_3$ to the third portion supports this inference.	

Contd...

Class of Drugs	Procedure	Inference	Observation (Positive/Negative)
Lead acetate test	Mix test solution with lead acetate solution.	White precipitate	
Bromine water test	Mix test solution with bromine water.	Discoloration of original solution	
Dilute iodine test	Mix test solution with dilute iodine solution.	Red color to solution	
Triterpenoids			
Liebermann–Burchard's test	Mix 2 ml test extract with 1 ml chloroform, 1 ml acetic anhydride, and add one drop concentrated H_2SO_4.	Blue-green to red-orange color. A bluish-green or blue color indicates presence of steroids, and a pink-violet color indicates terpenoids.	
Noller's test	Mix 2 ml test extract with small quantity of tin and thionyl chloride.	Pink coloration indicates the presence of triterpenoids.	
Sannie test	Mix 2 ml extract with stannous chloride, acetic acid and carbon tetrachloride (6:50:50). Heat at $100^{O}C$	Brown color	
Steroids			
Liebermann test	Mix 2 ml test extract with 2 ml acetic anhydride. Boil and add 0.5 ml of H_2SO_4.	Blue color.	
Zimmermann test	Mix 2 ml test extract with 1 ml of 2N KOH in alcohol and 1 ml 1% dinitrobenzene in alcohol. After 10 min add this mixture to 8 ml alcohol.	Violet color	
Salkowoski reaction	Dissolve 1–2 mg of the sample in 1 ml of $CHCl_3$ and add 1 ml concentrated H_2SO_4.	Chloroform layer shows red color and acid layer shows green fluorescence	
Saponins			
Foam test	Shake aqueous solution of a saponin containing sample producing foam, which is stable for 15 minutes or more.	Foam lasts for more than 15 seconds	
Hemolysis test	Mix red blood sample with sufficient quantity of extract solution. Shake and observe.	Clear red solution	
Anthraquinone Glycosides			
Borntrager's test	Take a little quantity of aqueous solution of sample; add H_2SO_4, then add CCl_4 or ether in it. Separate the organic layer and shake with dilute ammonia.	Rose pink color of ammonia layer.	

Contd...

Class of Drugs	Procedure	Inference	Observation (Positive/Negative)
Modified Borntrager's test for C-glycosides	Take little quantity of aqueous solution of sample; add ferric chloride solution, HCl, and then add CCl_4 or ether. Separate the organic layer and shake with dilute ammonia.	Rose pink color of ammonia layer	
Cyanogenetic Glycosides			
Sodium picrate test (Guignard picrate test)	Take the aqueous test solution of sample in test tube and add dilute H_2SO_4; suspend sodium picrate treated filter paper.	Hydrogen Cyanide (HCN) turns the paper to brick red color due to formation of sodium iso-perpurate.	
Mercurous nitrate test	Mix 2 ml test extract solution with 3% aqueous mercurous nitrate solution.	Formation of metallic mercury	
Guaiacum test	Dip strip of paper in guaiacum resin, then, moisten with dilute $CuSO_4$ and exposed to cut surface of crude drug.	Paper turns to blue due to HCN.	
Coumarin Glycosides			
Odour test	Take the odour of powder or extract.	Aromatic smell.	
Alkali test	Mix the test solution with alkali.	Blue green fluorescence	
Fluorescence test	Take the moist powder of drug in test tube, cover test tube with alkali moist filter paper. Heat the test tube and observe paper under UV light.	Yellow green fluorescence	
Gum	Take the powder of gum sample and add HCl to hydrolyze the polysaccharides. Now, perform Fehling's or Benedict's test.	Positive test.	
Mucilage			
Ruthenium red test	Treat the powder with ruthenium red.	Red color	
Swelling test	Dissolve the powder in water.	Powder swells	
Fatty Oil			
Filter paper test	Press the powder between filter paper.	Permanent oily spot.	
Solubility test	Mix oil in alcohol.	Insoluble	
Essential Oil			
Sudan red III test	Treat the test solution with Sudan red III.	Red color	
Tincture alkana test	Treat the test solution with tincture alkane.	Red color	
Solubility test	Dissolve the oil in alcohol.	Completely soluble	

Result: Preliminary phytochemical screening of following sample crude drug was performed and following phytochemical class constituents are found present:

Questions

1. What are the chemical tests for identification of steroids?
2. What are the chemical tests for identification of triterpenoids ?
3. What are the chemical tests for identification of tannins ?
4. What is difference between Borntrager's and modified Borntrager's test?
5. What are the chemical tests for identification of saponins?
6. What is c-glycoside?
7. What is Shinoda test?

Aim: 3: To determine alcohol content of Asava and Arista

Requirements: Distillation assembly, Distilled water, and Pumice powder.

Theory: Asava and Arishta are medicinal preparations made by soaking the drugs, either in coarse powder or in the form of decoction (kasaya), in a solution of sugar or jaggery, as the case may be, for a specified period of time, during which it undergoes a process of fermentation generating alcohol, thus facilitating the extraction of the active principles contained in the drugs. Alcohol, so generated, also serves as a preservative. It should not be more 12 %.

Draksharishta or Drakshasava is a liquid Ayurvedic medicine with dry grapes (raisins) as its main ingredient. It contains 5-10% self-generated alcohol that helps deliver water and alcohol-soluble herbs to the body. It is mainly used in the treatment of respiratory and intestinal or digestive issues and is packed with essential nutrients and medicinal properties. It provides overall strength to the body and is a good remedy to cure weakness after a chronic disease.

Procedure

Take accurately measured 25ml of the Asava or Arishtha preparation being examined at 24.9°C to 25.1°C and transfer to the distillation flask. Add 150ml of water and a little pumice powder. Now start distillation until not less than 90ml of the distillate is collected into a 100 ml volumetric flask.

Dilute this distillate to 100 ml volume with distilled water at 24.9° to 25.1°. Measure the relative density at 24.9° to 25.1°and calculate the alcohol content from the density table given in Indian Pharmacopoeia/standard density table.

Observation

Relative density of Drakshasva:

Relative density of Draksharishta:

Density of Ethanol and Water Mixtures (20 °C)

Ethanol (%)	Density (g/cm^2)	Ethanol (%)	Density (g/cm^2)	Ethanol (%)	Density (g/cm^2)
0	0.998	34	0.947	68	0.872
2	0.995	36	0.943	70	0.868
4	0.991	38	0.939	72	0.863
6	0.988	40	0.935	74	0.858
8	0.985	42	0.931	76	0.853
10	0.982	44	0.927	78	0.848
12	0.979	46	0.923	80	0.843
14	0.977	48	0.918	82	0.839
16	0.974	50	0.913	84	0.834
18	0.971	52	0.909	86	0.828
20	0.969	54	0.905	88	0.823
22	0.966	56	0.900	90	0.818
24	0.964	58	0.896	92	0.813

Contd...

Ethanol (%)	Density (g/cm^2)	Ethanol (%)	Density (g/cm^2)	Ethanol (%)	Density (g/cm^2)
26	0.960	60	0.891	94	0.807
28	0.957	62	0.887	96	0.801
30	0.954	64	0.882	98	0.795
30	0.950	66	0.877	100	0.789

Results:

The percentage of alcohol content in Drakshasva and draksharishta estimated and found …..

Questions

1. What is difference between Asava and Aristha?
2. Which is the main ingredient responsible for fermentation during preparation of Asava and Aristha?
3. What is role of fermented alcohol in Asava and Aristha?
4. What is kasaya?

Aim 4 : To evaluate excipients of natural origin: Agar, Tragacanth, Beeswax, Castor oil

Requirements: All Pharmacognosy chemical tests reagents, test tubes, Gas burners, water bath

Theory:

Natural excipients are generally safe as it is biodegradable, biocompatible and non-toxic – chemically, economic, safe, devoid of side effects and easily availability. But they also possess some disadvantage like Microbial contamination, Batch to batch variation, the uncontrolled rate of hydration, slow process and heavy metal contamination. Excipients are expected to be inert and should not exert any therapeutic or biological action or modify the biological action of the drug substance but excipients can potentially influence the rate and/or extent of absorption of a drug. As herbal excipients are non toxic and compatible, they have a major role to play in pharmaceutical formulation. Following are Sources of natural excipients:

Animal	Beeswax, Cochineal, Gelatin, Honey, Lactose, Spermaciti, Lanolin, Musk, Suet.
Vegetable	Kokum butter, Pectin, Starch, Peppermint, Cardamon, Vanilla, Tumeric, Saffron, Guar-gum
Minerals	Bentonite, Kieselghur, Kaolin, Paraffins, Talc, Calamine, Fuller's earth, Asbestos
Marine	Agar, Carrageenans, Alginic acid, Laminarin.

Following are examples of natural excipients based on phytochemical class

Phytochemical class	Examples
Carbohydrates	Acacia, agar, aliginate, gaur gum, caraggenan, cellulose derivatives, pectin, honey, aloe mucilage, tragacanth
Fixed oil	Almond oil, arachis oil, castor oil, cod liver oil, sesame oil, olive oil, jojoba oil,
Fats	Cocca butter, coconut oil, kokum butter, lard, palm oil, suet
Waxes	Bees wax, wool fat, carnauba wax, spermaceti
Volatil oils	Clove oil, cardamom oil, lemon oil, lavender oil, orange oil, peppermint oil, sandalwood oil, vetiver oil, musk oil
Resins	Asafoetida, ginger and capsicum resin, myrrh, peru balsam tolu balsam, shellac, storax,
Proteins	Casein, gelatin, thaumatin
Enzymes	Diastase, papain, pepsin, pancreatin, rennin
Tannins	Amla, behera, catechu, hirda, tannic acid
Pigments	Chlorophyll, cochineal, annatto, carotene
Polyphenols	Curcumin, gallic acids
Saponins	Soapnut, shikakai, quillaja bark saponins

Procedure:

Excipient	Morphology and Chemical analysis tests	Observation
Agar/ Agar – agar/ Japanese Isinglass ***Biological Source:*** Dried gelatinous substance,	Morphology: Strips: Colourless, slender, translucent, 4 mm wide Bands: Yellowish, 4 cm wide Sheets: 45-60 cm long and 10-15 cm wide Flakes or Course Powder: Greyish white, Odour:	

Contd...

<table>
<tr><td rowspan="7">obtained from Gelidium amansii, G. Cartilagineum, G. Pristodes, Gracilaria confervoides, pteocladialucida, P. Capollacea and other closely allied members of Family. Rhodophyceae

Uses: Bulk laxative, Pharmaceutical aid , in the preparation of culture media</td><td colspan="2">Odourless
Taste : mucilaginous
Solubility: practically insoluble in cold water, but swells to gelatinous mass. Soluble in boiling water.</td><td></td></tr>
<tr><td>Take aqueous solution and add ruthenium red.</td><td>Red color</td><td></td></tr>
<tr><td>Take aqueous solution and add N/50 iodine.</td><td>Deep crimson to brown color</td><td></td></tr>
<tr><td>Take 5% aqueous solution; and add 5 ml of dilute hydrochloric acid and heat on water bath for 30 min. Add to the first part, 3 ml of 10% caustic soda solution and 2 ml of Fehling solution. Heat on water bath.</td><td>Reduction takes place due to galactose</td><td></td></tr>
<tr><td>Take 5% aqueous solution and add 5 ml of dilute hydrochloric acid, and heat on water bath for 30 min. Add barium chloride solution (10%) to second part.</td><td>White precipitate of barium sulphate</td><td></td></tr>
<tr><td>Prepare ash of Agar, add dilute hydrochloric acid, and observe under microscope.</td><td>Skeleton and sponge spicules of diatoms will be observed.</td><td></td></tr>
<tr><td>Take 5% aqueous solution and add tannic acid to it.</td><td>No precipitate</td><td></td></tr>
<tr><td rowspan="5">Gelatin
Biological Source:
A protein extracted by partial hydrolysis of animal collagenous tissue like skin, tendons, ligaments and bones with boiling water

Uses: Pharmaceutical aid, capsule shell preparation; in pessaries, plasters etc</td><td colspan="2">Morphology
Colour: Colourless or pale yellow
Odour: Very slight
Taste: Characteristic and bouillon like.
Shape: Translucent sheets, flakes, shred or a course to fine powder.
Solubility: Insoluble in cold water but swells and softens, absorbs water but soluble in hot water forms jelly on cooling.</td><td></td></tr>
<tr><td>Heat a small quantity of gelatin with soda lime.</td><td>Ammonia is evolved</td><td></td></tr>
<tr><td>Take 0.5% aqueous solution and add a few drops of 10% tannic acid.</td><td>White precipitate</td><td></td></tr>
<tr><td>Take 0.5% aqueous solution and add Millon's Reagent.</td><td>White precipitate which becomes red on heating</td><td></td></tr>
<tr><td>Take 0.5% aqueous solution and add 10% picric acid solution to it.</td><td>Yellow precipitate</td><td></td></tr>
</table>

Contd...

Acacia/ India Gum/ Acasia, Babul or kikar gond(Hindi) ***Use:*** Pharmaceutical aid, binding, emulsifying agent, suspending agent, demulcent	Colour: Tears are cream brown to red in colour, powder is light brown in colour Odour: Odourless Taste: Bland and mucilaginous Size and shape: Irregular brown tears of varying size Extra features: Tears with minute fissures, brittle in nature, glossy and occasionally iridescent		
	Take 5 ml of 2% w/v solution and add 1 ml of strong lead sub-acetate solution.	Flocculent white precipitate	
	Take 5% aqueous solution; add 0.5 ml hydrogen peroxide solution and 0.5 ml of 1% alcoholic benzidine. Shake well and allow to stand for 5 minutes.	Deep blue color peroxidase enzyme	
	Treat powder with ruthenium red solution and examine microscopically.	No red color indicates that it is different from agar	
	Take 10 ml of 2% w/v solution and add 0.2 ml of 20% w/v lead acetate solution.	No precipitation indicates it is different from agar and tragacanth	
	Take 0.1 g of powder and add 1 ml of N/50 iodine to it.	No crimson color indicates that it is different from agar and tragacanth	
	Take 1 ml of solution, add 4 ml of water, and dilute hydrochloric acid; boil for few min. Add Fehling's solution and heat.	Red precipitate of cuprous oxide	
Tragacanth/ Gum ***Biological Source:*** Tragacanth Dried gummy exudation obtained by incision from stems and branches of *Astrogalus gummifer* Labill and other species of Astragalus Family : Leguminosae ***Uses:*** Pharmaceutical aid; Demulcent, emollient, laxative.	**Morphology** Colour : White or pale yellowish - white flakes. Odour : Odourless Taste: Tasteless Shape: Thin flattered ribbon like flakes Size: Flakes are 25 × 12 × 2 mm. Solubility : Partly soluble in water, swells, insoluble in alcohol		
	Take 4 ml of 0.5% w/v solution; add 0.5 ml of hydrochloric acid and heat it for 30 min on a	Red precipitate	

Contd...

	water bath; add 1.5 ml of sodium hydroxide solution and Fehling's solution, Heat solution using water bath.		
	Take 4 ml of 0.5% w/v solution; add 0.5 ml of hydrochloric acid and heat for 30 min on a water bath; add 10% barium chloride solution.	No precipitate indicates it is different from agar	
	Take 0.5% w/v solution of the gum and add 20% w/v solution of lead acetate.	Flocculent precipitate is obtained which indicates it is different from acacia	
	Treat powder with ruthenium red solution and examine microscopically.	No pink color (distinction from Indian tragacanth)	
	Treat powder with N/50 iodine solution.	Olive green color (distinction from acacia and agar)	
	Warm powder with 5% aqueous caustic potash (KOH).	Canary yellow color	
Beeswax/ Yellow Bees wax/ White or bleached yellow bees wax. ***Biological Source:*** : The purified wax obtained from the honeycomb of the bees *Apis dorsata* Linn. And other species of Apis Family : Apidae *Uses*:Pharmaceutical aid in preparation of semi-solid dosage forms	Morphology: Colour : Yellow bees wax : Yellow to greyish – brown solid White Beeswax: Yellowish white solid Odour Yellow Beeswax: Agreeable and honey like White Beeswax: Faint and characteristic Extra Features : Breaks with granular fracture Solubility : Insoluble in water, Slightly soluble in alcohol, soluble in chloroform		
	Heat wax with aqueous sodium hydroxide, cool and acidify	No turbidity	
	1g drug + 10 ml alcoholic KOH solution +10 ml alcohol, reflux for one hour, stir	Cloudy liquid between 60°C	

Contd...

Castor oil /Ricinus oil ***Biological Source:*** The fixed oil obtained by cold expression from kernels of seeds of Ricinus communis Linn Family : Euphorbiaceae	Colour: Pale yellow or almost colourless liquid Odour : Nauseating Taste: First bland, then slightly acrid and usually nauseating Extra features : A viscous and transparent liquid		
	Completely miscible with half of its volume of light petroleum ether		
	Oil +equal volume of alcohol Clear liquid. Cool at 0°C	Clear liquid for three hours.	
	Acidified pet.ether +oil shake, add a drop of ammonium molybdate	white turbidity	
Honey Madhu (Hindi)Honey purified, Mel. ***Biological Source:*** A sugar secretion deposited in honey comb by the bee, Apis dorsata, and other species of Apis Example- A Indica, A florea etc Family: Apidae *Uses*: Sweetening agent	Colour: Pale yellow or yellowish brown. Odour: Characteristic , Pleasant Taste: sweet and faintly acrid Extra features: Syrup thick liquid translucent when fresh, then opaque and granular due to the crystallization of glucose		
	Fehling solution test	Red ppt	
	Fiehe's test: It is used to detect adulteration of honey with invert sugar (Acid hydrolyzed sugar). It actually detects the presence of HMF (Hydroxymethyl furfural) content in honey. Invert sugar has high HMF content whereas, honey has lesser HMF content (around 10 mg/kg). Fiehe's reagent (seliwanoff reagent) which contains Resorcinol and HCL gives Cherry Red colour on reacting with Furfural.	Cherry Red colour	
Wool fat/ Anhydrus lanolin **Biological source:** The purified wax prepared from the wool sheep *Ovis aries* Family : Bovidae **Use:** Pharmaceutical aid, Ointment base	**Morphology**: Color: Whitish Yellow, Odour; Faint and characteristic, Taste: bland, Solubility: Insoluble in water and soluble in chloroform		
	0.5 gm wool fat in 5 ml of chloroform, add 1 ml of acetic anhydride, 2 drops of sulfuric acid	Deep green color	

Results: All given excipients of natural origin evaluated for morphology and chemical tests.

Questions

1. Which chemical test differentiates between Agar and acacia?
2. How Fiehe's test helps in identification of Pure Honey?
3. Which chemical test differentiates between Agar, tragacanth and acacia?
4. Explain benzidin test for acacia?
5. How tannic acid helps to differentiate Agar and Gelatin?
6. What is biological source of Agar, Acacia, Tragacanth, Gelatin, Honey, Beeswax, Castor oil and wool fat?
7. How to identify adulteration in Honey by chemical tests?
8. What is odor of Agar, acacia and Tragacanth?
9. How to obtain yellow and white beeswax?
10. What is chemical test for Woolfat?

Aim 5: To prepare and evaluate skin lightening cream containing standardized licorice extract

Requirements: Licorice root powder, alcohol, Silica Gel G, Methanol, Standard Glycyrrhizin, TLC plates, Stearic acid, Cetyl alcohol, Almond oil, Glycerin, Methyl paraben, Propyl paraben, Triethanolamine, P^H meter, homogenizer

Theory: Skin whitening is a term used for lightening the complexion of the skin through artificial means like creams, lotions, soaps and injections. Unfortunately the appeal of these skin bleaching products is based on the obsession of people across the world with skin color. Melanins are produced by specialized cells, termed melanocytes, which are located primarily in the skin, hair bulbs, and eyes. The melanins can be of two basic types: eumelanins, which are brown or black, and phaeomelanins, which are red or yellow, in mammals typically there are mixtures of both types. Increased production and accumulation of melanins characterize number of skin diseases, which include hyperpigentation such as melanoma, post-inflammatory melanoderma, solar lentigo, etc. Depigmentation can be achieved by (i) regulating the transcription and activity of tyrosinase, (ii) regulating the uptake and distribution of melanosomes in recipient keratinocytes and (iii) interference with melanosomes maturation and transfer.

Licorice extract is obtained from the root of Glycyrrhia Glabra Linnera. It is cultivated extensively in India. Licorice extract improves hyperpigmentation by dispersing the melanin, inhibition of melanin biosynthesis and inhibition of cyclooxygenase activity thereby decreasing free radical production. Glabridin, a polyphenolic flavonoid is the main component of licorice extract. Studies have shown that glabridin prevents Ultraviolet B (UVB) induced pigmentation and exerts anti-inflammatory effects by inhibiting superoxide anion and cyclooxygenase activity. However, more studies are needed to prove its de-pigmenting action.

Procedure

Preparation and evaluation of standardized licorice extract: Yasti Dry Extracts is obtained by extracting Yasti with water or aqueous ethanol or any other suitable solvent. Yasti dry extracts contains not less than 9.0 percent w/w and not more than 120.0 percent w/w of the stated amount of glycyrrhizinic acid. It is used as expectorant, antiulcer, stomachic, anti-inflammatory, kasa. Flavonoids- Liquiritin, iso-liquiritin, glabridin.	
Evaluation	
Appearance	A yellowish-brown to dark powder
Thin-layer chromatography Identification	Stationary Phase: Silica gel GF254. Mobile Phase: butanol: acetic acid : water. (7:1:2) Test Solution: Dissolve 200 mg of the extracts under examination with 50 ml of methanol(70 percent) and filter. Reference solution: A 0.1 percent w/v solution of glycyrrhizin ammonical hydrate R in methanol (70 percent). Procedure: Apply to the plate 10 µl of each solution as bands 10 mm by 2 mm. Allow the mobile phase to rise 8 cm. Dry the plate in air and examine under ultraviolet light at 254 nm and 366 nm. Spray the plate with anisaldehyde sulphuric acid reagent and heat at 105° for 10 minutes and examine the plate in day light. The chromatogram obtained with test solution shows a band corresponding to the band obtained with the reference solution indicating the presence of glycyrrhizin.

Contd...

Acid insoluble ash	Not more than 2.0 percent.
Heavy metals:	1.0 g complies with the limit test for heavy metals, Method B (20ppm)
Loss on drying	Not more than 5.0 percent determine on 1.0 g by drying in an oven at 105°.
Microbial Contamination	Complies with the microbial contamination test. No growth
Assay: (Spectroscopy/ Chromatography)	**HPLC** **Test solution**: Dissolve about 500 mg of the extract or a quantity containing 7 mg of glycyrrhizinic acid and dissolve in the mobile phase by mixing for 30 minutes with the aid of ultrasound and dilute to 100.0 ml with the mobile phase and filter. **Reference solution**: A 0.01 percent w/v solution of glycyrrhizin ammonical hydrate RS in the mobile phase. - A stainless steel column 25 cm × 4.6 mm, packed with octadecylsilane bonded to porous silica (5 µm), - Mobile phase: a mixture of 1 volumes of glacial acetic acid, 67 volumes of methanol and 33 volumes of 0.2 M ammonium acetate in water. - Flow rate- 1 ml per minute, - Spectrophotometer set at 250 nm, - Injection volume: 20 µl.

Preparation and evaluation of skin lightening cream : An extract of **Glycyrrhiza glabra** is rich of natural antioxidants. The best natural antioxidants in extract of Glycyrrhiza glabra are glycyrrhizin (glycyrrhizic acid) and flavonoids. Glycyrrhiza glabra extract is obtained from the roots of Glycyrrhiza glabra by solvent extraction method and then concentrating the extract by rotary evaporator. Glycyrrhiza glabra extract is preserved by refrigeration and/or freezing. The role of Glycyrrhiza glabra extract on skin is mainly attributed to its antioxidant activity particularly to its potent antioxidants triterpene saponins and flavonoids. Skin whitening, skin depigmenting, skin lightening, antiaging, anti-erythemic, emollient, anti-acne and photoprotection effects are mainly attributed to Glycyrrhiza glabra extract.

Method of preparation: Oil in water (O/W) emulsion-based cream (semisolid formulation) :. Dissolve the emulsifier (stearic acid) and other oil soluble components (Cetyl alcohol, Mineral oil) in the oil phase (Part A) and heat to 75°C. Dissolve the preservatives and other water soluble components (Methyl paraban, Propyl paraban, Triethanolamine, glycerin and extract of liquorice (Glycyrrhiza glabra) in the aqueous phase (Part B) and heat to 75°C. After heating, add the aqueous phase in small portions to the oil phase with continuous trituration in porcelain mortar until a smooth cream is formed.

Ingredient	Quantity	Ingredient	Quantity
Licorice Extract	1 gm	Licorice Extract	1 gm
Stearic acid	5 gm	Glycerin	18 ml
Cetyl alcohol	3 gm	Paraffin oil	20 ml
Almond oil	2 ml	Coconut oil	02 ml
Glycerin	2 ml	Beeswax	05 gm
Methyl paraben	0.02 gm	Cetomacrogol 1000	1.8 gm
Propyl paraben	0.02 gm	Cetostearyl Alcohol	6.0 gm
Triethanolamine	q.s.	-----------------	-----

Evaluation: Evaluate the cream for standard parameters.

- **Appearance, feel and homogeneity:** Determine the color, odor and homogeneity of the lotion visually.
- **P^H:** Prepare 10% solution of lotion measure pH with a digital pH meter.
- **Viscosity:** evaluate viscosity using Brookfield viscometer using LV-64 spindle at rotation rate to 25 RPM. Immerse the spindle into formulated lotion and measure the viscosity.
- **Spreadability:** Determine the spreadability of lotion by the parallel plate method. Select two glass slides of 20/20 cm. Place about 1 g of the lotion formulation over one of the slides. Place the other slide upon the top of the lotion such that the lotion is sandwiched between the slides and 125 g weight is placed upon the upper slide so that lotion between the two slides is pressed uniformly to form a thin layer. Remove the weight and measure the spread diameter.
- **Sensitivity Test:** Apply a portion of lotion on the forearms of 6 volunteers and keep for 20 minutes. After 20 minutes, note if any kind of irritation or redness occurrs.
- **Stability Test:** Store the formulated lotion at different temperatures and humidity conditions of 25±2°C / 60±5% RH (at room temperature), 40±2°C/ 75±5% RH (accelerated temperature) for a period of three months and studied for pH, viscosity and spreadability.

Observation and Results:

Evaluation Parameters	Results/Observations
Appearance	
Feel	
Homogeneity	
p^H	
Sensitivity	
Viscosity	
Spreadability	
Extrudability	
Brightness level or spot pigmentation score by Skin Analyzer	
Stability	

Questions

1. What is meaning of standardized extract?
2. Which analysis parameters are used to evaluate standardized extract?
3. What is difference between simple extract and standardized extract?
4. What is mechanism of action of Skin lighting herbal compounds?
5. What is role of triethanolamine in cream formulation development?

6. What is permissible limit of quantity of Methyl paraben and Propyl paraben in cosmetic formulations?
7. Which chemical constituents of Licorice extract are responsible for skin lightening and how?
8. What is meaning of "1000" in Cetomacrogol 1000?
9. Explain the working of instrument skin analyser?
10. Why spredability is important parameter in cream evaluation?

Aim 6: To prepare and evaluate skin lightening lotion containing standardized licorice extract

Reference: Khadabadi, Deore, Baviskar "Experimental Phytopharmacognosy', Nirali prakashan, Pune. 2nd Edition, 2013: 6.12

Requirements: Licorice root powder, alcohol, Silica Gel G, Methanol, Standard Glycyrrhizin, TLC plates, Stearic acid, Cetyl alcohol, Methyl paraben, Propylene glycol , Propyl paraben, Triethanolamine, homogenizer, P^H meter

Theory:

Lotions are typically lighter and less greasy than creams. With higher water content, lotions is quickly absorbed by the skin and is good for normal to lightly dry skin. Creams tend to feel greasier than lotions because they contain more oil than lotions. Creams are best for very dry skin. It is also an ideal skin care product for winter and cold months.

Procedure:

Ingredients	Quantity	Method of preparation:
Licorice extract	100mg	Prepare the lotion by adding non-polar phase to the polar phase with rapid stirring to avoid separation of water and oil phase. Melt non-polar phase first together and then slowly add to the preheated mixture of polar phase.
Mineral oil	12 ml	
Stearic acid	10 mg	
Cetosteryl alcohol	2 ml	
Propylene glycol	2 ml	
Triethanolamine	3 ml	
Methyl paraben sodium	2mg	
Propyl paraben sodium	0.2mg	
Purified Water Vehicle	Qs to 100 ml	

Pharmaceutical Evaluation of lotion

- **Appearance, feel and homogeneity:** Determine the color, odor and homogeneity of the lotion visually.
- **P^H:** Prepare 10% solution of lotion measure pH with a digital pH meter.
- **Viscosity:** evaluate viscosity using Brookfield viscometer using LV-64 spindle at rotation rate to 25 RPM. Immerse the spindle into formulated lotion and measure the viscosity.
- **Spreadability:** Determine the spreadability of lotion by the parallel plate method. Select two glass slides of 20/20 cm. Place about 1 g of the lotion formulation over one of the slides. Place the other slide upon the top of the lotion such that the lotion is sandwiched between the slides and 125 g weight is placed upon the upper slide so that lotion between the two slides is pressed uniformly to form a thin layer. Remove the weight and measure the spread diameter.
- **Sensitivity Test:** Apply a portion of lotion on the forearms of 6 volunteers and keep for 20 minutes. After 20 minutes, note if any kind of irritation or redness occurrs.

- **Stability Test:** Store the formulated lotion at different temperatures and humidity conditions of 25±2°C / 60±5% RH (at room temperature), 40±2°C/ 75±5% RH (accelerated temperature) for a period of three months and studied for pH, viscosity and spreadability.
- **Washability Test:** Apply a portion of lotion over the skin of hand and allow to flow under the force of flowing tap water for 10 minutes. Note the time when the lotion is completely removed.
- **Type of emulsion test:** Conduct dye solubility and dilution test t determine the type of emulsion formed

Observation and Results:

Evaluation Parameters	Results/Observations
Appearance	
Feel	
Homogeneity	
p^H	
Viscosity	
Spreadability	
Extrudability	
Brightness level or spot pigmentation score by Skin Analyzer	
Stability	
Sensitivity	

Questions:

1. What is meaning of standardized extract?
2. Which analysis parameters are used to evaluate standardized extract?
3. What is difference between simple extract and standardized extract?
4. What is difference between cream and lotion?
5. What is mechanism of action of Skin lighting herbal compounds?
6. What is role of triethanolamine in cream formulation development?
7. What is permissible limit of quantity of Methyl paraben and Propyl paraben in cosmetic formulations?
8. Which chemical constituents of Licorice extract are responsible for skin lightening and how?
9. What is difference between mineral oil and vegetable oil?
10. Explain the working of instrument skin analyser?
11. Why spredability is important parameter in cream evaluation?
12. What should be ideal P^H of skin cosmetic products?

Aim 7: To prepare and evaluate herbal shampoo containing standardized extract of Reetha (*Sapindus mukorosii*) fruit

Requirements: Soapnut fruits powder, Silica gel GF254, chloroform, methanol, water, Amla extract, Lemon juice, Methyl paraben, Gelatin solution, Citric acid, Essential oil, homogenizer, P^H meter

Theory: Soapnut is known for its fruit, which contains triterpenoid saponins (10.1%) in the pericarp. Saponin is a natural detergent for washing the body, hair, and clothes, and it is used as a natural surfactant. There are more than 40 wild species in the genus Sapindus (family Sapindaceae). Among these species, Sapindus mukorossi (*S. mukorossi*) and *Sapindus trifoliatus* (*S. trifoliatus*) are the two main varieties. S. mukorossi is composed of about 56% pericarp, with the balance being the hard, black, smooth seed that contains the kernel inside. The seed kernel of *S. mukorossi* contains 23% oil in the pulp, of which almost 90% are triglycerides.

Procedure:

Standardized extract preparation	Take accurately weighed 100 gm powder of soapnut fruits. Extract with 500 ml water for 3 hours. Filter and evaporate filtrate to dry mass. Determine total saponins by Gravimetry. Evaluate extract by TLC and HPLC for presence of Sapinoside-B. It should contain 10-12 % total saponins.
TLC	Stationary Phase: Silica gel-GF^{254}. Mobile Phase: chloroform: methanol: water Detection: 630 nm.
HPLC	Column: C-18 (non-polar) Mobile phase : Acetonitrile-water gradient (Polar) Detection: 215 nm
Total saponins	Weigh accurately 5 gm of the extract and dissolve it into 100 ml of water. Partition the solution 3 times with 50 ml benzene each time. Discard the benzene fractions. Partition the aqueous layer further 3 times with 50 ml n-butanol each time. Collect the butanol fractions and shake it with 50 ml of water. Collect the butanol layers and filter to remove the traces of water. Dry the butanol fractions under vaccum and keep it in desiccators for three hour and weigh. % of total saponins = weight of residue / weight of extract taken X 100

Shampoo:

Ingredients	Quantity	Method of Preparation:
Reetha extract (10-12 % total saponins)	4.5 g	Add Herbal extracts to 10% gelatin solution and mix by shaking for 20 min. Add Lemon juice (1 mL) and Methyl paraben with stirring. Adjust the pH of the solution by adding sufficient quantity of 1% citric acid solution. Add few drops of rose essential oil to impart aroma to the prepared shampoo and made the final volume to 100 mL with gelatin solution.
Amla extract	2.5 g	
Lemon juice	1 mL	
Methyl paraben	1 mL of 0.05% solution	
Gelatin solution	q.s	
Citric acid	q.s	
Essential oil	0.1 mL	

Evaluation:

- **Physical appearance/visual inspection:** Evaluate the shampoo for the clarity, color, odor and foam producing ability.
- **Determination of pH:** Measure the pH of 10% v/v shampoo solution in distilled water by using pH meter at room temperature.
- **Determination of % of solid contents:** Place 4 grams of shampoo in a previously clean, dry and weighed evaporating dish. Weigh the dish and shampoo again to confirm the exact weight of the shampoo. Evaporate the liquid portion of the shampoo by placing the evaporating dish on the hot plate. Calculate the weight and thus % of the solid contents of shampoo left after complete drying.
- **Dirt dispersion test:** Add two drops of shampoo to 10 mL of distilled taken in a large test tube. To this solution, add one drop of India ink and the stopper the test tube and shake ten times. The amount of ink in the foam will be indicated by the rubric such as None, Light, Moderate or Heavy.
- **Surface tension measurement:** Measure the surface tension of 10% w/v shampoo in distilled water using Stalagmometer at room temperature.
- **Foaming ability and foam stability:** Determine foaming ability by using cylinder shake method. Place 50 mL of the 1% commercial or formulated shampoo solution into a 250 mL graduated cylinder; cover with one hand and shake 10 times. Record the total volume of the foam content after 1 min of shaking. Evaluate foam stability by recording the foam volume after 1 min and 4 min of shake test.
- **Wetting time test:** Cut a canvas paper into 1-inch diameter discs having an average weight of 0.44 g. Place the smooth surface of disc on the surface of 1% v/v shampoo solution and start the stopwatch. The time required for the disc to begin to sink is noted down as the wetting time.
- **Evaluation of conditioning performance:** Take the hair tress of an Asian woman from a local salon. Cut it into four swatches of the tresses with approximately the length of 10 cm and the weight of 5 g. A swatch without washing served as the control. Wash other three tresses with the formulated shampoos in an identical manner. For each cycle, shake each tress with the mixture of 10 g of a sample and 15 g of water in a conical flask for 2 min and then rinse with 50 mL water. Afterward, dry each tress at room temperature. Wash the tresses for maximum ten cycles. Evaluate the conditioning performance of the shampoos i.e. smoothness and softness, by a blind touch test, by twenty randomly selected student volunteers. All the students should blind folded and asked to touch and rate the four tresses for conditioning performance from score 1 to 4 (1 = poor; 2 = satisfactory; 3 = good; 4 = excellent).
- **Total saponins determination:** Determine total saponins by Gravimetry. It should contain 10-12 % total saponins.
- **TLC/HPLC Analysis:** Evaluate extract by TLC and HPLC for presence of Sapinoside-B.

Observation and Results:

Evaluation Parameters	Results/Observations
Physical appearance/visual inspection	
Determination of pH:	
Determination of % of solid contents	
Dirt dispersion test:	
Surface tension measurement:	
Foaming ability and foam stability:	
Foaming ability and foam stability	
Wetting time test	
Evaluation of conditioning performance	
Total saponins determination:	
TLC/HPLC Analysis:	

Questions:

1. What is meaning of standardized extract?
2. Which analysis parameters are used to evaluate standardized extract?
3. What is difference between simple extract and standardized extract?
4. What is biological source of Reetha?
5. What is use of reetha fruit powder and extract?
6. List famous reetha containing marketed shampoos?
7. Explain the foaming ability and wetting time test?
8. Explain dirt dispersion test?

Aim 8: To prepare and evaluate standardized Licorice extract containing cough syrup

Requirements: Licorice root powder, alcohol, Silica Gel G, Methanol, Standard Glycyrrhizin, TLC plates, P^H meter, homogenizer, Sugar, Methyl paraben

Theory:

Glycyrrhiza glabra (family Fabaceae), commonly known as licorice, is a herbaceous perennial that has been used as a flavoring agent in foods and medicinal remedies for thousands of years. Licorice root has been widely used around the world to treat cough since ancient times. It contains several active compounds including glycyrrhizin, glycyrrhetinic acid, flavonoids, isoflavonoids, and chalcones. Glycyrrhizin and glycyrrhetinic acid are considered to be the main active components and are potent inhibitors of cortisol metabolism, due to their steroid-like structures. The root of this plant has been used for treatment of coughs, colds, asthma, and COPD. Glycyrrhizin is a triterpene glycoside, a major active constituent obtained from the plant G. glabra. Glycyrrhizin alleviated allergic asthma in an ovalbumin-induced experimental mouse model of asthma as evidenced by increased IFNγ level, while it decreased IL-4, IL-5 levels, and eosinophil count in bronchoalveolar lavage (BAL). It also reduced OVA-specific IgE levels and also upregulated total IgG2a in serum. These results indicated that glycyrrhizin interfered with the production of IgE by decreasing the IgE-stimulating cytokines.

Procedure:

Mix 66.7% w/w of sucrose in required quantity of distilled water to prepare a concentrated solution of simple syrup. Mix 50 mg of licorice dry extract (Refer Experiment 5- for standardized licorice extract preparation) in 100 of simple syrup. Add 0.1% of methyl paraben as preservative, to the above mixture. Mix well to get visibly clear solution.

Evaluation

- **Organoleptic Properties:** Evaluate syrup for various organoleptic parameters such as colour, odour, and taste, consistency, uniformity
- **Determination of pH:** Measure pH by digital pH meter.
- **Specific gravity:** Determine the specific gravity using pycnometer by dividing the weight of the syrup contained in the pycnometer by the weight of water contained, at 25^0C.
- **Stability Testing:** Carry out stability testing of the prepared syrup by keeping the samples at room and accelerated temperature conditions. Take final syrup in six different amber colored glass bottles and keep three bottles at room temperatures (37^0C) and three bottles at accelerated temperatures (47^0C). Examine the samples for all the physicochemical parameters, turbidity and homogeneity at the interval of 24 hr, 48 hr and 72 hr for any change.
- **Assay:** Perform the assay as discussed in experiment of standardized licorice extract preparation

Observation and Results:

Evaluation Parameters	Results/Observations
Organoleptic Properties	
p^H	
Viscosity	
Specific gravity	
Stability	
Assay/TLC	

Questions:

1. What is meaning of standardized extract?
2. Which analysis parameters are used to evaluate standardized extract?
3. What is difference between simple extract and standardized extract?
4. What are different methods to prepare syrup?
5. How licorice relieves cough?
6. Which are major chemical constituents of licorice responsible to relieve cough?

Aim 9: To prepare and evaluate Senna syrup containing standardized Senna fluid extract

Requirements: Senna leaves powder, water, alcohol, Silica Gel G, Methanol, Standard Glycyrrhizin, TLC plates, P^H meter, homogenizer, Sugar, Methyl paraben, Fennel Essence

Theory:

The cough it is a most common problem are face by the all people. There are two types of cough one is the Dry cough and second is wet cough. The dry cough is a no mucous and secretion while in wet cough there is cough mucous or secretion. The syrup is most commonly used and popular dosage form there is used in cure the cough and cold because it having ease of patients compliance.

Procedure:

Senna Fluid extract Extraction method: Mix 1000 g of Senna, in coarse powder, with a sufficient quantity (600 mL to 800 mL) of menstruum consisting of a mixture of 1 volume of alcohol and 2 volumes of water to make it evenly and distinctly damp. After 15 minutes, pack the mixture firmly into a suitable percolator, and cover the drug with additional menstruum.

Macerate for 24 hours, then percolate at a moderate rate, adding fresh menstrum, until the drug is practically exhausted of its active principles. Reserve the first 800 mL of percolate, and use it to dissolve the residue from the additional percolate thAt has been concentrated to a soft extracts at a temperature not to exceed 60°. Add water and alcohol to make the product measure 1000 mL., and mix. Preserve in tight, light-resistant containers, and avoid exposure to direct sunlight and to excessive heat.

Evaluation:

Appearance	A light greenish brown to dark brown liquid.
Alcohol content	Between 23.0 % and 27.0 of C_2H_5OH
Thin-Layer Chromatography Identification	**Stationary Phase**: Silica gel GF254. **Mobile Phase**: A mixture of 40 volumes of n-propyl alcohol: 40 volumes of ethyl acetate: 20 volumes of water and 1 volumes of glacial acetic acid. **Test solution:** Shake well 0.1 gm of the extract under examination with 5 ml of a mixture of equal volumes of methanol and water for 5 minutes, heat to 60°, cool and allow to settle. Use the supernatent liquid. **Reference solution:** Dissolve 10mg of calcium sennosides RS in 1 ml of a mixture of equal volumes of methanol and water. **Procedure**: Apply 10 µl of each solution to the plate as 10 mm band separated by 2 mm. Allow the mobile phase to rise 10 cm. Dry the plate in ir and examine under ultraviolet light at 254nm and 366 nm, soray the plate with 20 percent v/v of nitric acid solution. Heat the plate at 110° for 10 minutes and examine the plate in day light. Allow to cool and spray with a 5 percent w/v solution of potassium hydroxide in ethanol (50 percent v/v) until the zone appears. The chromatographic profile of the test solution is similar to that of the reference solution.

Contd...

	A. To about 25 mg of the extract add 50 ml of water and 2 ml of hydrochloric acid. Heat in the water bath for 15 minutes. Cool and shake with 40 ml of ether. Separate ether layer, dry over anhydrous sodium sulphate and evaporate 5 ml to dryness. To the cooled residue add 5 ml of the dilute ammonia. A yellow or range colour develops. Heat on a water bath for 2 minutes. A reddish-violet colour develops.
Microbial Contamination	Total aerobic viable count is not more than 10° CFU per g and total fungal count is not more than 10^2 CFU per g. is free from *Escherichia coli* and 10gm is free from *salmonella.*
Assay (HPLC)	**Solvent mixture:** A 0.3 percent of acetic acid with the pH adjusted to 5.9 with 1 M sodium hydroxide. **Test Solution:** Dissolve an accurately weighed quantity of substance under examination containing about 10 mg of calcium sennosides in 50.0 ml of the solvent mixture. **Reference Solution:** Dissolve an accurately weighed quantity of calcium sennoside RS containing 10 mg of calcium sennosides in 50.0 ml of the solvent mixtures. **Chromatographic system:** - A stainless steel column 25 cm × 4.6 mm packed with octadecylsilane bonded to porous silica (5µm), - Mobile phase: a mixture of 83 volumes of 1 percent v/v solution of glacial acetic acid and 17 volumes of acetonitrile, - Flow rate: 1 ml per minute. - Spectrophotometer set at 350 nm, - Injection volume: 10 µl. **Procedure**: Inject the reference solution. The test is not valid unless the relative standard deviation for replicate injections is not more than 2.0 percent. Inject the reference solution and test solution. Calculate the total sennosides from the peak area of sennosides A and B using declared content of total sennosides is calcium sennosides. 1 mg of sennoside is equivalent to 1.044 mg of calcium sennoside.

Senna syrup formula

Ingredient	Quantity	**Method of Preparation:** Mix well all ingredients and evaluate for various pharmaceutical parameters.
Senna Fluid Extract	120 ml	
Fennel Essence	04 ml	
Syrup	360 ml	
Dose: 1.5 to 3 ml		

Evaluation of syrup

- **Organoleptic Properties:** Evaluate syrup for various organoleptic parameters such as colour, odour, and taste.
- **Determination of pH:** Measure pH by digital pH meter.

- **Specific gravity:** Determine the specific gravity using pycnometer by dividing the weight of the syrup contained in the pycnometer by the weight of water contained, at 25^0C.
- **Stability Testing:** Carry out stability testing of the prepared syrup by keeping the samples at room and accelerated temperature conditions. Take final syrup in six different amber colored glass bottles and keep three bottles at room temperatures (37^0C) and three bottles at accelerated temperatures (47^0C). Examine the samples for all the physicochemical parameters, turbidity and homogeneity at the interval of 24 hr, 48 hr and 72 hr for any change.
- **Assay:** Perform the assay as discussed in above experiment of standardized senna extract preparation

Observation and Results:

Evaluation Parameters	Results/Observations
Organoleptic Properties	
p^H	
Viscosity	
Specific gravity	
Stability	
Assay	

Questions:

1. What is fluid extract?
2. What is meaning of standardized extract?
3. Which analysis parameters are used to evaluate standardized extract?
4. What is difference between simple extract and standardized extract?
5. What are different methods to prepare syrup?
6. What is use of senna syrup?
7. Which is more efficient and should be preferred: Senna powder in the form of churna or senna syrup?
8. What should be ideal P^H of syrup?

Aim 10: To prepare and evaluate Senna mixture containing standardized senna fluid extract

Requirements: Fluid extract of senna, Fluid extract of Jalap, Fluid extract of Ginger, Sulphate of Magnesia, Alcohol (50%), Water

Theory:

Herbal drug preparations are obtained by subjecting herbal drugs to treatments such as extraction, distillation, expression, fractionation, purification, concentration or fermentation. These include comminuted or powdered herbal drugs, tinctures, extracts, essential oils, expressed juices and processed exudates.

Standardized extracts (also referred to as guaranteed potency extracts) refer to an extract guaranteed to contain a "standardized" level of active compounds or key chemical marker. Stating the content of active compounds or key chemical marker rather than the concentration ratio allows for more accurate dosages to be made. However, the complex composition of an herbal medicine makes it unwise to ignore the other constituents. **Fluid extract** is an alcoholic liquid extract produced by percolation of herbal material(s) so that 1mL of the fluidextract contains the extractive obtained from 1g of the herbal material(s). **Soft extract** is a semi-solid preparation obtained by total or partial evaporation of the solvent from a liquid extract. **Dry extract** is a solid preparation obtained by evaporation of the solvent from a liquid/fluid extract. Dry extract can also be prepared by spray-drying with or without the use of an adsorbent (such as methyl cellulose), or by drying and milling to produce a powder. This may be further processed by compression or with use of a binding agent or granulation liquid to produce multiparticulate granules.

Procedure:

Ingredient	Quantity	**Method of Preparation:** Mix well all ingredients and evaluate for various pharmaceutical parameters.
Fluid extract of senna	2 ml	
Fluid extract of Jalap	1 ml	
Fluid extract of Ginger	0.8 ml	
Sulphate of Magnesia	15 ml	
Alcohol (50%)	4 ml	
Water	30 ml	

Evaluation of mixture

- **Organoleptic Properties:** Evaluate mixture for various organoleptic parameters such as colour, odour, and taste.
- **Determination of pH:** Measure pH by digital pH meter.
- **Specific gravity:** Determine the specific gravity using pycnometer by dividing the weight of the syrup contained in the pycnometer by the weight of water contained, at 25^{0}C.
- **Stability Testing:** Carry out stability testing of the prepared mixture by keeping the samples at room and accelerated temperature conditions. Take final syrup in six different amber

colored glass bottles and keep three bottles at room temperatures (37^{0}C) and three bottles at accelerated temperatures (47^{0}C). Examine the samples for all the physicochemical parameters, turbidity and homogeneity at the interval of 24 hr, 48 hr and 72 hr for any change.

- **Assay:** Perform the assay as discussed in above experiment of standardized senna extract preparation

Observation and Results:

Evaluation Parameters	Results/Observations
Organoleptic Properties	
p^H	
Viscosity	
Specific gravity	
Stability	
Assay	

Questions:

1. What is fluid extract?
2. What is meaning of standardized extract?
3. Which analysis parameters are used to evaluate standardized extract?
4. What is difference between simple extract and standardized extract?
5. What are different methods to prepare syrup?
6. What is use of senna mixture?
7. What is jalap and why it is used to prepare senna mixture?

Aim 11: To determine total phenolic content in given crude drug sample

Requirements: Dilute Folin-Ciocalteu reagent with equal volume of distilled water, 20% sodium carbonate in water, and Gallic acid.

Theory: The Folin-Ciocalteu reagent (FCR) or Folin's phenol reagent or Folin-Denis reagent or Gallic Acid Equivalence method (GAE) uses a mixture of phosphomolybdate and phosphotungstate for the colorimetric assay of phenolic and polyphenolic antioxidants. It works by measuring the amount of the substance needed to inhibit the oxidation of the reagent. However, this reagent does not only measure total phenols but will react with any reducing substance. The reagent, therefore, measures the total reducing capacity of a sample, not just the level of phenolic compounds. This reagent forms part of the Lowry protein assay and will also react with some nitrogen-containing compounds such as hydroxylamine and guanidine.

Procedure

1. Prepare calibration curve of standard Gallic acid (10-100 μg/ml in water).
2. Prepare 1 milligram/ml of extract solutions. (sample /s)
3. Mix 1 ml of each sample with 0.25 ml of Folin–Ciocalteu reagent and 1.25 ml of 20% sodium carbonate solution.
4. Allow the mixture to react for 40 min. at room temperature.
5. After the reaction period, mix the contents and measure the blue color at 725 nm in comparison with standards. Calculate the amount of total phenols from calibration curve as a Gallic acid equivalent by the following formula:

$$T = \frac{C * V}{M}$$

Where, T = total content of phenolic compounds, (milligram per gram of plant extract), C = the concentration of gallic acid established from the calibration curve(milligram per milliliter), V = the volume of extract(milliliter), M=the gram weight of plant extract.

Observations:

Standard Gallic acid)		Sample (Extract)	
Concentration (ug/ml)	**Absorbance**	**Concentration (ug/ml)**	**Absorbance**
20		---	
40		---	
60			
80			
100			

Results: Percentage of total phenol in ------------------ sample found to be........

Questions:

1. What is principle of Folin-Ciocalteu method to estimate total phenolic compounds?
2. Which wavelength is used to estimate total phenolic content by Folin-Ciocalteu method?

Aim 12: To determine total alkaloid content in given crude drug sample

Requirements: **BCG Solution** (Dissolve 69. 8 mg BCG in 3 ml 2N NaOH and 5 ml distilled water. Make up the volume up to 100 ml), Phosphate Buffer Solution (pH 4.7), and **Standard Atropine Solution** (Dissolve 1 mg atropine in 10 ml distilled water).

Theory: Bromocresol green (BCG) reacts with alkaloids having nitrogen atom within ring and forms yellow colored complex which can be easily measured colorimetrically. BCG doesn't reacts with alkaloids having nitrogen in side chain, and thus, this method is not useful to determine amine or amide alkaloids.

Procedure

1. Take 0.4. 0.6, 0.8, 1.0, and 1.2 ml atropine solution in a separate test tube.
2. Add 5 ml of Phosphate Buffer Solution (pH 4.7) and 5 ml of BCG solution.
3. Shake well and extract the yellow colored complex with chloroform.
4. Separate chloroform and make up the volume to 10 ml.
5. Measure the absorbance at 470 nm against blank.
6. Now prepare the methanolic extract of plant material. Dry and dissolve in 2N HCl. Filter and wash with chloroform. Adjust the pH neutral with 0.1 N NaOH.
7. Now add 5ml of Phosphate Buffer Solution (pH 4.7) and 5 ml of BCG solution.
8. Shake well and extract the yellow colored complex with chloroform.
9. Separate chloroform and make up the volume to 10 ml and measure the absorbance at 470 nm.
10. Calculate concentration of total alkaloids from calibration curve of atropine standard.

Observations:

Standard (Atropine)		Sample	
Concentration (ug/ml)	**Absorbance**	**Concentration (ug/ml)**	**Absorbance**
0.4		---	
0.6		---	
0.8			
1.0			
1.2			

Results: Percentage of total alkaloid in ------------------ sample found to be........

Questions:

1. What is principle of Bromocresol green (BCG) method to estimate total alkaloid content?
2. Which wavelength is used to estimate total total alkaloid content by Bromocresol green (BCG) method?
3. What is meaning of Beer–Lambert law obeying concentration?

Aim 13: To perform monograph analysis (Indian Pharmacopoeia, 2018) of Castor Oil

Requirements: TLC plates, Silica Gel GF254, Refractometer, Polarimeter, blue litmus paper, Sulfuric acid, Potassium Hydroxide

Theory:

Monographs articulate the quality expectations for a medicine including for its identity, strength, purity, and performance. They also describe the tests to validate that a medicine and its ingredients meet these criteria. The Good Pharmacopoeial Practices (GPhP) guidance published by the World Health Organization states, "A pharmacopoeia's core mission is to protect public health by creating and making available public standards to help ensure the quality of medicines" (8). The GPhP guidance continues, "Pharmacopoeial monographs provide an important tool for assurance of the quality of marketed pharmaceutical ingredients and products through testing of their quality." These monographs are generally available for excipients, drug substances, and drug products, providing the tests, analytical procedures, and acceptance criteria that enable assessment of the quality of the material. Taken together with the other requirements contained in the pharmacopoeia, these monographs can help safeguard the health of patients around the world through the availability of public quality standards.

Castor oil is the fixed oil obtained by cold expression from the seeds of *Ricinus comminis* Linn. (Fam. Euphorbiaceae). It may contain suitable antioxidants.

Procedure:

Analysis: Perform analysis of castor oil for below mentioned parameters given in Monograph as per standard procedures.

Description:	A pale yellowish or almost colourless, transparent, viscid liquid, odour, slight and characteristics.
Storage:	Store protected from light and moisture at a temperature not exceeding 15°.
Light absorption:	**Absorbance** of a 1.0 percent w/v solution in ethanol (95 percent) at the maximum at about 269 mm, not more than 1.0.
Weight per ml:	0.0945 g to 0.965 g
Refractive index:	1.4758 to 1.4798
Optical rotation:	+3.5° to +6.0°
Peroxide value:	Not more than 5.0
Acid Value:	Not more than 2.0
Acetyl value:	Not less than 143
Hydroxyl value:	Not less than 150.
Saponification Value:	176 to 187
Iodine Value:	82 to 90.
Foreign fatty substances	• A mixture of 2 ml of the substance under examination and 8 ml of ethanol (95 percent) is clear. • Shake 10.0 ml with 20.0 ml of light petroleum (60° to 80°) and allow to separate; the volume of the lower layer is not less than 16.0 ml.
Labeling	The label states (1) the name and quantity of any added antioxidant; (2) whether the contents are suitable for use in the manufacturer of parenteral preparations.

Observation and Results:

Evaluation parameter	Results
Description:	
Storage:	
Light absorption:	
Weight per ml:	
Refractive index:	
Optical rotation:	
Peroxide value:	
Acid Value:	
Acetyl value:	
Hydroxyl value:	
Saponification Value:	
Iodine Value:	
Foreign fatty substances	

Questions:

1. What is monograph?
2. What is principle of acid value, acetyl value and peroxide value?
3. What is use of castor oil?

Aim 14: To perform monograph analysis (Indian Pharmacopoeia, 2018) of Clove oil

Requirements: TLC plates, Silica Gel GF254, Refractometer, Polarimeter, blue litmus paper, Sulfuric acid, Potassium Hydroxide

Theory: Clove oil is the oil distilled from the dried flower buds of *Syzygiumaromaticum* (Linn.) Merrill and Perry *Eugenia caryophyllus* (Spreng.)Bull. And Harr. (Fam. Myrtaceae).

Procedure:

Analysis: Perform analysis of castor oil for below mentioned parameters given in Monograph as per standard procedures.

Description:	A clear, colourless, or pale yellow liquid when freshly distilled, becoming darker and thicker by ageing or exposure to air, odor as of clove. Clove Oil contains not less than 85.0percent w/w of phenolic substances, chiefly eugenol, $C_{10}H_{12}O_2$.
Storage	Store protected from light in well- filled containers at a temperature not exceeding 30°.
Thin layer chromatography	• Stationary phase: silica gel *GF254.* Mobile phase: Toluene • Test Solution: Dissolve 20 µl of the substance under examination in 2 ml of toluene. • Reference solution: Dissolve 20 µl of eugenol RS in 2ml of toluene. • Apply to the plate 20 µl of the test solution and 10 µl of the reference solution as bands 20 mm separated by 3 mm. Use an unlined tank, develop the chromatogram immediately after pouring the mobile phase into the tank and allow the mobile phase to rise 10 cm. Dry the plate, allow to stand for 5 minutes and again allow the mobile phase to rise 10 cm under the same conditions. Following the second development, dry the plate in air, examine in ultraviolet light at 254 nm and mark the quenching band. In the chromatogram obtained with the test solution there is a quenching band in the middle of the plate corresponding to quenching band due to eugenol in the chromatogram obtained with the reference solution. A weak quenching band may also be seen in the chromatogram obtained with the test solution with test solution with an Rf value slightly lower than that of the band corresponding to eugenol (acetyleugenol). Spray the plate with about 10 ml of the anisaldehyde solution, heat at 100° to 105° for 10 minutes and examine in daylight. In the chromatogram obtained with the test and reference solutions the bands corresponding to eugenol are strongly coloured brownish-violet abd any band corresponding to acetyleugenol in the chromatogram obtained with test solution, in particular a faint red band in the upper part (Caryophyllene).
Optical Rotation:	0° to -1.50°.
Weight per ml:	1.038g to 1.060 g.
Refractive index:	1.527 to 1.535, determined at 20°.
Heavy metals:	0.5 g complies with the limit test for heavy metals, Method B (40 ppm).
Phenol:	Shake 1 ml with 20 ml of hot water, the mixture shows not more than a scarcely perceptible acid reaction with blue litmus paper. Cool the mixture, pass the aqueous layer through a wetted filter and treat the clear filtrate with 1 drop of ferric chloride test solution. The mixture has only a transient greyish-green colour but not a blue or violet colour.

Contd...

Alkali-Soluble Matter:	Place 80 ml of a 5 percent w/v solution of potassium hydroxide in a 150-ml flask with a long neck which is graduated in tenths of a ml and is of such a diameter that not less than 15 cm in length has a capacity of 10 ml. clean the flask with sulphuric acid and rinse well with water before use. Add 10 ml of the oil and shake thoroughly at 5 minutes intervals for 30 minutes at ambient temperature. Raise the undissolved portion of the oil into the graduated part of the neck of the flask by the gradual addition of more of the potassium hydroxide solution; allow to stand for not less than 24 hours and read off the volume of the undissolved portion of the oil which measures between 1.0 and 1.5 ml.
Assay (gas chromatography)	Test solution (a): A 0.2 percent w/v solution of the oil under examination in ethanol (95 percent). Test solution (b): A 0.2 percent w/v solution of the oil under examination and 0.15 w/v of 1-decanol (internal standard) in ethanol (95 percent). Reference solution: A solution containing 0.2 percent w/v solution of eugenol RS and 0.15 w/v of the internal standard in ethanol (95 percent). Chromatographic Condition: - A glass column 1.5 m × 4mm, packed with 3 percent w/w of dimethyl silicon fluid on acid-washed diatomaceous support (120 mesh), - Temperature: column: 110° for 118 minutes, then increased to 170° at a rate of 12° per minute and maintained at this temperature for 2 minutes, - Inlet port at 220° and detector at 300°, - Flow rate 40 ml per minute of the carrier gas. Calculate the eugenol content in the oil under examination using the ratios of the area of the peak corresponding to eugenol to the area of the peak due to internal standard in the chromatogram obtained with test solution (b) and the reference solution.

Observations and Results:

Evaluation parameters	Results
Description	
Storage	
Thin layer chromatography	
Optical Rotation	
Weight per ml	
Refractive index	
Heavy metals	
Phenol	
Alkali-Soluble Matter	
Assay (Gas Chromatography)	

Questions:

1. What is principle of Gas chromatography?
2. What is major chemical constituent of clove oil?
3. How optical rotation, refractive index and specific gravity is useful to evaluate clove oil?

Aim 15: To evaluate herbal drug (Licorice) as per Monograph analysis from recent Pharmacopoeias [*Indian Pharmacopoeia 2018, The Ayurvedic Pharmacopoeia of India,* 2001, *British Pharmacopoeia 1993, USP 26, NF 21 2003*]

Requirements: Magnifying glass, Glass slide, Watch glass, Brush, Pholoroglucinol-HCl reagent, butanol, acetic acid, TLC plates, Muffle furnace

Theory: Herbal monograph is a summary of the scientific findings of a crude drug and should include: Title, Definition, Limits of active ingredients, Marker compounds, Description, Category, Identification, Chemical Tests, Assay of the marker constituents, Contaminants, Specific Tests, and Additional Requirements if any.

Perform the tests as mentioned in various monographs.

YASTI (INDIAN PHARMACOPOEIA 2018)

Liquorice root; Mulethi; *Glycyrrhizaglabra.* Yasti consists of the dried, unpeeled roots and stolons of *Glycyrrhizaglabra.* Linn. (Fam. Leguminosae). Yasti contains not less than 3.0 percent w/w of glycyrrhizinic acid.

Category: Expectorent, antiulcer, stomachic, anti-inflammatory, kasa.

Description	Odour, characteristics and slightly aromatic, taste, very sweet and faintly astringent; the bark is not bitter.
Identification	
Macroscopic	Root with few branches, up to 1 m long and 0.5 to 3 cm in diameter. Bark, brownish-grey to brown with longitudinal striations, bearing traces of lateral roots. Stolons, cylindrical, 1 to 2 cm in diameter and up to several meters long, but may be cut into length of 10 to 15 cm; similar in external appearance to the root but with occasional small buds. Fracture of the root and stolon, granular and fibrous. Cork layer, thin; secondary phloem region, wide, light yellow with radial striations; xylem, compact, yellow, with radiate structure. The stolon has a central pith, which is absent from the root.
Microscopic	Cork and phelloderm are narrow Phloem consisting of bundles of thick-walled, yellow fibers with narrow lumina surrounded by cells each containing a calcium oxalate prism, alternating in the external layers with areas of strongly hyaline keratenchyma; functional sieve tissue near the cambium. Medullary rays parenchymatous, widening towards the exterior, 3 to 12 cells wide. Xylem composed of radial rows of tracheids and vessels alternating with bundles of lignified fibres with crystals sheaths similar to those of the secondary phloem; vessels 30 µm to 150 µm in diameter with thick walls (5 µm to 10 µm) having reticulate thickenings or numerous bordered pits with slit-shaped openings associated with lignified xylem parenchyma . medullary rays, 2 to 5 cells wide. Parenchymatous cells throughtout containing simple, round, oval or fusiform starch granules 2 µm to 20 µm, mostly 5 µm to 12 µm, in diameter; parenchymatous pits present solely in the stolon
Thin layer chromatography	**Stationary Phase:** Silica Gel GF 254. **Mobile Phase:** A mixture of 70 volumes of butyl alcohol, 20 volumes of water and 10 volumes of acetic acid.

Contd...

	Test Solution: Add 10 ml of 70 percent v/v methanol to 1 g of dried yasti powder, heat by shaking on a water bath for 5 minutes, cool and filter. **Reference solution:** Add 10 ml of 70 percent v/v methanol to 1 g of dried yasti powder, heat by shaking on a water bath for 5 minutes, cool and filter. Apply to the plate 10 µl of each solution as bands, 10mm by 2 mm. allow the mobile phase to rise 8 cm. dry the plate in air and examine under ultraviolet light at 254 nm and 360 nm, spray with *anisaldehyde sulphuric acid reagent.* Heat the plate at 105° for 10 minutes and examine the plate in day light. The chromatographic profile of the test solution is similar to that of the reference solution. Mix a small quantity, in powder, with 0.05 ml of sulphuric acid; the powder particles become orange-yellow and some fragments change, more slowly, to pinkish red.
Water-soluble extractive	It should not be not less than 20 percent, determined by the following method. Mix 2.5 g of the finely powdered drug with 50 ml of water and allow to stand for 2 hours, shaking frequently, filter, evaporate 10.0 g of the filtrate to dryness on a water-bath, dry the residue at 105° and weigh.
Acid-insoluble ash	Not more than 2.0 percent
Sulphated ash	Not more than 10.0 percent
Assay	Liquid chromatography **Test solution:** Weigh accurately 1.0 g of the coarsely powdered substance under examination in a 250 ml conical flask, add 100 ml of 0.1 M ammonia and mix with the aid of ultrasound for 30 minutes. Centrifuge a part of the supernatant liquid and dilute 1.0 ml to 5.0 ml with 0.1 M ammonia. Filter the solution through a membrane filter ~~dis~~ with an average pore diameter not greater than 1.0 µm and use the filtrate. **Reference solution:** A 0.005 percent w/v solution of *glycyrrhizinic acid RS* in 0.1 M ammonia. **Chromatographic System:** - A stainless steel column 25 cm × 4.6 mm, packed with octadecylsilane bonded to porous silica (5 µm), - Mobile phase: a mixture of 6 volumes of glacial acetic acid, 30 volumes of acetonitrile and 64 volumes of water, - Flow rate- 1.5 ml per minute, - Spectrophotometer set at 254 nm, - Injection volume: 20 µl. Inject the reference solution. The test solution is not valid unless the relative standard deviation for replicate injections is not more than 2.0 percent. Inject the reference solution and test solution. Calculate the content of glycerrhizinic acid.
Storage	Store protected from light and moisture

YASTI (THE AYURVEDIC PHARMACOPOEIA OF INDIA, 2001)

Yasti consists of dried, unpeeled, stolon and root of Glycyrrhizaglabra Linn, (Fam. Leguminosae); a tall perennial herb, upto 2 m high found cultivated in Europe, Persia, Afghanistan and to little extent in some parts of India.

Synonyms-

Sansk. : Yastimadhuka, Yastika, Madhuka, Madhuyasti, Yastyahva.

Assam. : Jesthimadhu, Yeshtmadhu.

Beng. : Yashtimadhu

Eng. : Liquorice root

Guj. : Jethimadha, Jethimard, Jethimadh

Hindi :Mulethi, Mulathi, Muleti, Jethimdhu, Jethimadh.

Kan. :Jestamadhu, Madhuka, Jyeshtamadhu, Atimadhura

Kash. : Mulethi

Mal. :Irattimadhuram

Mar. :Jesthamadh

Ori. : Jatimmadhu, Jastimadhu.

Punj. : Jethimadh, Mulathi.

Tam. : Athimadhuramu

Urdu. : Mulethi, Asl-us-sus

Description:	
Macroscopic-	Stolon consist of yellowish brown or dark brown outer layer, externally longitudinally wrinkled, with occasional small buds and encircling scale leaves, smoothed transversely, cut surface shows a cambium ring about one-third of radius from outer surface and a small central pith; root similar without a pith; fracture, coarsely fibrous in bark and splintery in wood; odour, faint and characteristics; taste, sweetish.
Microscopy	Stolon- transverse section of stolon shows cork of 10-20 or more layers of tubular cells, outer layers with reddish-brown amorphous content, inner 3 or 4 rows having thicker, colourless walls; secondary cortex usually of 1-3 layers of radially arranged parenchymatous cells containing isolated prisms of calcium oxalate; secondary phloem a broad band, cells of inner part cellulosic and outer lignified, radially arranged groups of about 10-50 fibres, surrounded by a sheath of parenchyma cells, each usually containing a prism of calcium oxalate about 10-35 μ long; cambium form tissue of 3 or more layers of cells; secondary xylem distinctly radiate with medullary rays, 3-5 cells wide, vessels about 80-200 μ diameter with thick, yellow, pitted, reticulatelythickend walls; groups of lignified fibres with crystals sheath similar to those of phloem; xylem parenchym of two kinds, those between the vessels having thick pitted walls without inter-cellular spaces, the remaining with thin walls; pith of parenchymatous cells in longitudinal rows, with inter-cellular spaces. Root- Transverse section of root shows structure closely resembling that of stolon except that no medulla is present; xylem tetrarch; usually four principal medullary rays at right angles to each other; in peeled drug cork shows phelloderm and sometimes without secondary phloem; all parenchymatous tissue containing abundant, simple, oval or rounded starch grains, 2-20 μ in length.
Identity, Purity and Strength-	
Total ash	Not more than 10 percent
Acid-insoluble ash-	Not more than 2.5 percent
Alcohol-soluble extractive	Not less than 10 percent
Water-soluble extractive	Not less than 20 percent
Constituents	Glycyrrhizin, glycyrrhizic acid, glycyrrhetinic acid, asparagine, sugar, resin and starch.

Contd...

Properties and action	**Rasa :**Madhura **Guna :**Guru, snigdha **Virya :**Sita **Vipika :**Madhura **Karma :**Vatapittajit, Raktaprasadana, Balya, Varnya, Vrsya, Carksusya : .
Important Formulations	**Eladigutika; Yastimadhuka tails; Madhuyastyaditaila**
Therapeutic Uses	Kasa;Svarabheda; Ksaya; Vrana; Vatarakta
Dose	2-4 g of the drug in powder form

LIQUORICE (BRITISH PHARMACOPOEIA 1993)

Definition

Liquorice consists of the dried,unpeeled rots and stolons of *Glycyrrhizaglabra*L. It contains not less than 4.0 % of glycyeehizinic acid.

Characteristics	Odour, characteristics and slightly aromatic. Taste, very sweet, faintly astringent; the bark is not bitter.
Microscopical	Root with few branches, up to 1 m long and 0.5 to 3 cm in diameter. Bark, brownish grey to brown with longitudinal striations, bearing traces of lateral roots. Stolon, cylindrical, 1 to 1 cm in diameter and up to several meters long, but may be cut into length of 10 to 15 cm, similar in external appearance to the root but with occasional small buds. Fracture of the root and stolon, granular and fibrous. Cork layer, thin; secondary phloem region, wide, light, with radial striations; xylem, compact, yellow, with radiate structure. The stolon has a central pith which is absent from the root.
Microscopical	Cork and phelloderm narrow. Phloem consisting mainly of radially arranged bundles of thick- walled, yellow fibres 700 to 1200 µm long and 10 to 20 µm wide with a narrow lumen surrounded by cells each containing a prism of calcium oxalate crystals, 10 to 35 µm long and 2 to 5 µm wide, alternating in the external layers with areas of strongly hyaline keratenchyma; normal sieve tissue near the cambium. Xylem of radial rows of tracheids and vessels alternating with bundles of partially lignified fibers with crystals sheaths similar to those of the secondary phloem; vessels 30 to 150 µm in diameter with walls 5 to 10 µm thick having numerous bordered pits with slit- shaped openings, associated with lignified xylem parenchyma. Medullary rays, two to five cells wide. Parenchymatous cells throughout containing simple, round or oval starch granules 2 to 20 µm, mostly 5 to 12 µm, in diameter; Parenchymatous pith present only in the stolon.
Identification	
Thin-layer chromatography	Carry out the method for, using silica GF_{254} as the coating substance and as the mobile phase the upper layer, even if turbid, of a mixture of 60 volumes of ethyl acetate, 27 volumes of 1 M ammonia and 13 volumes of absolute ethanol, shaken together and allowed to stand for 5 minutes. Prepare the following for solutions (1) shake 1.0 g, in No. 180 powder, with 20 ml of chloroform for 15 minutes, filter and reserve the extracted powder for the preparations of solution (2). Evaporate the filtrate to dryness and dissolve the residue in 2 ml of mixture of equal volumes of chloroform and methanol. For solution (2) add the extracted powder 30 ml of 0.5 M sulphuric acid and heat under a reflux condensor for 1 hour, allow to cool and extract with two 20-ml quantities of chloroform; dry the combined chloroform extracts with anhydrous sodium sulphate, filter, evaporate

Contd...

	to dryness and dissolve the residue in 2 ml of a mixture of equal volumes of glycyrrhizinic acid in 2 ml of a mixture of equal volumes of chloroform and methanol. For solution (3) dissolve 10 mg of glycyrrhetinic acid in 2 ml of a mixture of equal volumes chloroform and methanol. Apply separately to the plate in three bands, each 20 mm long and not more than 3 mm wide, 10 µl of solutions (1) and (2) and 20 µl of solution. After the removal of the plate, allow it to dry in air for 5 minutes and examine under ultraviolet light (254 nm). The chromatogram obtained with solution (3) exhibits a band corresponding to ß-glycyrrhetinic acid with an Rf value of about 0.1. the chromatogram obtained with solution (2) exhibits a corresponding band but this is not seen in the chromatogram obtained with solution (1). Spray the plate with anisaldehyde solution, using about 10 ml for a plate 200 mm × 200 mm in size , heat at 100° to 105° for 10 minutes and examine in daylight. The ß-glycyrrhetinic acid bands become violet blue. One or two bands with an Rf value of about 0.6, visible in daylight before spraying, become orange-yellow and several other violet-blue bands appear in the chromatogram obtained with solutions (1) and (2). The band corresponding to ß-glycyrrhetinic acid in the chromatogram obtained with solution (3).
	Mix a small quantity, in powder, with 0.05 ml of sulphuric acid. The powder particles become orange-yellow and some fragments change, more slowly, to pinkish red.
Water-soluble extractive	Mix 2.5 g, in No. 180 powder, with 50 ml of water and allow to stand for 2 hours, shaking frequently, filter, evaporate 10.0 g of the filtrate to dryness on a water bath and dry the residue at 100° to 105°. The residue weighs not less than 0.1 g (20%).
Acid Insoluble Ash	Not more than 2.0 %.
Sulphated Ash	Not more than 10.0%. Use 1 g, in powder
Assay	Carry out the method for thin-layer chromatography, using silica gel GF_{254} as the coating substane and as the mobile phase the upper layer, even if turbid, of a mixture of 60 volumes of ethyl acetate, 27 volumes of 1M ammonia and 13 volumes absolute ethanol, shaken together and allowed to stand for 5 minutes. Apply separately and quantitatively to the plate two 60- µl quantities of each of the following solutions as bands 20 mm long and not more than 3mm wide, but ensuring that part of the plate remains free from the solutions being examined. For solution (1) mix 1 g, in No 180 powder, with 25 ml of 1M hydrochloric acid and 2.5 ml of 1,4-dioxane.Heat under reflux condenser in a water bath for 2 hours, allow to cool, filter through a hardened filter paper 9 cm in diameter and discard the filtrate. Rinse the flask and filter with five 20-ml quantities of water and discard the rinsings. Dry the flask and filter at 105° foe 20 minutes, transfer the filter paper to the flask and add 50 ml of chloroform. Boil under a reflux condenser in a water bath for 5 minutes and filter the warm chloroform solution through a filter paper 9 cm in diameter. Repeat the extraction with two 25 ml quantities of chloroform using the same filter each time. Transfer the filter paper to the flask, extract with 25 ml of chloroform and filter through another filter paper 9 cm in diameter. Evaporate the combined filtrates to dryness, dissolve the residue in a mixture of equal volumes of chloroform and methanol and transfer to 10-ml graduated flask. Rinse with two 10-ml quantities of chloroform and evaporate the rinsings until 2 ml remains. Transfer this solution to the graduated flask and dilute to 10 ml with a mixture of equal volumes of chloroform and methanol. For solution (2) mix 50mg of glycyrrhizinic acid EPCRS with 25 ml of 1 M hydrochloric acid and 2.5 ml of 1,4-dioxan and proceed as described for solution (1) beginning at the words 'Heat under a reflux condensior…'. Develop the chromatogram twice, allowing the plate to dry in air after each development. Examine the plate under ultraviolet light (254 nm) and mark the areas corresponding to ß-glycyrrhizinic acid in all four chromatograms. Carefully scrape off the coating substance

Contd...

	from the marked areas and treat each separately in the following manner. Shake with 5 ml of absolute ethanol for 15 minutes and filter through a small sintered-glass filter (BS porosity No. 4). Rinse the filter with absolute ethanol and dilute the filtrate to 10 ml with the same solvent. Measure the absorbance of each of the four solutions at 250 nm, using in the reference cell a solution prepared by treating in the same manner an area of the corresponding in position and size to the marked areas of ß-glycyrrhizinic acid but taken from the part of the plate that has remained free from the solutions being examined. Calculate the content of ß-glycyrrhizinic acid from the absorbance of solution (1) and (2) and the declared content of ß-glycyrrhizinic acid in ß-glycyrrhizinic acid EPCRS.
Storage	Liquorice should be kept in an airtight container and protected from light
Action and use:	Flavour.

LICORICE (USP 26, NF 21)

Licorice consists of the roots, rhizomes, and stolons of *Glycyrrhiza glabra* Linne or *Glycyrrhizauralensis* Fisher (Fam. Leguminosae). It contains not less than 2.5 percent of glycyrrhizic acid ($C_{42}H_{62}O_{16}$), calculated on the dried basis.

Packaging and Storage	Preserve in well-closed containers. Store in a cool, dry place.
Labeling-	the label states the Latin binomial name and, following the official name, the part of the plant contained in the article.
USP Reference standards	*USP Glycyrrhizic Acid RS*
Botanical Characteristics	
Macroscopic	The terrestrial stem is nearly cylindrical, 0.5 to 3.0 cm in diameter, and over 1 m in length; it is extremely dark brown to red-brown and longitudinally wrinkled. It often has lenticels, small buds, nd scaly leaves. The transverse section a rather clear border between the phloem and the xylem, and a radial structure that often has radiating splits.
Microscopic	The transverse section reveals several yellow-brown cork layers, and a layer of phelloderm that is 1 to 3 cells thick. The cortex exhibits medullary rays, and obliterated sieve portions radiate alternatively. The phloem exhibits groups of phloem fibres, which are surrounded by crystal cells, with thick but incompletely lignified walls. The vessels are accompanied by xylem fibers, which are surrounded by crystals cells, and by xylem parenchyma cells. The parenchyma cells contains starch grains and often contains single crystals of calcium oxalate.
Thin-layer chromatographic identification test	Test solution- Add 10 mL of a mixture of alcohol and water (7:3) to 2.0 g of pulverized licorice, heat by shaking on a water bath for 5 minutes, cool, and filter. Standard solution- Dissolve 5 mg of USP Glycyrrhizic Acid RS in 1 mL of a mixture of alcohol and water (7:3) Application volume: 2 µL. Developing solvent system: a mixture of butyl alcohol, water, and glacial acetic acid (7:2:1). Procedure: Proceed as directed in the chapter, except to develop the chromatogram in an unsaturated chamber to a length of about 10 cm. Examine the plate under UV light at a wavelength of 254 nm. The chromatograms show a dark purple zone, among other spot, due to glycyrrhizic acid at an Rf value of about 0.4.

Contd...

Loss on drying	Dry it at 105° for 6 hours: it loses not more than 12.0 % of its weight
Foreign organic matter	not more than 2.0 %
Total ash	not more than 7.0 %
Acid-insoluble ash	Not more than 2.0 %
Alcohol-soluble extractives	Not less than 25.0%.
Pesticides residues	Meets the requirements
Heavy Metals:	0.003%.
Content of glycyrrhizin acid-	Solvent: a mixture of alcohol and water (1:1). Mobile Phase: a filtered and degassed mixture of diluted acetic acid (1 in 15) and (3:2). Standard solution- Dissolve an accurately weighed quantity of USP Glycerrhizic Acid RS in solvent to obtain a solution having a known concentration of about 0.25mg per mL. Test Solution- Transfer about 500 mg of licorice, reduced to a powder and accurately weighed, to a powder and accurately weighed, to a suitable flask, add 70 mL of solvent, shake for 14 minutes, centrifuge, and decant the supernatant into a 100–mL volumetric flask. Mix the residue with 25 mL of solvent, shake for 15 minutes, centrifuge, and add the supernatant to the volumetric flask. Dilute with solvent to volume, mix and pass through a membrane filter having a 0.45-µm porosity. Chromatographic System-The liquid chromatography is equipped with a 254-nm detector and a 4,6 mm×15-cm column that contains packing L1. The flow rate is about 0.6 mL per minute. Chromatograph the standard solution, and record the peak areas as directed for procedure: the column efficiency determined from glycyrrhizic acid is not less than 5000 theoretical plates; the tailing factor for the glycyrrhizic acid peak is not more than 2.0; and the relative standard deviation for replicate injections is not more than 2.0%. Procedure: Separately inject equal volumes (about 20 µL) of the standard solution and the test solution into a chromatograph, record the chromatograms, and measure the peak areas. Calculate the percentage of glycyrrhizic acid ($C_{42}H_{62}O_{16}$) in the portion of Licorice taken by the formula: 10,000 (C/W) (r_u/r_s), where in which c is the concentration in mg per mL, of USP Glycyrrhizic Acid RS in the standard solution; W is the weight, in mg, of licorice taken to prepare the test solution; and r_u and$r_s$are the peak areas for glycyrrhizic acid obtained from the Test solution and the Standard solution, respectively.

Results:

Complies	Indian Pharmacopoeia 2018	The Ayurvedic Pharmacopoeia of India	British Pharmacopoeia 1993	USP 26, NF 21
Identification Macroscopic				
Microscopic				
Thin layer chromatography		NA		
Water-soluble extractive				NA
Alcohol-soluble extractive	NA		NA	
Total ash	NA		NA	
Acid-insoluble ash	Not More Than 2%	Not More Than 2.5%	Not More Than 2%	Not More Than 2%
Sulphated ash		NA		NA
Pesticides residues	NA	NA	NA	
Loss on drying	NA	NA	NA	
Foreign organic matter	NA	NA	NA	
Assay	HPLC	NA	TLC	HPLC
Heavy Metals	NA	NA	NA	

Questions:

1. What is difference observed between Licorice monograph of Indian Pharmacopoeia 2018, The Ayurvedic Pharmacopoeia of India, British Pharmacopoeia 1993, USP 26, NF 21?
2. How monograph analysis helps in quality control of herbs and derived products?
3. What is total ash value of licorice mentioned in monograph of different Pharmacopoeias?
4. Which mobile phase, stationary phase and detection agent of licorice mentioned in monograph of different Pharmacopoeias?

Further Reading

1. A.N.M. Alamgir. Therapeutic Use of Medicinal Plants and Their Extracts: Volume 1
2. Alice Kurian, M. Asha Sankar Medicinal Plants. New India Publishing Agency. 2007
3. Anjoo Kamboj, Moronkola Dorcas Olufunke Practical Pharmacognosy. Scitus Academics LLC. Thomas Edward Wallis. Practical Pharmacognosy. Churchill. 2018
4. Ashutosh Kar. Pharmacognosy And Pharmacobiotechnology. New Age International (P) Limited. 2003
5. Biren Shah, Avinash Seth. Textbook of Pharmacognosy and Phytochemistry. Elsevier Health Sciences. 2014
6. S. Shah, J. S. Qadry. A Textbook of Pharmacognosy. Messrs B.S. Shah 1971
7. C.K. Kokate, Purohit, Gokhlae. Text book of Pharmacognosy, 37th Edition, Nirali Prakashan, Pune. 2007
8. Christophe Wiart, Ashok Kumar. Practical Handbook of Pharmacognosy-Preliminary Techniques of Identification of Crude Drugs of Plant Origin. 2000
9. Deore SL. Pharmacognosy and Phytochemistry: A Companion Handbook. PharmMed Press, Hyderabad. . 2nd Edition, 2017.
10. Deore SL, Khadabadi SS, Baviskar BA. Pharmacognosy and Phytochemistry-A Comprehensive Approach. PharmMed Press, Hyderabad. 2nd Edition, 2018.
11. GS Kumar. KN Jayaveera. A Textbook of Pharmacognosy and Phytochemistry. S CHAND & Company Limited. India. 2014.
12. Gunnar Samuelsson. Drugs of Natural Origin-A Textbook of Pharmacognosy. Apotekarsocieteten. 1999
13. H. Ansari. Essentials of Pharmacognosy. Second edition, Birla publications, New Delhi, 2007
14. James Bobbers, Marilyn KS, VE Tylor. Pharmacognosy & Pharmacobiotechnology. Williams & Wilkins. 1996.
15. Jean Bruneton. Pharmacognosy, Phytochemistry, Medicinal Plants. Technique & Documentation. 1999
16. Joshi Saroja, Vidhu Aeri. Practical Pharmacognosy. Frank Brothers. 2009.
17. Khadabadi SS, Deore SL, Baviskar BA. Experimental Phytopharmacognosy. Nirali prakashan, Pune. 1st Edition, 2019.

18. K. Mangathayaru. Pharmacognosy: An Indian perspective. Pearson Education India. 2013
19. K. R. Khandelwal. Practical Pharmacognosy. Nirali Prakashan, Pune. 2008
20. Kaliya.A. Text Book of Industrial Pharmacognosy. CBS Publishers & Distributors, Delhi. 2009
21. Kendall Jefferson. Pharmacognosy and Phytotherapy. Foster Academics.2019
22. Kokate CK. Practical Pharmacognosy. Vallabh Prakashan, Delhi. 2005
23. Luqi Huang. Molecular Pharmacognosy. Springer Netherlands. 2012
24. M A Iyengar, S G K Nayak. Pharmacognosy Lab Manual. PharmaMed Press. 2019
25. M A Iyengar. Pharmacognosy of Powdered Crude Drugs. PharmaMed Press. 2017
26. M A Iyengar. Study of Crude Drugs. PharmaMed Press. 2016
27. Michael Heinrich, Elizabeth M. Williamson, Joanne Barnes, Simon Gibbons, Jose Prieto-Garcia Fundamentals of Pharmacognosy and Phytotherapy E-Book. Elsevier Health Sciences. 2017
28. Michael Heinrich, Joanne Barnes, Simon Gibbons. Fundamentals of Pharmacognosy and Phytotherapy. Churchill Livingstone/Elsevier. 2012
29. Mohammad Ali. Pharmacognosy and Phytochemistry, CBS Publishers & Distribution, New Delhi.
30. N P S Sengar, Ashwini Singh, Ritesh Agrawal. A Textbook of Pharmacognosy. PharmaMed Press. 2018
31. Nilambari S. Gurav, Shailendra S. Gurav Indian Herbal Drug Microscopy. Springer New York. 2013
32. Rangari VD. Pharmacognosy& Phytochemistry. Career Publication, Nashik. 2008
33. S. S. Agarwal, M. Paridhavi. Herbal Drug Technology. Universities Press. 2012
34. S. S. Handa. Pharmacognosy. Vallabh Prakashan, New Delhi. 1989
35. Saikat Sen, Raja Chakraborty Herbal Medicine in India-Indigenous Knowledge, Practice, Innovation and Its Value. Springer Singapore. 2019
36. Simone Badal Mccreath. Rupika Delgoda. Pharmacognosy-Fundamentals, Applications and Strategies. Elsevier Science. 2017
37. Steven E. Ruzin. Plant Microtechnique and Microscopy.1999
38. T. C. Denston. A Textbook of Pharmacognosy. Read Books. 2012

39. Vidhu Aeri, D.B. Anantha Narayana, Dharya Singh. Powdered Crude Drug Microscopy of Leaves and Barks. Elsevier Science. 2019

40. W.C.Evans, Trease and Evans Pharmacognosy, 16th edition, W.B. Sounders & Co., London, 2009.

41. The British Pharmacopeia. London: Medicines and Healthcare Products Regulatory Agency; 1993.

42. Indian Pharmacopeia 2018, Ghaziabad: Indian Pharmacopeia Commission; 2018.

43. United States Pharmacopoeia and National Formulary, USP 25 NF 19/National Formulary 20, Rockville, MD, U. S. Pharmacopoeial Convention, Inc. 2002.

44. Ayurvedic pharmacopoeia of India Part-I vol.I, 2001.

45. Arbab Ahmed, Eltahir Mahmoud. Review on Skin Whitening Agents. Khartoum Pharmacy Journal. 2010;13(1).

46. Sarkar R, Arora P, Garg KV. Cosmeceuticals for Hyperpigmentation: What is Available?. J Cutan Aesthet Surg. 2013;6(1):4-11.

47. Ramesh C. Gupta, Rajiv Lall and Ajay Srivastava. Nutraceuticals Efficacy, Safety and Toxicity. Academic Press. Second Edition • 2021

www.ingramcontent.com/pod-product-compliance
Lightning Source LLC
LaVergne TN
LVHW082019150826
845671LV00005B/208

* 9 7 8 9 3 9 1 9 1 0 9 9 0 *